Research Techniques
for the Health Sciences

Research Techniques for the Health Sciences

LAURNA RUBINSON
University of Illinois at Urbana-Champaign

JAMES J. NEUTENS
University of Tennessee at Knoxville

Macmillan Publishing Company
New York

Collier Macmillan Publishers
London

Macmillan Publishing Company
866 Third Avenue, New York, New York 10022

Collier Macmillan Canada, Inc.

Library of Congress Cataloging-in-Publication Data

Rubinson, Laurna.
  Research techniques for the health sciences.

  Includes bibliographies and index.
  1. Public health—Research—Methodology.   2. Health
education—Research—Methodology.   3. Health promotion—
Research—Methodology.   4. Medicine—Research—
Methodology.   I. Neutens, James J.   II. Title.
RA440.85.R83   1987   362.1'072   86–8638
ISBN 0–02–404540–3

Printing: 1 2 3 4 5 6 7   Year: 7 8 9 0 1 2 3

ISBN   0-02-404540-3

To
Jayne and my parents
L.R.

To
Mary and my parents
J.J.N.

Foreword

The history of experimental science is far too short to permit an adequate perspective of its true relation to human welfare and to the understanding of the universe.

> —Rene Dubos (1901–   )
> *Louis Pasteur, Free Lance of Science*
> Chapter One

I'm frequently tempted to ask my research colleagues whether among their most musty memories of undergraduate training they can recall Philosophy 101. I wonder whether they, like I, as freshmen consequently were compelled, and stretched to the limits of their young abstract abilities, to fathom some notion called *epistemology*. I wonder whether they were as intrigued as I, and also whether they were as sure as I that there was no useful application for such a notion beyond the contemplative, elbow-patched lives of the literati.

Epistemology, you will recall, is the study of the origin, nature, methods, and limits of knowledge. Granted, I may be slower than many, but it took me nearly twenty more years to discover how central and practical epistemology is in any effort to improve the well-being of human societies—truth (knowledge) being an elusive but essential prerequisite for the success of such efforts. While Plato and Aristotle laid far-reaching conceptual foundations for seeking truth more than two thousand years ago, it's been a mere twenty years since Campbell and Stanley published more specific, operational methods for discerning fact from illusion in their text on *Experimental and Quasi-Experimental Research Designs*. It will be interesting to learn the extent to which future historians glean that Campbell and Stanley influenced the course of science and human events.

Certainly during the past twenty years the process and conceptual tools of scientific inquiry—the process and tools by which truth is determined—have evolved at a rate unprecedented in history. The tools themselves continuously have been studied, applied, refined, debated, re-applied, elaborated, and codified. Today, virtually every collective social endeavor is shaped and guided with knowledge generated by these tools, or those responsible for such endeavors decry the lack of such knowledge. From these tools, the lifegiving seeds of modern agronomy are fashioned; vaccines that eradicate disease are formulated; the effect of Papal policies on birth control, and the consequence of those policies on Catholicism, are determined; ever more powerful weapons of war are forged; and techniques to market toothpaste are devised.

The book that you have opened thus is at the same time a treatise on epistemology, as well as a treasure-chest of some of the most sophisticated tools yet to be developed by human ingenuity. Herein lie the tools of reason, developed collectively by the brightest thinkers of our age—tools that still are bright and shiny, tools that are dynamic and continually evolving. By enabling you to become familiar with and skilled in using these tools, *Research Techniques for the Health Sciences* offers you the opportunity to understand and to participate in the process by which humankind comes to know. You can learn how to form a hypothesis, construct an appropriate experimental or quasi-experimental design, draw a representative sample, generate quantitative or qualitative data, analyze your data with descriptive or inferential statistical techniques (using a calculator or a computer), and present your findings not only to reflect truth, but to have an impact on the course of human events influenced by that truth.

Importantly, by describing a comprehensive range of tools, the authors have eliminated the need for you to reference multiple sources. In this one volume you have access to four separate types of tools usually found only in four separate texts: (1) a guide to writing theses and dissertations; (2) quantitative research methods; (3) qualitative research methods; and (4) basic statistics. More importantly, by addressing these four types of tools together, the authors have enabled you to understand their interrelationships and how they can be used together. Most importantly, by writing about these tools in language that is clear and concise, the authors have enabled almost anyone to understand and use them.

Don't be misled by the title. *Research Techniques for the Health Sciences* is not just for those who aspire to conduct research. Anyone who plans to *use* knowledge (certainly educators, physicians, lawyers, psychologists, politicians, and other professionals) should be able to analyze how the specific knowledge they use has been developed and thus should be able to determine the extent to which that knowledge approximates truth (its internal and external validity, as you will learn). The text, then, also is not necessarily just for those who plan to work in the health sciences: the process and tools for developing knowledge are virtually the same across disciplines.

Those involved in health education and health promotion, however, will be most rewarded by studying this text. The authors have prefaced each relevant chapter with a case study that describes how a different health education or health promotion *program* could be improved with specific additional knowledge. The authors then employ that case study to describe both a given research tool and how that tool can be applied to generate the specific knowledge that would improve the program. Thus, the authors illuminate the critical juncture between the development of knowledge and its use—between research and action—as they simultaneously illustrate the principles and practice of health education and health promotion.

These few words are written with the hope that you will approach this text with all the excitement and gusto it warrants. For here are the techniques by which humankind unveils the universe—comes to discover, comes to know techniques that can be employed constantly over a lifetime by anyone gifted with an inquiring mind and the drive to master them.

LLOYD J. KOLBE, Ph.D.
Center for Health Promotion and Education
Centers for Disease Control
Atlanta, Georgia

Preface

Until recently, research conducted in the health sciences was done by those in related professions. Concomitantly, to learn about research in our profession, it was necessary to employ textbooks from other disciplines and adapt them to the health sciences. This void in self-contained health science research literature was the principal reason for writing this text. It is intended to assist: (1) upper-level undergraduates and graduate students in the health sciences; (2) practitioners in the fields of health education, public health, nursing, medicine, and allied health; and (3) related professionals.

This book focuses on the pragmatic aspects of health science research with a basis in theory. In concert with the theme, the theory is explained in a commonsense fashion so that the reader is not overwhelmed at the expense of how to do research. Each chapter that deals with a particular research technique begins with a case study which is addressed throughout the chapter to offer both unity and practicality. At the end of each chapter are more case studies and activities that illustrate different health science settings.

Chapter 1, What Is Research, presents an overview of health science research that introduces the characteristics of the research process as well as the interrelationship of science and theory. The spectrum of basic to applied research is shown as are the steps involved in conducting a research project.

Chapter 2, Developing the Research Proposal, offers guidance in selecting a research problem and how to state the problem in a research manner. Employing illustrations, subproblems are derived, and the problem setting—limitations, delimitations, assumptions, definition of terms, hypothesis formulation—is discussed. Problem significance and related literature are introduced. An example time schedule shows the dissertation or thesis student how a flow plan can be established. Finally, and perhaps most importantly, a research proposal checklist is provided to ensure appropriate development of the research proposal.

Chapter 3, Review of the Literature and Information Sources, covers the purposes of the review, how to complete a review, and sources that are applicable to the health sciences. Computer searches are discussed also.

Chapter 4, Conducting Experimental Research, begins the use of a case study that demonstrates a real situation requiring an experimental approach in a school setting. Variables and control thereof, including advantages and disadvantages, are presented using the case study. Each design contains pragmatic detail.

Chapter 5, Survey Research, uses a community mental health center setting as the introductory case study. The characteristics of survey research are tendered, and much of the chapter is devoted to sampling techniques. A survey flow plan shows the overall steps in doing survey research, and the section on questionnaire design and construction provides greater detail for each step. The advantages, disadvantages, and procedures of mail surveys, face-to-face interviews, and telephone interviews with and without computer assistance are furnished. The Delphi technique is briefly addressed as it applies to the health sciences.

Chapter 6, Qualitative Research, commences with a research consortium case study in a hospital setting. Qualitative research is compared to quantitative research efforts, and theoretical foundations are provided. Several qualitative methodologies, including ethnomethodology, are discussed in a realistic manner. Techniques in collecting qualitative data are detailed, followed by a presentation of analyzing and coding such data.

Chapter 7, Evaluating Research, provides a case study in a school setting with the research conducted by a university Department of Health Behavior. The purposes of evaluation research and numerous evaluation models provide the reader with a comprehensive approach to this type of research. Steps are outlined in sequence varying with the nature of evaluation research. Cost analysis also is discussed.

Chapter 8, Carrying Out Historical Research, introduces a case study about a master's student who wants to trace the foundations of the wellness movement. Historical research is presented through the meaning of historical events, problem defining and hypothesis formulation, historical sources, and the systematizing and evaluation of historical data. Caveats of historical research are identified, and suggestions for the historical thesis are given.

Chapter 9, Analyzing and Interpreting Data, involves a case study of a public health professional working with acquired immune deficiency syndrome (AIDS) data. Descriptive and inferential data analysis techniques are discussed, with elaboration on testing for statistical significance. Exploratory data analysis is introduced, and the use of the computer for data reduction and analysis is addressed.

Chapter 10, Presenting the Data, starts with a senior health science student facing a research study assignment. A detailed discussion of table and figure presentations, as well as the use of graphs, charts, and photographs, is included. As would be expected, part of the discussion is about computer graphics.

Chapter 11, Scaling, is based on a case study of a patient education coordinator who is developing a sexuality scale for spinal-cord injury patients. In addition to the three major scales—Likert, Guttman, and Thurstone—semantic differential and factor scaling are offered in detail, including advantages and disadvantages of each. This chapter ends with suggestions for using a combination of techniques.

Chapter 12, Considering Ethics in Research, provides a situation in which a doctoral candidate is placed in a rather precarious position. This chapter shows the ethical decisions that must be made by the health science researcher from inception to the production of a manuscript. Several illustrations of past research efforts are given to help develop an awareness on the part of the researcher. Numerous questions are raised that can be valuable for group discussion.

Chapter 13, Ex Post Facto Research, opens with two case studies. One involves a health care professional at a large long-term care facility; the second involves a dentist at a large university clinic. Both cause-to-effect and effect-to-cause research procedures are explored. Techniques of control are developed for ex post facto research, and common errors are identified.

Chapter 14, Writing a Research Report, employs the perception of the report as a communication document. Explicit directions offer the student a step-by-step approach to develop a sound report for acceptance by other health care professionals.

Appendix A, Manuscript Considerations, delineates issues regarding publication of the research effort from journal selection through the review process. It also lists references for writing assistance.

Appendix B, Guidelines for Authors, is taken from the *Journal of School Health* as an example for prospective authors.

The authors wish to thank all of those people who were instrumental in the development of this text and, in particular, those students in our research methodology classes who tested this material over time. We are especially grateful to the reviewers and to those special secretaries who helped type the manuscript.

L.R.
J.J.N.

Contents

CHAPTER 1

What is Research?

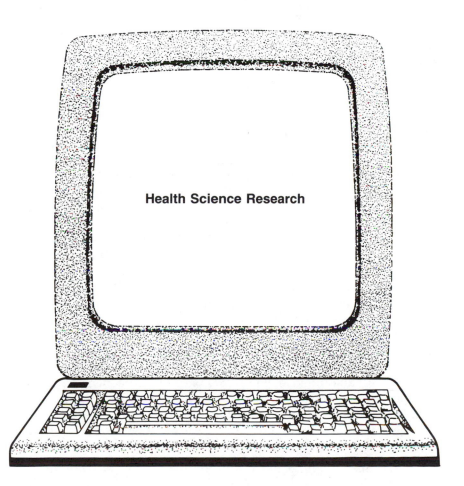

Health Science Research

Human beings possess the ability to think rationally and logically, which in turn leads to curiosity. You may have heard of the Philosophy 101 final examination that contained just one question: *"Why?"* Students wrote up to twenty pages, quoting philosophers ranging from Aristotle to Buber, but the correct answer was *"Because."* Research, or the process thereof, answers the question *Why?* There are multiple reasons for a myriad of questions, but how can we know what the best answer is? *Research* and the application of scientific method will enable us to answer such questions.

Health Science Research

The health science profession had its beginnings at the start of the nineteenth century, when improvement of the health of school-age children provided impetus for the new discipline. In addition, we health science professionals have strived to provide information to those populations of high risk. These have been our primary goals and we have attempted to use research and evaluation to improve our ability to meet these objectives. However, the profession has been criticized for its lack of research and evaluation activity and for its many studies conducted by graduate students that appear to give little or no new information to the profession (Iverson & Hosokowa, 1975). With these general criticisms in mind, you might be asking, why study health science research? What can it do? What can we expect?

These questions will be answered as you progress through the text and get better acquainted with the process and product of research in the health sciences. Even though the discipline has been criticized, research in the health sciences has proven to be valuable. In the school setting alone, research has shown that children have increased their knowledge and altered their attitudes in such areas as smoking, human sexuality, dental health, cardiovascular diseases, drug and alcohol abuse, and driver education.

Research endeavors in the schools can inculcate good and acceptable health behaviors in youths if the programs being tried allow for decision-making and problem-solving skills, improve self-concept and self-esteem, and provide additional social interactions. Such programs, under the auspices of rigorous research, can lead to a reduction of risk factors associated with well-being.

Research in the community can lead to baseline information regarding needs assessments in relationship to health status studies. In addition, public health policies are developed through research in the community. The determination of effective policy strategies can best be accomplished through rigorous and thorough research studies.

Patient education has been the setting for many research projects, including studies on diabetes, hypertension, postsurgical procedures, nutrition, and weight reduction. Many studies have led to major advances in diabetes control, where patients are able to self-medicate and be relatively free of the hospital regimen. Determination of how overweight patients react to specific weight control programs has had an influence in proper nutrition and exercise for both youth and adults.

For students to gain a thorough understanding of research and its place in the health sciences, they must have a working knowledge of science, scientific inquiry, and the importance of theory in research.

Using Science in the Quest for Knowledge

Knowledge may be gained or accumulated in many ways. Pierce explained four general ways of "fixing belief," or knowing: (1) the method of finality, (2) the method of authority, (3) the a priori method; and (4) the method of science. We are concerned with the scientific method, or science, and how this science helps us to know.

> To satisfy our doubts, . . . therefore, it is necessary that a method should be found by which our beliefs may be determined by nothing human, but by some external permanency, by something upon which our thinking has no effect. . . . The method must be such that the ultimate conclusion of every man shall be the same. Such is the method of science. Its fundamental hypothesis . . . is this: There are real things, whose characters are entirely independent of our opinions about them (Buchler, 1955).

Scientists, in their quest for knowledge and truth, use self-correcting devices that serve as built-in checking methods to assure that the conclusions they may reach are factual. Hypotheses are formulated but so too are alternate hypotheses to test the objectivity of the experiment and experimenter. In addition, by publishing the experiment and its results scientists allow for others to replicate and inspect their work.

Each scientific field (physics, engineering, psychology, health) has a method for arriving at knowledge, which will be discussed later as the scientific approach. Science can be considered a method to solve problems or answer questions that investigators find to be of interest. Scientists acquire specific attitudes that enable them to think and act in a scientific manner. These attitudes are best described by Ary, et al. (1985, p. 14).

1. Scientists are essentially doubters, who maintain a highly skeptical attitude toward the data of science. Findings are regarded as tentative and are not accepted by scientists unless they can be verified. Verification requires that others must be able to repeat the observations and obtain the same results. Scientists want to test opinions and questions concerning the relationships among natural phenomena. Furthermore, they make their testing procedures known to others in order that they may verify, or fail to verify, their findings.
2. Scientists are objective and impartial. In conducting observations and interpreting data, scientists are not trying to prove a point. They take particular care to collect data in such a way that any personal biases they may have will not influence their observations. They seek truth and accept the facts even when they are contrary to their own opinions. If the accumulated evidence upsets a favorite theory, then they either discard that theory or modify it to agree with the factual data.
3. Scientists deal with facts, not values. They do not indicate any potential moral implications of their findings; they do not make decisions for us about what is good or what is bad. Scientists provide data concerning the relationship that exists between events, but we must go beyond these scientific data if we want a decision about whether or not a certain consequence is desirable. Thus, while the findings of science may be of key importance in the solution of a problem involving a value decision, the data themselves do not furnish that value judgment.
4. Scientists are not satisfied with isolated facts but seek to integrate and systematize their findings. They want to put the things known into an orderly system. Thus scientists aim for theories that attempt to bring together empirical findings into a meaningful pattern. However, they regard these theories, as tentative or provisional, subject to revision as new evidence is found.

Science as Static and Dynamic. Conant (1951) describes science in two ways: the dynamic and the static. The emphasis in the *static view* is on the present state of knowledge, and of scientists contributing to that state. In addition, the extent of knowledge and the present theories, hypotheses, and principles are considered. In this view science may be used to explain observations and to discover new facts that contribute systematized information to the existing body of knowledge.

The actions of scientists are considered to be the *dynamic view* of science. In this view, the present state of knowledge serves as a base for further inquiry. The *heuristic view* of science (a subset of the dynamic view) means science that discovers or reveals, including the idea of self-discovery. The emphasis here is on discovery of something new that can add to the present base or body of knowledge. In the heuristic method of scientific inquiry, the actual emphasis is on the investigator being imaginative in his or her approach for answering a question or solving a problem.

Science and Theory. The ultimate goal of scientific inquiry is to formulate theories. Theories provide a way to conceptualize, organize, integrate, and classify the facts that scientists accumulate. A theory can describe a tentative explanation of some phenomenon. As scientists, when we ask the question, Why? and attempt to answer it, we are formulating a theory. It is then verified through evidence either by observation or experimentation, and thus uses the gathered facts to verify the theory.

Several characteristics of a sound theory serve to illustrate the constraints that scientists must work within when formulating a theory:

1. A theory should be able to explain the observed facts relating to a particular problem; it should be able to propose the "why" concerning the phenomena under consideration. This explanation of events should be in the simplest form possible. A theory that has fewer complexities and assumptions is favored over a more complicated one. This statement is known as the principle of parsimony.
2. A theory should be consistent with observed facts and with the already established body of knowledge. We look for the theory that provides the most probable or the most efficient way of accounting for the accumulated facts.
3. A theory should provide means for its verification. This is achieved for most theories by making deductions in the form of hypotheses stating the consequences that one can expect to observe if the theory is true. The scientist can then investigate or test these hypotheses empirically in order to determine whether the data support the theory. It must be emphasized that it is inappropriate to speak of the truth or falsity of a theory. The acceptance or rejection of a theory depends primarily upon its *utility*. A theory is useful or not useful, depending upon how efficiently it leads to predictions concerning observable consequences, which are then confirmed when the empirical data are collected. Even then, any theory is considered tentative and subject to revision as new evidence accumulates.
4. A theory should stimulate new discoveries and indicate further areas in need of investigation (Ary, et al. 1985, p. 18).

The health sciences have been very slow in achieving theoretical bases, probably because health, along with many other social sciences, is a young science. For the past forty years, health professionals have been collecting data to gather empirical evidence and build toward theoretical constructs. While several models (the Health Belief Model, the Precede Model) have been developed for and by health

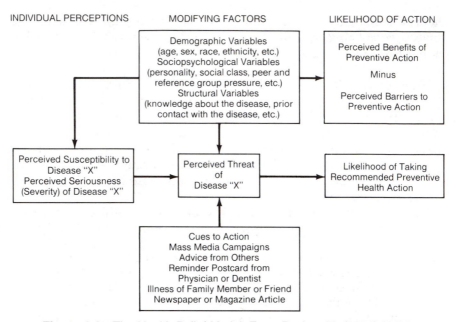

INDIVIDUAL PERCEPTIONS   MODIFYING FACTORS   LIKELIHOOD OF ACTION

Figure 1.1 The Health Belief Model. From Becker, M. (1974) *H.Ed. Monographs* **2**: 409–419. Copyright © 1974. Reprinted by permission of John Wiley & Sons, Inc.

educators, theories that could be directly attributed to the health sciences have been nonexistent.

It must be understood that there is a difference between a model and a theory. Theories provide an understanding of a phenomenon and provide prediction and control. Theories also can provide a way for conceptualizing the world. However, *models* provide perhaps a better way of conceptualizing. Some models are replicas, such as miniature toys; others are symbolic, such as the diagram of The Health Belief Model (see Figure 1.1). Models also can be used in computers, as scientists have been able to program computers to behave in a human-like manner when solving problems. Models provide us with a simplistic way of looking at complex problems or phenomena.

Basic and Applied Research

When we think about research, our initial image is of a laboratory with animals and scientists in white coats. This image is generally true when basic researchers are at work. *Basic research* aims to expand the knowledge base by formulating, evaluating, or expanding a theory. Research in the medical sciences is usually of this type, because biochemistry, biology, and microbiology fall into this pattern.

Hence, the primary purpose of basic research is discovering knowledge for the sake of knowledge alone; the practical side of the issue is considered at a later time.

Applied research aims to solve practical problems, although it uses the same characteristics as basic research. Here theoretical concepts are tested in real situations. Laboratories cannot be the scene for investigations, but rather the real world, i.e., classrooms, hospitals, clinics, become the laboratory for applied health researchers. Most research in the health sciences is applied, because it is concerned with testing the processes of health behavior in a real-life situation.

Several major health science projects have used the applied research approach. These include the Chicago Heart Association's *Body Power Program,* The American Health Foundation's *Know Your Body* Curriculum, and the University of Minnesota smoking prevention program. These projects use similar conceptual and theoretical approaches in schools: the real world. However, whether basic or applied research is being conducted by health scientists, one type of research must depend on the other for the proper research process to take place. Applications of theories help solve some practical problems, such as when social learning theory is used to attempt to explain why children adopt healthful behaviors. This can work the other way as well, where theoretical concepts are advanced by the practical uses of the theory. As in the example just mentioned, new light could be shed on social learning theory if it were found to be useful in classroom situations.

The Scientific Approach

There are several characteristics of the scientific approach (or research process) that future researchers should be attuned to in order to become familiar with the method of scientific inquiry. Rather than reiterate the major traits associated with research, we will use the excellent list provided by John Best in *Research in Education* (1981, p. 20).

1. Research is directed toward the solution of a problem. The ultimate goal is to discover cause-and-effect relationships between variables, though researchers often have to settle for the useful discovery of a systematic relationship, for lack of enough evidence to establish one of cause-and-effect.
2. Research emphasizes the development of generalizations, principles, or theories that will be helpful in predicting future occurrences. Research usually goes beyond the specific objects, groups, or situations investigated and infers characteristics of a target population from the sample observed. Research is more than information

retrieval, the simple gathering of information. Although many school research departments gather and tabulate statistical information that may be useful in decision making, these activities are not properly termed research.

3. Research is based upon observable experience or empirical evidence. Certain interesting questions do not lend themselves to research procedures because they cannot be observed. Research rejects revelation and dogma as methods of establishing knowledge and accepts only what can be verified by observation.

4. Research demands accurate observation and description. Researchers use quantitative measuring devices, the most precise form of description. When this is not possible or appropriate, they use qualitative or nonquantitative descriptions of their data-gathering procedures and, when feasible, employ mechanical, electronic or psychometric devices to refine observation, description, and analysis of data.

5. Research involves gathering new data from primary or first-hand sources or using existing data for a new purpose. Teachers frequently assign a so-called research project that involves writing a paper dealing with the life of a prominent person. The students are expected to read a number of encyclopedias, books, or periodical references, and synthesize the information in a written report. This is not research, for the data are not new. Merely reorganizing or restating what is already known and has already been written, valuable as it may be as a learning experience, is not research. It adds nothing to what is known.

6. Although research activity may at times be somewhat random and unsystematic, it is more often characterized by carefully designed procedures, always applying rigorous analysis. Although trial and error are often involved, research is rarely blind, shotgun investigation—trying something to see what happens.

7. Research requires expertise. The researcher knows what is already known about the problem and how others have investigated it. He or she has searched the related literature carefully, and is also thoroughly grounded in the terminology, the concepts, and the technical skill necessary to understand and analyze the data gathered.

8. Research strives to be objective and logical, applying every possible test to validate the procedures employed, the data collected, and the conclusions reached. The researcher attempts to eliminate personal bias. There is no attempt to persuade or to prove an emotionally held conviction. The emphasis is on testing rather than on proving the hypothesis. Although absolute objectivity is as elusive as pure righteousness, the researcher tries to suppress bias and emotion in his or her analysis.

9. Research involves the quest for answers to unsolved problems. Pushing back the frontiers of ignorance is its goal and originality is frequently the quality of a good research project. However, previous important studies are deliberately repeated, using identical

or similar procedures, with different subjects, different settings, and at a different time. This process is replication, a fusion of the words repetition and duplication. Replication is always desirable to confirm or to raise questions about the conclusions of a previous study. Rarely is an important finding made public unless the original study has been replicated.

10. Research is characterized by patient and unhurried activity. It is rarely spectacular and researchers must expect disappointment and discouragement as they pursue the answers to difficult questions.

11. Research is carefully recorded and reported. Each important term is defined, limiting factors are recognized, procedures are described in detail, references are carefully documented, results are objectively recorded, and conclusions are presented with scholarly caution and restraint. The written report and accompanying data are made available to the scrutiny of associates or other scholars. Any competent scholar will have the information necessary to analyze, evaluate, and even replicate the study.

12. Research sometimes requires courage. The history of science reveals that many important discoveries were made in spite of the opposition of political and religious authorities. The Polish scientist Copernicus (1473–1543) was condemned by church authorities when he announced his conclusion concerning the nature of the solar system. His theory that the sun, not the earth, was the center of the solar system, in direct conflict with the older Ptolemaic theory, angered supporters of prevailing religious dogma, viewed his theory as a denial of the story of creation as described in the book of Genesis. Modern researchers in such fields as genetics, sexual behavior, and even business practices had personal convictions, experiences, or observations that were in conflict with some of the research conclusions.

Upon reading the above list, you may get a view of researchers that is not realistic but ideal: imaginative, honest, hard-working, very rigid, and probably boring—because all they may know is the subject they are so relentlessly pursuing. We can argue that this description is not accurate, especially for the health science researcher. The health professional is usually people oriented and thus conducts research in real-world settings: hospitals, schools, places of worship, community centers, and so on. However, the good health researcher seeks to be rigorous and to adhere to scientific standards at all times.

Because we have set as one of the goals of this text to provide a basis from which students could conduct research, we will list and briefly explain the stages of the research process. Consideration here should be given to the nature of the research process, i.e., that one component is integral to all others and that good research becomes almost cyclical. Figure 1.2 points out the various stages of the research process and attempts to show its cyclical nature.

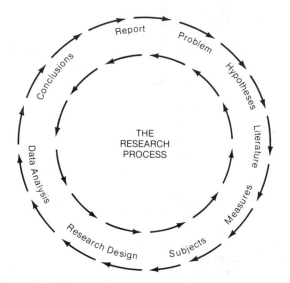

Figure 1.2 The cyclical stages of the research process.

Selecting a Problem. The health science student will probably decide on a subarea of interest to focus his/her research upon. The problem is usually phrased as a question.

1. To what extent can the Health Belief Model explain contraceptive behavior among sexually active females? (Robertson, 1983)
2. What are the long term effects of a cardiovascular curriculum? (Hoadley, 1982)
3. What are the effects of a health education self-management intervention as measured by the glycosylated hemoglobin level? (Isdale, 1983)

See Chapter 2 for an in-depth analysis of problem selection.

Formulating Hypotheses. The hypothesis is the researcher's tentative explanation that will predict the significant results of the research study or process. However, the hypotheses are always supported by theory and/or previous research. Examples of hypotheses that relate to the problems in the previous section are

1. Females who are adequate contraceptive users feel more susceptible to pregnancy than those who are inadequate users.
2. Students exposed to the cardiovascular curriculum will demonstrate superior scores on all of the subscale sets of questions, as compared to the students in the control group.

3. Subjects exposed to the self-management program will exhibit normal or lower glycosylated hemoglobin levels than measured prior to the intervention program.

Chapter 2 will illuminate the specifics of hypothesis formulation.

Reviewing the Literature. Relevant literature provides the hypotheses and initial problem selection. In addition, a thorough review of material may lead to suggested investigative methods.

Listing the Measures. Identifying all the possible measures enables the researcher to tighten the hypotheses by eliminating and rethinking those that have no available measure or none that can be developed for use in the study.

Describing the Subjects. The researcher carefully describes and considers the types of subjects necessary for the project. Particular attention should be given to the number and availability of the subjects.

Constructing a Research Design. The research design should be fully explained so that the researcher is sure that the design will allow the student to test the stated hypothesis. Chapter 4 will discuss the various types of experimental designs.

Constructing and Identifying Measurement Devices. The adoption and/or construction of appropriate instruments is used to measure the selected variables. There are some standardized instruments in the health sciences; however, modification of these instruments, construction and pilot testing of new ones, or construction of questionnaires and interview schedules may be necessary.

Analysis of the Data. A plan to analyze the data should be carefully considered, so that the number of subjects, the instruments, and the method of recording the data all coincide to fit the analysis procedure. This is an extremely important part of the stages of the research process, because all too often the instrumentation is not geared for appropriate data analysis, therefore rendering results improper or inadequate.

Generating Conclusions. The data should reveal several conclusions that are directly related to the hypotheses.

Writing the Report of Research. Chapter 14 details report writing where instruction is offered for each section of the report.

Research Methodologies in the Health Sciences. There are several methodologies that are utilized by health science investigators, each of which will be described in detail in subsequent chapters. These methods, in brief, are:

1. **Experimental** research is a study in which the investigator controls and manipulates one or more variables. The focus of experimental research is on the relationships between the variables. The major purpose of this type of research is to determine what will happen.
2. **Survey, interview, and observational** research are considered descriptive *methodologies* in which the results reveal what is happening in a particular occurrence. This research involves recording, describing, analyzing, and interpretating conditions that presently exist. Comparisons and contrasts are attempted to reveal relationships between the nonmanipulated variables.
3. **Evaluation** research is a method of evaluating a process to enable judgments to be more accurate and objective (Weiss, 1982). Evaluation may establish clear and specific criteria for success. Evidence is collected from a sample of the population, translated into quantitative terms, and compared with the previously set criteria. Conclusions are then drawn about the effectiveness, merit, and success of the program that was studied.
4. **Historical** research describes what has occurred in the past. "The process involves investigating, recording, analyzing, and interpreting the events of the past for the purpose of discovering generalizations that are helpful in understanding the past, understanding the present, and to a limited extent, in anticipating the future" (Best, 1981).

The type of methodology used is most often determined by the questions asked and the kinds of data that will be collected. Too often, inexperienced investigators will attempt an inappropriate methodology for their convenience. A thorough discussion of these methodologies can be found in Chapters 4 to 8.

The health sciences have grown at a very fast pace since the early 1950s, when they became a separate and valued part of the educational process. During this time, the health field has become increasingly sophisticated in its approach to research. From the early days of one-group, no-control studies, to today's Solomon Four-Group designs, which include the correlation of biomedical data, we have seen health science researchers publish and present their work in prestigious journals and meetings.

Summary_____

Human beings possess the ability to think rationally and logically, which in turn leads to curiosity. *Why?*, the most-asked question, leads researchers to conduct studies to find answers to questions, sometimes simplistic and at other times complex.

Research in the health sciences is still in its early years, because the profession is relatively young. Even though they have their critics, and most of them are on target, health scientists have dramatically advanced the field's research and evaluation efforts in the 1970s and 1980s. Using science in the quest for knowledge, health scientists have become imaginative, rigorous, and conscientious in their approach to research.

The method of science has enabled us to accumulate knowledge in many ways. Scientists assure themselves and the public that their conclusions are based on fact by having built-in checking mechanisms to ensure accuracy, replication, and inspection of their work. Scientists have very specific attitudes about their work that set them apart from the layperson attempting research. Science has two broad views: static and dynamic, where the latter describes the actions of scientists—how they think and behave to solve intricate problems.

The ultimate goal of scientific inquiry is to formulate theories. Theories enable us to conceptualize the facts that investigators accumulate. Several characteristics are inherent in a sound theory, each depicting the constraints under which scientists work. The health sciences have been slow in developing their own theories, but rely on those of other social sciences: psychology, sociology, anthropology, and education. Researchers in the health field have developed several models (the Health Belief Model and the Precede Model), which are different from theories. Models provide a simplistic way of looking at complex problems.

There are distinct differences between basic and applied research. However, each may complement the other. Professionals in the health sciences have concentrated upon applying principles and theories for real-world situations. It is difficult to conduct basic research in the settings that are available to health educators: schools, nursing homes, clinics, hospitals, and so on.

The scientific approach is the process investigators use in the quest for knowledge. Several important characteristics of the process enable standards to be scientific and rigorous. Stages of the scientific process begin with the selection of a problem and proceed through the writing of the research report.

Four general methodologies are used in health science research: experimental, survey, interview, and observational, evaluation, and historical. The type of methodology required is dictated by the questions that need to be asked and the data that are collected.

Suggested Activities⎯⎯⎯⎯⎯⎯⎯⎯⎯⎯⎯⎯⎯⎯⎯

1. Revise each of the following research topics so that they would be feasible for a research project. Indicate if the statement is in the form of a hypothesis or a statement of the problem.
   a. Smoking among adolescents.
   b. Diabetes control at home.
   c. Hypertension of the elderly.
   d. Fitness among aphsics.
   e. Cardiovascular rehabilitation for angina patients.
   f. Dental health for pregnant teenagers.
   g. Alcohol abuse among housewives.
2. Describe in one sentence each of the following characteristics of the research process:
   a. Research is directed toward the solution of a problem.
   b. Research emphasizes the development of generalizations, principles, or theories that will be helpful in predicting future occurrences.
   c. Research is based on observable experience or empirical evidence.
   d. Research demands accurate observation and description.
   e. Research involves gathering new data from primary or firsthand sources or using existing data for a new purpose.
   f. Although research activity may be at times somewhat random and unsystematic, it is more often characterized by carefully designed procedures.
   g. Research requires expertise.
   h. Research strives to be objective and logical.
   i. Research involves the quest for answers to unsolved problems.
   j. Research is characterized by patient and unhurried activity.
   k. Research is carefully recorded and reported.
   l. Research requires courage.
3. Devise your own definition of research, and defend it.
4. Discuss how the health sciences have contributed to the body of knowledge concerning one aspect of health behavior.

Bibliography⎯⎯⎯⎯⎯⎯⎯⎯⎯⎯⎯⎯⎯⎯⎯⎯⎯⎯

Ary, D., Jacobs, L., and Razevieh, A. (1985) *Introduction to Research in Education,* New York: Holt, Rinehart, and Winston.

Becker, M. (1974) The health belief model and personal health behavior, *H.Ed. Monographs* 2:409–419.

Best, J. (1981) *Research in Education,* New Jersey: Prentice-Hall.

Buchler, J. (ed.) (1955) *Philosophical Writings of Pierce,* New York: Dover.

Conant, J. (1951) *Science and Common Sense,* New Haven: Yale University Press.

Hoadley, M. (1982) An evaluation of the effects of a cardiovascular health education program. Unpublished doctoral dissertation, University of Illinois.

Isdale, L. (1982) Diabetes self-management through educational intervention. Unpublished doctoral dissertation, University of Illinois.

Iverson, D. and Hosokawa, M. (1975) Health education research: accomplishment or exercise, *J. Sch. Health* 45(3):154–156.

Robertson, N. (1983) The health belief model and contraceptive behavior among college females. Unpublished doctoral dissertation, University of Illinois.

Weiss, C. (1982) *Evaluation Research,* New Jersey: Prentice-Hall.

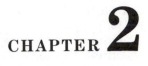

CHAPTER 2

Developing the Research Proposal

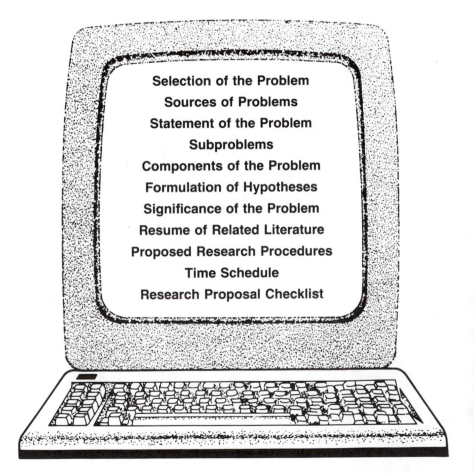

Selection of the Problem

Sources of Problems

Statement of the Problem

Subproblems

Components of the Problem

Formulation of Hypotheses

Significance of the Problem

Resume of Related Literature

Proposed Research Procedures

Time Schedule

Research Proposal Checklist

Much research ends in futility because the neophyte rushes into research activity—choosing a sample, collecting data, deriving conclusions—with only a meager plan at best. To be successful, the researcher must have a detailed plan as well as an overall conceptualization. The research proposal allows the investigator to specify the problem and related components, to elaborate on the significance of the research to the health profession, to review related literature, and to outline the appropriate methodology within an equitable time frame.

The sequence employed throughout this chapter is the format used in most theses and dissertations, although each university, not unlike most requests for proposals in funded research, will have modifications that must be followed by the researcher.

Selection of the Problem

One of the most difficult tasks confronting the beginner is to select a researchable problem. More often than not, the newcomer has a proclivity to tackle an exotic issue making the problem too broad or too narrow in scope. Some of the factors that should be involved in the ultimate selection are listed here (Tuckman, 1978; Bailey, 1982):

1. **Interest.** The researcher should be interested in pursuing the problem area. It should relate to the background and career interests of the student as well as develop useful skills for the future.
2. **Operability.** The nature of the problem should be such that the researcher has both the resources and time available to complete the project.
3. **Scope.** While the research problem should not attempt to solve all the health dilemmas of the world, neither should it be so small as to negate the variables necessary for adequate results.
4. **Theoretical and practical values.** The research should contribute to the health field, perhaps through publication, and be of benefit to health practitioners.
5. **Health paradigm.** This is the school of thought or model employed by the researcher. For example, Hoyman's ecological model of health (1975) or the PRECEDE paradigm of Green et al. (1980) could serve as a source to a problem or as a methodological direction.
6. **Values of the researcher.** The myth of value-free research is just that, a myth. The student of research should be aware that

in addition to being untestable, values may prejudice the research effort to the degree that all objectivity is lost. Note that
even the selection of a problem is value laden.

7. **Research Methodology.** Every researcher has a philosophy of
research that affects procedure. Herein the student must be certain that hypotheses are well written and that appropriate criteria are used to interpret the data to reach conclusions.

8. **Reactivity.** The method of data collection should be scrutinized
for reactivity. That is, a reactive technique brings about a reaction on the part of those being studied in a way that affects
that data with the reactive effect commonly labeled the Hawthorne effect from the study of the Hawthorne Plant of the
Western Electric Company in Chicago. It was found that
worker productivity increased simply because the personnel
were being observed.

9. **Unit of analysis.** In health research the unit of analysis may
be an individual or an entire population, such as in a study of
the health habits of a single anorexic patient or seeking patterns among the hospital anorexic population. The researcher
must ascertain which is most appropriate and whether resources are available to collect the data.

10. **Time frame.** This is particularly important to the student because only a limited amount of time is usually available. In a
cross-sectional study a particular population is involved at a
single point in time whereas a longitudinal time frame involves
data gathered over an extended period of time such as months
or years.

The student should apply all of these criteria to the potential problem
to determine the feasibility of the research effort.

Sources of Problems

Now that we have developed some criteria for selecting a problem,
the next step is to commence the hunt. It should be kept in mind that
the problem must be researchable; i.e., it must meet the requirements
of the research process characteristics outlined in Chapter 1.

At the outset, the beginner should look around at the immediate
environment; it teems with researchable problems. Many problems in
the classroom, the hospital, or the community lend themselves to investigation. Which teaching technique is most likely to bring about a

change in smoking behavior? How does the community feel about the establishment of a wellness clinic at the hospital? Does presurgical education reduce the use of analgesics and the number of days of hospitalization?

Technological advances in medicine require continual revision in patient education, as do studies to measure their effectiveness. Similarly, in school health education the advent of specialized curricula demands research into presentation format, teacher usage, cost benefits, and evaluation. The community health educator can turn in almost any direction to find new drugs, industrial hazards, environmental pollutants, and health fads that need investigation.

The academic experience of college juniors, seniors, and graduate students should serve as a catalyst for a research project. Textbooks, periodicals, seminar reports, and conference proceedings can inaugurate the mind into the research world. Indexes and abstracts such as *Cumulative Index To Nursing and Allied Health Literature, Completed Research in Health, Physical Education and Recreation, Social Sciences Index, Hospital Literature Index,* and *Dissertation Abstracts* provide valuable sources for research ideas. Chapter 3 discusses review of the literature and offers suggestions for additional library sources.

If possible, the student should attend workshops, national and state conventions, and government-sponsored programs to gather ideas and more importantly meet current researchers in the field of health education. Closer to home, university faculty can be an impetus for health research. Although topics themselves may not be provided, consultation with experienced faculty is desirable to check operability, significance, and value.

To stimulate thinking in the direction of health education research, the following list is provided from which problems may be defined. It is important to realize that this is simply a list of ideas, not of properly expressed research problems.

1. Drug abuse in schoolchildren.
2. Patient education and reduction of health care costs.
3. Competency-based education in health education.
4. Marketing of health education.
5. Patient adherence to drug regimens.
6. Media effectiveness in health education.
7. Evaluation of health education programs.
8. Autonomy of school health educators.
9. Health policy and health education organizations (e.g., ASHA, APHA, SOPHE).

10. Patient education and ethics (e.s., informed consent, confidentiality).
11. Health career objectives of students.
12. Internship experiences of community health education students.
13. Health promotion.
14. Content areas (e.g., sex, drug, nutrition, and self-help education).
15. Health locus of control.
16. Behavior change techniques.
17. Safe transportation of toxic wastes.
18. Health advocacy.
19. Employee assistance programs and health education.
20. Physical educators and health education.
21. Health education concerns of rural populations.
22. Motivation in health-conscious individuals.
23. The promotion of wellness.
24. Mental health education in a clinical setting.
25. Computer-assisted instruction in health education.

Statement of the Problem

The statement of the problem offers focus and direction in the research proposal. The problem statement can be written either as a question or as a declarative statement. In either case, it must be written clearly and concisely. That means each word of the statement should be definitive, indispensable, and expressive. On completion, the statement of the problem should be such that it can be read and understood by anyone without the researcher's presence.

Listed here are some examples of poorly written statements that only imply the actual problem.

- *School setting:* "Drugs and School Children"
- *Clinic setting:* "Hypertensive Drugs and Patients"
- *Community setting:* "The Fear of Toxic Wastes"

This indicates to the student that the researcher does not have the problem clearly in mind or at least has not expressed it completely. Needless to say, this would be an inappropriate way to commence a research report.

These three meaningless statements could be refined to show a complete statement of the problem.

- *From the school setting:* What drug is most frequently abused by those students enrolled in the junior high schools of Chatham?
- *From the clinic setting:* The purpose of this study is to ascertain what factors play a role in the low compliance rate among males at an East Tennessee hypertension clinic.
- *From the community setting:* What are the health fears of residents living near a proposed New Jersey toxic waste dump site?

It should be realized that these statements are specific as to topic and to population. In other words, the parameters have been established within the statement of the problem. No one can divine thoughts from the researcher, thus the need for clarity. Cliches, colloquialisms, slang, and professional jargon obscure thought and should be avoided when research writing is edited.

Subproblems

Frequently, the main problem has inherent components that if extracted would serve as minor, related research projects. These are called *subproblems* and as such could be investigated separately; however, the subproblems must add up to the totality of the principal problem. Further, each subproblem must be written in such a manner as to show that the data will be interpreted. Employing these two characteristics, totality and interpretation of data, the researcher may distinguish between two subproblems and apparent subproblems.

To identify subproblems, first examine the problem statement itself for the components it contains. For example, inspect the following problem statement:

> The purpose of this study is to analyze the wellness practices of Kent County high school health teachers in contrast to the wellness practices they teach in the classroom.

The next step is to demarcate the subproblem areas within the problem statement. This can be accomplished by underlining or "boxing off" the appropriate sections of the statement. Keep in mind that each subproblem must contain a word or words that imply data interpretation by the researcher.

> The purpose of this study is *(to analyze the wellness practices of Kent County high school health teachers) (in contrast)* to the *(wellness practices they teach in the classroom).*

Now the subproblems may be written out thus:

1. What are the personal wellness practices of Kent County high school health teachers?
2. What wellness practices are taught in the classroom by Kent County high school health teachers?
3. What will analysis of the wellness practices of these teachers indicate when contrasted with the wellness practices taught in the classroom?

It should be noted that each subproblem implies interpretation of the data and that the subproblems add up to the totality of the principal problem.

Components Comprising the Setting of the Problem

Though the problem statement offers focus and direction and the subproblems provide a means to stay on course, further delineation is necessary. It is important to indicate what limitations, delimitations, and assumptions surround the problem as well as to define terms that may be new to the reader. Also, if the researcher is making any assumptions, they must be pointed out.

Limitations

Limitations are the boundaries of the problem established by factors or people other than the researcher. For example, in the preceding problem statement the researcher may have wished to investigate five separate counties. However, permission may have been granted by only three of the five counties and subsequently the data limited to those participating counties. Other limitations could be available resources, time, survey forms completed, and honesty of the respondents.

Delimitations

Delimitations deal with boundaries also, but they are set by the researcher. Though the problem statement indicates what the researcher will investigate, it is important to know what will not be included. In other words, the delimitations are an answer to the inquiry, what are the precise limits of the problems? This is particularly salient to the novice researcher, who is most likely to attempt to solve every problem imaginable. Delimitations rule out the peripheral considerations to allow the researcher to concentrate on the central effort. The study mentioned may require the researcher to delimit the population to high school teachers who have a bachelor's degree in health education, not just anyone who teaches health. The researcher may delimit the study by geographical location, the size of the population, a central issue, or similar considerations.

Assumptions

An assumption is a condition that is taken for granted and without which the research effort would be impossible. An assumption is believed to be fact, but cannot be verified as one. In the Kent County study on wellness, the researcher may make the assumption that the teachers will answer the questionnaire honestly and thereby submit appropriate data.

Definition of Terms

Many research studies employ terms that may have special meaning to the study itself. To understand the usage of such terms, the researcher must define each term as it relates to the project at hand. Dictionary definitions are usually not adequate or helpful, because they fail to provide the true meaning intended by the researcher. The meaning of "wellness practices" would have to be defined from the Kent County problem statement. It is recommended that the reader review theses and dissertations to observe the role of the section on definition of terms.

Formulation of Hypotheses

While hypotheses may be included in components that comprise the setting of the problem, they are considered separately because of their significance to the research problem. Simply put, a hypothesis is a logical supposition, a reasonable guess, or a suggested answer to a problem or subproblem. A hypothesis provides further direction for the research effort by setting forth a possible explanation for an occurrence. For example, when the monitor of a personal computer fails to work, the following tentative reasons may be posited:

1. The monitor is not plugged in.
2. The interface cable is not connected.
3. The monitor is not turned on.
4. The picture tube is malfunctioning.

Each of these "guesses" can be tested by checking the plug, the interface cable, the on-off switch, and the picture tube.

Hypotheses are derived from the subproblems, and often a one-to-one correspondence is found. However, on other occasions, just one hypothesis may be developed from either the problem statement itself or from a single subproblem. Generally, a hypothesis should (1) be stated clearly and concisely, (2) express the relationship between two or more variables, and (3) be testable. Hypotheses are neither proved or disproved. The purpose of testing a hypothesis is to ascertain the probability that it is suggested by fact. In other words, the acceptance or rejection of a hypotheses is based on fact rather than a preconcerned bias.

In the early stages of a study, researchers state a scientific or research hypothesis as a prediction of the outcome of the test. For example, in the medical community it was predicted that as the number of cigarettes smoked increased so would the incidence of lung cancer. This concise statement expresses the relationship between smoking and lung cancer. Of course, a linear relationship could also be expressed to state that as one variable increases the other will decrease. The public health educator would predict that as the usage of contraceptives increases in teenagers the incidence of teenage pregnancy would decrease. In some studies there may be a nonlinear relationship between the variable, e.g., as one variable increases the other increases, then levels off. It might be predicted that as anxiety increases the ability to perform increases and then plateaus.

While research hypotheses demarcate the observations to be made, it is difficult to obtain unequivocal support for them. Subsequently, they are usually rephrased into a negative or null form. This negative or no-differences format is called a *null hypothesis*. The null hypothesis asserts that minor differences between the variables can occur because of chance errors and thus are not real significant differences. In other words, the testing of a null hypothesis reveals that either some force or factor has resulted in a statistical difference or that it has not resulted in such a difference. When the null hypothesis is rejected, indicating that a statistical difference does in fact exist between the variables, the competent researcher sees this as a red flag and will probe deeper into the problem to discover what has caused the difference and how. For example, a health educator may find that a particular program alters the attitudes of those exposed to it, thereby rejecting the null hypothesis that the effect of the program would make no difference. This finding leads to another research question: what caused the program to bring about the change, and could this factor or factors be employed in other programs? Note that if the researcher rejects the null hypothesis, then the research hypothesis is accepted.

Returning to the problem of the wellness practices of Kent County high school health teachers at both a personal and teaching level, the null hypothesis may be written as:

> *There are no differences in those wellness practices personally employed or taught in the classroom.*

Examination of this null hypothesis shows that it is derived from the third subproblem and that it expresses the relationship between two variables—practices personally employed and practices taught in the classroom. It is stated concisely and is testable. If the research hypothesis—that there are differences in personal practices and what is being taught—is accepted, then the next step is to explore the dynamics underlying the differences. The research effort should not stop with rejection of the null hypothesis.

Significance of the Problem

In this section of a research proposal the researcher has an opportunity to explain why the research effort is so important. The fledgling researcher frequently believes that the significance of the study is self-explanatory, or that because it is of personal interest it must be of interest to everyone. Needless to say, that is not usually the case. The relevance of the undertaking to one's school or community, or to patient health education needs to be stated in a way that the average citizen will comprehend. Although some health researchers may be solely concerned with theory, most health educators will demand pragmatic value from the research endeavor. Further, with so many areas of health education requiring research, there is no justification for the expenditure of efforts that fail to contribute to the profession.

Resume of Related Literature

Those who conduct an initial research project frequently regard the review of literature as wasted time, because they believe they could more appropriately be collecting data. Skilled researchers, however, realize that the more one knows about similar research the more likely the study can be conducted in an intelligent, comprehensible fashion.

As a general guide, keep in mind that the problem statement is central and that everything to be reviewed should serve as an aid in confronting the problem. Similar studies should be checked for population and sampling techniques; study design, including data gathering instruments; variables measured; extraneous variables that influenced findings; recommendations for future research; and of course, the findings and conclusions. Though the related literature section of the report follows several others, it is important to commence a literature review early so that it can help to define the problem statement, develop components that comprise the setting of the problem, justify the study, and plan the design. Research should be conducted with deliberate speed; otherwise, the only thing accomplished is proof of the adage, "Haste makes waste."

Proposed Research Procedures

Up to the point at which the research procedures are discussed, the report has dealt with the nature of the problems, the significance of the problem, and an explanation of what related studies have found. Now a detailed research plan must be outlined to include sample techniques, methodological steps, instruments employed, administration of instruments, data required, and method of analyzing data.

Time Schedule

Although a time schedule may not be a requirement of an advisor or funding agency, it is an invaluable device to assist in the budgeting of time and energy. Students are advised to develop a time schedule because their time is limited and academic deadlines are rarely negotiable. Moreover, dividing the research effort into operable portions with realistic dates helps organization and reduces procrastination. Table 2.1 demonstrates how a student may develop a time schedule for the Kent County problem statement:

The purpose of this study is to analyze the wellness practices of Kent County high school health teachers in contrast to the wellness practices they teach in the classroom.

TABLE 2.1 Time Schedule: Wellness Research Project

Study go-ahead

Dec. 1	Dec. 10	Feb. 5	Feb. 15	March 10
1. Obtain permission and develop working procedures with Kent County high schools		1. Develop instrument 2. Select pilot sample 3. Select study sample 4. Mail introductory letters to all participants	1. Committee review instrument 2. Mail to health teachers in pilot study	1. Revise instrument from pilot study

March 20	April 15	April 30	May 15	June 15
1. Mail instrument to health teachers in study 2. Revise/complete Chapters I, II and III	1. Questionnaire return 2. Data keypunched	1. Fund program 2. Begin data analysis and 3. Telephone contact with random sample of participants failing to return questionnaire	1. Write section on presentation and analysis of data 2. Write summary, conclusions, recommendations	1. Write, edit final report

Research Proposal Checklist_____

The research proposal is the initial step in developing the research project, and as such the investigator should check each area. The ckecklist in Table 2.2 offers a series of questions and statements that may be employed for this purpose. It is to serve as a guide and not a panacea for the research proposal.

TABLE 2.2 A Research Proposal Checklist

A. The Problem

1. The research problem should be able to meet the following criteria:

Universality	__Yes	__No
Replication	__Yes	__No
Control	__Yes	__No
Measurement	__Yes	__No

2. In addition, the following factors affecting problem selection must be considered and should be checked off once contemplated:

Interest	__Yes	__No
Operability	__Yes	__No
Scope	__Yes	__No
Values	__Yes	__No
Paradigm	__Yes	__No
Methodology	__Yes	__No
Reactivity	__Yes	__No
Unit of analysis	__Yes	__No
Time frame	__Yes	__No

B. Statement of the Problem

Write out the problem statement.

1. Is the problem statement clear and concise?	__Yes	__No
2. Does it focus on one research goal?	__Yes	__No
3. Does the problem statement set parameters?	__Yes	__No
4. Is interpretation of the data implied in the problem statement?	__Yes	__No

C. Subproblems

Underline or box off the problem statement and then construct and write out the subproblem(s).

1. Is each subproblem written in question form?	__Yes	__No
2. Is the writing clear and concise?	__Yes	__No
3. Can each subproblem be investigated separately?	__Yes	__No
4. Does each subproblem show that interpretation of the data will take place?	__Yes	__No
5. Do the subproblems add up to the totality of the principal problem?	__Yes	__No

D. Delimitations

Determine the precise boundaries of the problem and write out each.

1. Are all the peripheral considerations ruled out?	__Yes	__No
2. Is each delimitation established by the researcher?	__Yes	__No
3. Is each delimitation written clearly and concisely?	__Yes	__No

TABLE 2.2 (continued)   A Research Proposal Checklist

E. **Assumptions**
   Consider all the assumptions necessary to conduct the study.
   1. Is each assumption appropriate to the project? ___Yes ___No
   2. Are you assuming too much for the study to be done? ___Yes ___No
   3. Is each assumption really necessary to the study? ___Yes ___No
F. **Definition of Terms**
   Ascertain which terms require special interpretation.
   1. Is each term defined as it relates to the research project? ___Yes ___No
   2. Are the definitions clear and concise and do they avoid an
      abundance of professional jargon? ___Yes ___No
G. **Hypotheses**
   Apply the following questions to each hypothesis:
   1. Are the hypotheses written in an understandable fashion? ___Yes ___No
   2. Are they derived from the problem or subproblem(s)? ___Yes ___No
   3. Are they written in null form? ___Yes ___No
   4. Does each hypothesis express a relationship between two
      or more variables? ___Yes ___No
   5. Is each hypothesis testable? How? ___Yes ___No
H. **Significance of the Problem**
   This section is very important to justify a go-ahead for collecting data or to obtain
   research funding.
   1. To which of the following does the research apply?
      School health ___Yes ___No
      Patient health ___Yes ___No
      Community health ___Yes ___No
   2. List the ways in which the research project will contribute to health education.

      _____

      _____

   3. Do others concur that this would be a worthwhile project?
      Colleagues ___Yes ___No
      Faculty ___Yes ___No
      Major advisor ___Yes ___No
      Related personnel in the field ___Yes ___No
      Related literature ___Yes ___No
   4. Is this section written in a manner that shows why the study should be conducted
      without having to make the reader search for an answer?
      ___Yes ___No
I. **Related Literature**
   Whether this segment be brief or lengthy, it should meet the demands listed below.
   1. Have all the resources been reviewed? ___Yes ___No
   2. Does each section relate to the problem statement? ___Yes ___No
   3. Is this segment well organized? ___Yes ___No
   4. Is the related literature current? ___Yes ___No
J. **Research Procedures**
   All the steps of the research plan should be included in this segment.
   1. Where applicable, are the following included?
      Sample technique ___Yes ___No
      Methodological steps ___Yes ___No
      Instruments employed ___Yes ___No
      Administration ___Yes ___No

(continued)

TABLE 2.2 (continued)   A Research Proposal Checklist

Analysis techniques	__Yes	__No
2. Does this segment show the research plan in sequential order?	__Yes	__No
3. Is the information provided adequate enough that the study could be replicated?	__Yes	__No
K. Time Schedule		
This section is suggested for better organization.		
1. Is time available to complete the project?	__Yes	__No
2. Do all segments or sections surround the problem?	__Yes	__No
3. Is the proposal readable, concise, and cohesive?	__Yes	__No
4. Does the proposal represent a best effort?	__Yes	__No

Summary

An organized and concise research proposal shows that the researcher has a well-thought-out plan and that the project is likely to be worked through to completion. This chapter explains the factors that affect problem selection and suggests sources of problems suitable to research. Each section of the proposal is overviewed to include the statement of the problem, subproblems, components comprising the setting of the problem, hypotheses, significance of the problem, resume of related literature, research procedures, and time schedule. Review of the literature and information sources is a step in the process that assists all aspects of the research proposal.

Suggested Activities

1. Explain the errors in each of the following problem statements and rewrite each to meet the demands of a good problem statement.
   a. The purpose of this study was to examine the relationship between sexual experience and sexual and contraceptive attitudinal responses to a birth control film.
   b. The purpose of this study was to examine which of three different approaches aimed at helping to curb smoking among teenagers enrolled in public schools was most effective: the scare approach, the fact approach, or the attitude approach.
   c. To investigate the relationship between emotional maturity and accident involvement of male motorcycle operators in Michigan.
   d. What health education techniques could be used to reduce anxiety in pregnant women who face a cesarean section?

2. Once you have rewritten the problem statements from the first activity, demarcate and write out the subproblems of each.
3. Rewrite each of the following research hypotheses in the form of a null hypothesis.
   a. As patient involvement in their education increases, so will their knowledge in their health maintenance.
   b. As nutrition knowledge among fifth graders increases, their selection of junk foods will decrease.
   c. As more research information about AIDS is imparted to the community, the less anxiety there will be within the community.
4. Written below is a problem statement. Read it and then develop appropriate definitions, limitations, delimitations, and assumptions for such a study.

   What are the preabortion and postabortion attitudes of women experiencing problem pregnancies toward self, contraception, intercourse, and abortion?

Bibliography

Tuckman, B. (1978) *Conducting Educational Research,* New York: Harcourt, Brace, Jovanovich.

Bailey, K. D. (1982) *Methods of Social Research,* 2nd ed., New York: The Free Press.

Hoyman, H. (1975) Rethinking an ecologic system model of man's health, disease, aging, and death, *Journal of School Health* 45(9):509–18.

Green, L., Kreuter, M., Deeds, S., and Partridge, K. (1980) *Health Education Planning: A Diagnostic Approach,* Palo Alto, CA: Mayfield Publishing Company.

Roethlisberger, F. and Dickson, W. (1939) *Management and the Worker,* Cambridge: Harvard University Press.

CHAPTER 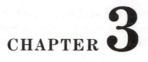 3

Review of the Literature and Information Sources

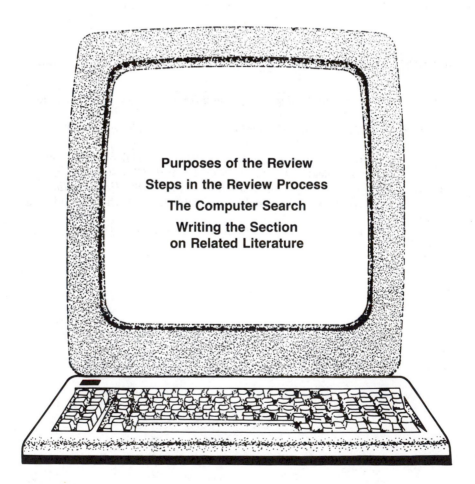

Purposes of the Review

Steps in the Review Process

The Computer Search

Writing the Section on Related Literature

A review of relevant literature provides a framework for the hypotheses and statement of the problem. It is usually required in the beginning chapters of a thesis or dissertation. This exercise in reviewing the literature will enable the researcher to formulate ideas and concepts from previous work. We can learn what other investigators have accomplished and failed at so that we can make a contribution to the knowledge of health sciences. Many first-time investigators find reviewing the literature a two-sided experience. On one hand it can be a challenging, interesting, and motivating exercise. On the other, it can be tedious and painstakingly slow, especially if one allows curiosity to take over: it is easy to get sidetracked into interesting areas that are peripheral to the project at hand.

Purposes of the Review_____

While the general purpose of reviewing the relevant literature is to gain an understanding of previous work and to generate new ideas and concepts, the process can additionally help the investigator to

1. Develop an understanding and grounding in theory.
2. Define the problem.
3. Review the procedures and instruments used.
4. Originate new ideas rather than repeat work already accomplished.
5. Use the recommendations for further research.

Understanding Of Relevant Theory

Too often investigators in the health sciences approach problems from an atheoretical perspective and therefore do not develop a well-defined set of hypotheses. By using the review of literature to search for relevant theoretical perspectives, investigators will gain additional knowledge and confirm hypotheses. This leads to an enrichment of the field in general and builds toward well-founded studies for the future.

Defining the Problem

While reviewing the health science literature, the investigator will be able to develop a concise plan for the study. Usually we begin with lofty ideas that are sometimes not workable in the real world of research. The review will enable the investigator to state quite narrowly the relevant hypotheses and research problem.

Reviewing Procedures and Instruments

The review of the literature provides information on and insight into proven and unproven methodologies and procedures previously used. Knowing that some research designs are inappropriate, sampling frames inadequate, and approaches unreasonable enables the investigator to improve on his or her research design. In the behavioral sciences, it is especially important to have reliable and valid instruments. The review provides insight into which measures are available and of those which will be useful in the present research study.

Originating New Ideas

Many experimenters have begun the literature search and deduced that their idea would not add any new knowledge or insight to their field of interest. A review of existing research can illuminate interest areas that need subsequent study and indicate useful applications, without reinventing the wheel. While some of us can create original ideas and concepts, they can be manifested by a thorough review of the literature.

Using Recommendations for Further Research

Authors of research studies usually include very specific recommendations for additional research. This is quite helpful to the investigator, because the suggestions provide the valuable insights of an experienced investigator in the same, or similar, area of research. The list that follows might provide impetus for you to formulate your own specific area of study.

Sample Research Ideas
1. Attitudes of parents toward sex education.
2. Behavior change and the use of self-efficacy.
3. The Health Belief Model and its utility in patient education.
4. A model for behavior change in anorexia nervosa.
5. Diffusion theory and its application in the health sciences.
6. The status of health education in Kentucky schools.
7. Hypertension screening in a small community.
8. Smoking cessation programs in the workplace.
9. Social learning theory and its application in dental health programs.
10. Evaluating health science programs in graduate schools.
11. Altering the attitudes of preschoolers toward family life education.

12. Diabetes education and its role in social modeling.
13. Using the PRECEDE model in planning an environmental hospital-based program.
14. Comparing the effects of an obesity program on middle- and low-income adults.
15. The effects of computer-assisted instruction as compared to classroom instruction on high school students enrolled in a nutrition course.
16. The effects of a cardiovascular intervention program on an adult population.
17. Determining the effectiveness of a cancer prevention program.
18. Decision-making skills in the health science curriculum.
19. Implementation of curricula: theory and strategy.
20. Expectancy value theory and its use in health science professional preparation programs.

Steps in the Review Process

You have decided to embark on a research study and now the time has arrived to begin searching the literature. A tentative problem statement, centered around a theory, has been determined. Now to the library!

The following is an outline of the steps to consider when beginning a review of the literature:

1. Read background information.
2. Gather the necessary tools.
3. List key words.
4. Use preliminary sources.
5. Conduct a computer search.
6. Read and take notes.

Reading Background Information

At this stage of your search *secondary sources* are generally used. These are usually textbooks or encyclopedias written by someone who has not directly observed the described event. A good textbook is written by an author who has searched the literature exhaustively and compiled a text based on her or his interpretation of other experiments or events. Of course, that same author may also report on experiments he or she has participated in or witnessed. This would be considered a *primary source,* because it was written by an author who observed or participated in an event. The importance of the secondary sources is that they usually have a bibliography, which provides the reader with the primary sources.

After reviewing the few textbooks devoted to your research problem, you realize that primary sources must be read. These include journals, final reports, or books that contain original research. In addition, government publications are good primary sources.

Gathering the Necessary Tools

You will need several tools for systematic data gathering. The *bibliography card* is used to reference each article or book that might be useful to the review. Use of either four-by-six-inch or five-by-eight-inch index cards is advisable. These cards become the cornerstone of the review of literature, as they will contain the information necessary for you to write your review of the literature and subsequently the entire first major section of your study.

The bibliography card should include the name of the author, the title of the reference, and a complete source listing. Any of several formats can be used. Investigators should check the required format for theses and dissertations at their institution so as not to have to recopy cards for bibliographical entry into the research report, thesis, or dissertation. Most health sciences journals use the American Psychological Association style (Figure 3.1).

Another necessary tool is to determine a *filing system* by which to order your bibliography cards. The most often-used systems are (1)

SMOKING AND SEXUAL BEHAVIOR

Zabin, L. (1984). The association between smoking and

sexual behavior among teens in US contraceptive clinics.

Am. J. of Pub. Health. 74, 261–263.

Figure 3.1 Sample bibliography card in American Psychological Association style.

alphabetized by author, (2) longituidinal (most recent first), and (3) subheading. We the authors order our cards by subtopic area, as this enables us to easily organize the writing of the report. However, you might find this system difficult at the beginning of your search because you have few ideas of what the subheadings might become. If that situation arises, use the alphabetical approach at first and reorganize into subtopics later.

The complete set of bibliography cards will enable you to compile your *list of references* at the end of the report, thesis, or dissertation. Each card should have a brief annotation (under title, author, and notation), to describe the entry. This enables the investigator to remember a reference quickly, and thus discern the usefulness of the reference.

Listing Key Words

After you have the background information, which is generally gathered from secondary source materials, you will have an idea of the topic area and be able to generate key words or phrases. Use of a thesaurus has proved valuable in this process. Consult the card catalogue and contact colleagues and professors who might have related interests.

Key words and phrases are necessary because almost all health science sources are organized by subject, and you should have a list of key words to begin looking in the indexes of these sources. As an example, your topic area may be patient education involving diabetes in outpatient settings. When you complete the general review, your first key word list might include patient education programs, outpatients, hospitals, diabetes, and nursing education. Such a list, although quite incomplete at this stage, will provide a starting point when you begin the actual search.

Checking Preliminary Sources

The second step in the search process is to check the *preliminary sources*. These include reference books, indexes, abstracts, guidebooks and periodicals that help the investigator locate primary sources. Most of the sources in the health sciences are available by computer search; we will discuss using the computer later in this chapter. Parts of the remainder of this section were written by Eileen Metress and appeared in *Health Education* (1982), vol. 13, no. 3, pp. 19–22 in an article entitled "Library Research in Health Education." Complete citations for books are in the following reference book indexes:

- *Books in Print*
- *Cumulative Book Index*
- *Library of Congress Catalog—Books*
- *National Union Catalogue*
- *Whitaker's Cumulative Book Index*

Strengths and weaknesses of books are critiqued in the following reference book reviews:

- Book review sections of specific journals
- *Book Review Digest*
- *Book Review Index*
- *Technical Book Review*

Indexing and Abstracting Services. Some indexing and astracting services are published monthly or quarterly. They enable the library researcher to keep up with newly published articles and can help in doing retrospective searches. Indexing services contain alphabetically arranged bibliographic citations, usually by subtopics. These services offer a published set of abstracts in a specialized or generalized field accompanied by a complete bibliographic citation. Abstract services enable the investigator to quickly ascertain the usefulness of an article and then obtain it, or to discard that piece of literature. Many of the following abstract services are available via computer, and may be obtained in library reference rooms for a manual search. The following is a list of index and abstract services that are most germane to the health sciences.

Abstracts on Health Effects of Environmental Pollutants. Contains references to material concerning the health effects of environmental pollutants, as well as general reviews, original research and reports of new analytical methods. It also includes reports on the use of lower vertebrates as toxicity indicators and the place of lower animal life in the biological amplification of pollutants through the food chain.

Bibliographic Index of Health Education Periodicals (BIHEP). BIHEP is a bibliographic tool that indexes articles in over 150 journals and an added 100 newsletters and regional publications. It was the first comprehensive index to the periodical literature in health education and is designed by and for health educators. A "Thesaurus of Descriptors" aids in finding specific terms relevant to a field, such as health education, risk-reduction projects or school health curriculum project. BIHEP is published quarterly (beginning with articles published in 1982) and is available in annual cumulative editions. Because BIHEP is so useful to the health sciences, your authors believe that is necessary to explain how to use the Index. Figures 3.2 and 3.3 are taken from BIHEP's introductory pages.

Instructions for Using BIHEP

1. Make Certain That *BIHEP* Is the Appropriate Index for Your Topic.

If your topic is about "health education," "health behavior," "health communication," or "health" as a social science, then *BIHEP* is the appropriate index to use.

If your topic is about "education" in general, or about the use of a particular educational technique or strategy, and not specifically about its use in health education, then an education index, such as *ERIC* or *Education Index* would be more appropriate.

If your topic is about a specific medical condition or therapy, or about a "subject matter" topic related to health, rather than about education/communication/behavior/social science, then a medical index, such as *Index Medicus* or *Excerpta Medica* would be more appropriate.

For Example

Topic: "The Use of Multimedia Techniques in Drug Education"
Index: *BIHEP* would be appropriate.
Topic: "The Use of Multimedia Techniques in the Classroom"
Index: An education index would be more appropriate as a primary source of information. *BIHEP* could provide additional information about this topic as it relates to health education.
Topic: "The Use of Narcotics in the Management of Chronic Pain"
Index: A medical index would be more appropriate as a primary source of information. *BIHEP* could provide some additional information on this topic.

2. If You Know the *Author,* and Want to Find the Items Published.

Use the AUTHOR INDEX (blue section) of *BIHEP* to locate the author, and find the item accession number after the author's name. Locate the item in the MAIN LISTING (white section).

3. If You Know the *Journal* that an Article was Published in.

Use the MAIN LISTING (white section) of *BIHEP* to locate the article, under the name of the journal. All indexed articles are listed, by journal, in order of publication.

4. If You Wish to Locate Information on a Given Subject.

Use the *BIHEP* THESAURUS OF HEALTH EDUCATION DESCRIPTORS (yellow section) of *BIHEP* to locate the correct subject matter descriptors used by *BIHEP*. Refer to the SUBJECT INDEX (green section) to locate all items on that topic by item accession number. Locate the item in the MAIN LISTING (white section).

Figure 3.2 Depiction of how the citations are listed in BIHEP.

Completed Research in Health, Physical Education and Recreation. Contains three sections that index according to subject headings, including a bibliography of published research, and list abstracts of research in alphabetical order according to the supervising institution.

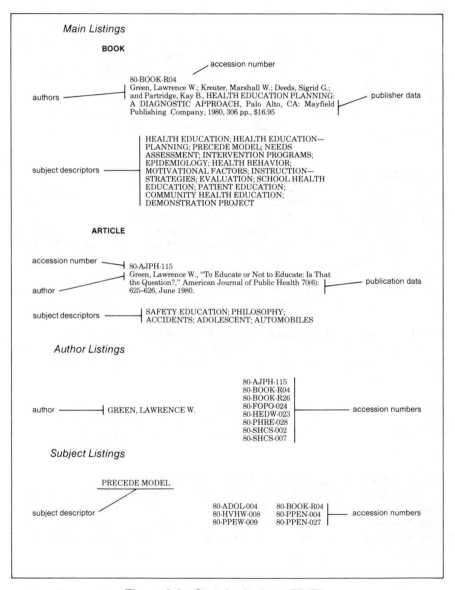

Figure 3.3 Sample citations, BIHEP.

Current Awareness in Health Education Abstracts (CAHE). Includes citations and abstracts of current journal articles, monographs, conference proceedings, reports and nonpublished documents acquired and selected by the U.S. Center for Health Promotion and Education. In addition to abstracts of published literature, CAHE also contains descriptions of ongoing programs in health education. Subject, author, and program title indexes are found in the back of each issue.

Current Literature in Family Planning. A monthly annotated review of the family planning literature in the United States. Part I lists books and Part II lists articles from 1,785 journals and a number of indexes, abstracts, bibliographies in the field. Each section is subdivided according to subject area.

Current Literature on Venereal Disease Abstracts and Bibliography (MEDLARS). Abstracts the current literature on veneral disease from the MEDLARS database.

Education Index. A cumulative index to publications in education. Health education and many subtopics can be found in this index. It is especially useful for retrospective work, as it has been published since 1929. Use a systematic approach here, as mentioned in the previous discussion concerning key words and checking each volume accordingly. You might find clues to other words, and eliminate key words you began using.

Education Resources Information Center (ERIC). Involves two indexes for which computer search systems are available. *Current Index to Journals in Education* is a source of articles concerning school health education. *Research in Education* lists titles of unpublished papers according to topic headings. Articles are usually stored on microfiche. After you have chosen the descriptors, you should search the monthly issues of Resources in Education. You can copy the ED number given at the end of the bibliographic entry (Figure 3.4). The ED number can then be found in the Document Resumes section, where a more complete description is available (Figure 3.5). By reading the Document Resume section you can decide whether you will need the entire document. If so, it can be ordered through the ERIC Document Reproduction Service or by computer.

Environmental Health Information Access. Indexes and abstracts articles published, as well as some unpublished articles, on air and water pollution, noise pollution, solid waste and food and drug problems.

Excerpta Medica. Includes a series of journals that abstract the major literature in a field. Journals in the series that are of interest to health workers include *Environmental Health, Gerontology and Geriatrics, Health Economics, Occupational Health, Hospital Man-*

Group Experience
The CORE Model to Student Organization Development.
ED 233 284

Group Homes
Community Residential Treatment of MR Adolescent Offenders.
ED 233 549

Group Unity
Black Solidarity: The Tie That Binds.
ED 234 117

Guidance Programs
ACT II: Adults in Career Transition.
ED 233 134
Individualized Career Education Plan (ICEP) K-12, and Comprehensive Career Guidance System. Second Edition.
ED 233 256

Guidelines
The Vocational-Technical Resource Consortia Serving Business and Industry in Ohio. Digest of Study: Operational Procedures for Successful Vocational-Technical Resource Consortia in Serving Business and Industry in Ohio.
ED 233 220

Handicap Identification
Public Law 94-142: Child Find/Serve, Project ACES, Related Services. Final Evaluation Report, 1981-1982. Document Number 82-272-877.
ED 233 513
Screening Withdrawn and Depressed Students in Public Schools: An Inservice Technique.
ED 233 523

Handicrafts
Arts and Crafts of the Mississippi Hills. ESEA, Title IV-C, 1982-83.
ED 233 944

Hawaii
Academic Crossover Study: Community Colleges, Fall 1981.
ED 233 747

Heads of Households
Women's Access to Agricultural Extension Services in Botswana.
ED 233 873

Health
Health and Humanity: Humanities 401 Syllabus.
ED 233 654

Health Programs
Child Survival/Fair Start. A Look at the Factors Threatening the Survival, Health, and Cognitive Development of the World's Disadvantaged Children, and the Ford Foundation's New Program to Help These Children Get a Fair Start in Life. Working Paper.
ED 234 135
A School Program for a Healthier America: Educator's Guide.
ED 233 837
*Toward a Healthy Community (Organizing Events for Community Health Promotion).
ED 234 134

Health Services
Psychotherapeutic Approaches to Dealing with Mentally Retarded Adolescents and Adults in Community Settings.
ED 233 551
Strategies for Promoting Health for Specific Populations.
ED 234 133

Hearing Impairments
Cognitive Education for the Hearing-Impaired Adolescent.
ED 233 511
Computer Graphics and Creativity/Problem Solving Skills with Deaf and Severely Language Disordered Students: Parts I, II, and III.
ED 233 517
Louisiana Statewide Assessment and Data Management System for Hearing Impaired, Visually Impaired, and Deaf-Blind Students. Final Report, 1981-82.
ED 233 520
Nebraska Survey of Sensory Impaired Children and Youth. Final Report, 1981-82.
ED 233 519
The Performance of Emotionally Disturbed, Hearing Impaired, and Visually Handicapped Children on the Vineland Adaptive Behavior Scales.
ED 233 542
Teaching Hearing-Impaired Children in Regular Classrooms. Language in Education: Theory and Practice, No. 54.
ED 233 590
Texas State Survey of Hearing Impaired Children and Youth. Final Report, 1981-82.
ED 233 521

Heat
Heat Problems.
ED 233 978

Figure 3.4 *Resources in Education*—subject index.

EDRS Price - MF01/PC03 Plus Postage.
Descriptors—*Achievement Gains, Attendance, *Bilingual Education Programs, Chinese, English (Second Language), Korean, *Mainstreaming, Outreach Programs, *Parent Participation, *Program Effectiveness, Self Concept, Social Studies, *Transitional Programs
Identifiers—New York City Board of Education, *Queens Chinese Korean Bilingual Language Arts NY
The Queens Chinese/Korean Bilingual Language Arts Resource Center operates at Newtown High School, in a multiethnic neighborhood in Queens, New York. The program, designed to provide bilingual educational services and curricular materials to Chinese and Korean students (grades 9-12) at Newtown, and ancillary services to students at Bryant High School, has several objectives: (1) to provide participants with the skills they need to function in mainstream classes; (2) to help students complete their high school education and pursue higher education; (3) to encourage the development of a positive self image; and (4) to eliminate or reduce content-area failures in social studies and in Chinese language arts (this objective is part of the Chapter 720-funded component). The program includes classroom instruction, curriculum development, supportive services (grade advisement and guidance, family assistance, extracurricular activities); staff development; and parental involvement efforts. This report describes program activities and objectives, and provides data on program results, including student achievement in all subject areas and parent achievement in English. (GC)

ED 234 129   UD 023 064
Reading and Math through the Community as Classroom, Summer 1982. Annual Evaluation Report. E.S.E.A. Title I.
New York City Board of Education, Brooklyn, N.Y. Office of Educational Evaluation.
Pub Date—82
Note—24p.
Pub Type—Reports - Evaluative (142)
EDRS Price - MF01/PC01 Plus Postage.
Descriptors—*Achievement Gains, Athletics, *Community Resources, Compensatory Education, Disabilities, *Disadvantaged Youth, Elementary Secondary Education, Mathematics Achievement, Program Effectiveness, Reading Achievement, Remedial Programs, *Special Education, *Summer Schools

Identifiers—New York City Board of Education, *Reading and Math through Community as Classroom NY
This report presents evaluation findings for the 1982 summer cycle of "Reading and Math Through the Community as Classroom," a Title I funded program operated by the Division of Special Education, of the New York City Public Schools. The program was designed to provide supplementary remediation to 1,197 mildly to moderately handicapped youngsters, and incorporate community experiences and sports activities into reading and math instruction. Results of analyses of pupil achievement data and program interviews and observations indicated that the summer program effectively met its proposed goals. Nearly all of the program participants mastered one or more new skills in reading (87.8 percent) and in math (91.9 percent). Students were also reported by teachers to have made social gains. Program sites were well-chosen and staff were enthusiastic. During 1982, the program made improvements over previous years in preparation, implementation, teacher appointments, and transportation services. However, attrition and the need to recruit new students posed problems. Based on evaluation findings, it is recommended (1) that preplanning be undertaken as early as possible to ensure optimal student recruitment, teacher assignment, and provision of materials and supplies, and (2) that difficulties with transportation be addressed, possibly by utilizing minibus services and by requiring preprogram trial runs. (Author/GC)

ED 234 130   UD 023 065
Torres, Judith A. And Others
Seward Park High School. Washington Irving High School. Chinese Bilingual Education Program, 1981-1982. O.E.E. Evaluation Report.
New York City Board of Education, Brooklyn, N.Y. Office of Educational Evaluation.
Pub Date—Apr 83
Grant—G00-800-6609
Note—80p.; For related document, see ED 223 759.
Pub Type—Reports - Evaluative (142)
EDRS Price - MF01/PC04 Plus Postage.
Descriptors—*Achievement Gains, Attendance, *Bilingual Education Programs, Bilingual Instructional Materials, Business Education, *Chinese, Curriculum Development, High Schools, Mathematics Achievement, Parent Participation, Program De-

Figure 3.5 *Resources in Education*—document resume section.

agement, Public Health, Social Medicine and Hygiene, and *Microbiology.*

Index Medicus (DIALOG MEDLINE). Lists biomedical literature from 2,000 journals published throughout the world. An abridged version that covers 100 major journals is available for individuals or small libraries (Figure 3.6).

Medical Care Review. Includes abstracts, chapter headings of books, literature reviews, and reprints of newspaper articles from public health economics and medical care literature. Topics covered are government health programs, insurance, medical facilities, and medical care organizations.

Nutrition Abstracts and Reviews. Abstracts prepared by specialists on various aspects of animal and human nutrition.

Pollution Abstracts. Major categories listed are air pollution, water pollution, solid wastes, noise, pesticides, radiation, and air environment quality. *(Allied Abstracts and Indexes of Health Resources)*

There are many other sources of indexes and abstracts that may be helpful:

Abstracts for Social Workers. The health professional should find various sections useful such as aging and aged, alcoholism and drug addiction, health and medical care, and housing and urban development.

Biological Abstracts (BIOCODES, Biosis Previews). Abstracts on a variety of fields are included. Subject headings of interest to the health professional are social biology, public health, nutrition, parasitology, and microbiology. The January issue includes the list of subject classifications, and the November issue contains a list of serials.

Bioresearch Index (Biosis Previews). A supplement to *Biological Aabstracts* that contains references to the literature in the life sciences. Available in specialized monthly subdivisions such as addiction, environmental pollution, food additives and residues, food microbiology, human and animal aging, human and animal parasitology, human ecology, industrial health and toxicology, pesticides, and population-fertility and birth control.

Current Contents. Lists the table of contents of important journals and appears in three editions that may be of interest to the health professional: (a) life sciences; (b) agriculture, biology and environmental sciences; and (c) social and behavioral sciences. It includes weekly listings and authors' addresses for reprint requests.

Dissertation Abstracts. Abstracts are arranged by subject and indexed by the author's name as well as by keywords. Abstracts prepared by the author provide a concise overview of the nature of the dissertation.

DIAGNOSIS

Head trauma evaluated by magnetic resonance and computed tomography: a comparison. Han JS, et al. **Radiology** 1984 Jan;150(1):71–7

PHYSIOPATHOLOGY

In-vitro head and neck response to impact. Kabo JM, et al. **J Biomech Eng** 1983 Nov;105(4):316–20

PREVENTION & CONTROL

[Modeling cranio-cerebral injury for evaluation and elaboration of the methods of protection of pilots from an impact] Barer AS, et al. **Kosm Biol Aviakosm Med** 1983 Sep-Oct;17(5):7–12 (Eng. Abstr.)
                                              (Rus)

PSYCHOLOGY

The behavioral sequelae of head injury. McLean A Jr, et al. **J Clin Neuropsychol** 1983 Dec;5(4):361–76

RADIOGRAPHY

Computed tomography in acute head injuries. Hryshko FG, et al. **CT** 1983 Nov;74(4):331–44
[What is the value of emergency cranial radiography in craniofacial injuries?] Bernard C, et al. **Sem Hop Paris** 1983 Oct 13;59(36):2567–9 (Eng. Abstr.)   **(Fre)**

REHABILITATION

Recovery trends of functional skills in the head-injured adult. Panikoff LB. **Am J Occup Ther** 1983 Nov;37(11):735–43

SURGERY

[Head injuries in patients with pre-existing skull defects] Sakai H, et al. **No Shinkei Geka** 1983 Oct;11(10):1093–6 (Eng. Abstr.)
                                              (Jpn)

THERAPY

Drug stop. Iatrogenic barbiturate coma in severe head injury. Ambielli M. **J Neurosurg Nurs** 1981 Dec;13(6):344–5

HEAD NURSES see NURSING, SUPERVISORY

HEAD PROTECTIVE DEVICES see under PROTECTIVE DEVICES

HEADACHE

Management of headaches in childhood. Barabas G. **Pediatr Ann** 1983 Nov;12(11):806–13 (26 ref.)
[New orientations in the diagnosis and therapy of headache in children] Lendvai D, et al. **Clin Ter** 1983 Sep 30;106(6):457–65 (Eng. Abstr.)   **(Ita)**

CHEMICALLY INDUCED

[Drug-induced headache] Kohl FV. **Med Welt** 1983 Nov 18;34(46):1294–7   **(Ger)**

DIAGNOSIS

Unilaterality of headache. Hauge's studies revisited. Sjaastad O, et al. **Cephalalgia** 1983 Dec;3(4):201–5
[Diagnostic methods in chronic and recurrent headache] Banach S, et al. **Neurol Neurochir Pol** 1983 May–Jun;17(3):361–5 (29 ref.)   **(Pol)**

ETIOLOGY

'Cervicogenic' headache. An hypothesis. Sjaastad O, et al. **Cephalalgia** 1983 Dec;3(4):249–56
[Acute spontaneous subdural hematoma. On the differential diagnosis of acute headache] Gerhard H, et al. **Med Welt** 1983 Oct 7;34(40):1116–8   **(Ger)**

OCCURRENCE

Migraine, headache, and survival in women. Waters WE, et al. **Br Med J [Clin Res]** 1983 Nov 12;287(6403):1442–3

PSYCHOLOGY

Sick—a way of life. Runnels GO. **J Miss State Med Assoc** 1983 Nov;24(11):301–4

THERAPY

Re: epidural blood patch [letter] Crawford JS. **Anaesth Intensive Care** 1983 Nov;11(4):384
Nonpharmacologic treatment of chronic headache: prediction of outcome. Blanchard ED, et al. **Neurology (NY)** 1983 Dec;33(12):1596–603

HEALTH

The effects of high voltage transmission lines on the health of adjacent resident populations. Haupt RC, et al. **Am J**

Figure 3.6 Example of entry from *Index Medicus,* March 1984.

Human Resources Abstracts. Contains valuable socioeconomic literature of significance to the public health professional. Sections are included on social conditions, social action, health and medical care, food and nutrition, and housing.

Industrial Hygiene Digest. Abstracts periodicals, pamphlets, and books that deal with industrial health.

Masters Abstracts. An author-prepared abstract of master's theses, published quarterly.

Oral Research Abstracts. Provides information on dental public health, nutrition, and social aspects of dental science.

Population Sciences: Index of Biomedical Research (MEDLARS). A monthly index of the periodical literature on various aspects of population science.

Psychological Abstracts. Various topics of importance to the health professional are included such as drugs, human sexuality, and human behavior.

Public Affairs Information Sources. Indexes publications dealing with public affairs. Provides information on the economics, politics and sociology of health care delivery.

Reader's Guide to the Periodical Literature. Provides an author/subject index to periodicals in the popular literature. A heading appears for health education.

Social Science Index. Selected popular and professional sources are listed under a variety of useful headings, such as disease, food, hospitals and medical care.

Sociological Abstracts. Sections on demography, human biology and the sociology of health and medicine are of significance to the health professional.

Government Documents. * Most large libraries have a government documents section, which contains valuable information pertinent to several areas in the health sciences. *The Monthly Catalogue of United States Publications* lists all government publications. The subject index in the back of the catalogue lists an entry number along with a special call number for library use. The publication will be filed according to its call number. The *National Health Information Clearinghouse,* which was established by the Office of Disease Prevention and Health Promotion, provides a publication called *Health Information Resources in the Department of Health and Human Services.* This is a directory that describes federal health information resources in the DHHS.

*Parts of this section are taken from Wilson, W. and Iverson, D. (1982) Federal data bases for health education resources, *Health Education, 13* No. 3: 33–34.

National Center for Health Statistics (NCHS). This arm of the government operates a survey and inventory program, with legislative authority to collect information concerning an array of health-related matters. The major surveys conducted by the NCHS are described below:

> *The National Health Interview Survey (NHIS)* is a continuous household survey, since 1957, of the civilian, noninstitutionalized population of the United States. It is based on an annual sample of about 40,000 households, providing data on approximately 110,000 individuals. The purpose of the survey is to provide national estimates of the incidence of acute illness and injuries; the prevalence of chronic conditions and impairments; the extent of disability; the use of health services and other health promotion areas, such as smoking behavior; and the use of preventive health services. Data are published in *Vital and Health Statistics* (Series 10) and the *AdvanceData* reports.

> *The National Health and Nutrition Examination Survey (NHANES)* is a periodic survey obtaining data from physical examinations, clinical and laboratory tests, and related measurement procedures on a national probability sample of the civilian, noninstitutionalized population. Data of particular interest to health education researchers include blood pressure distributions, levels of toxic agents in blood, prevalence of dental conditions, nutritional factors related to health, obesity, and physical activity levels. NHANES I provided data on persons 1 to 74 years of age for the period 1971–75, and NHANES II provides information on persons aged 6 months to 74 years for the period 1976–80. Earlier health examination surveys collected data (without the nutrition component) for adults in 1960–62, for children ages 6 to 11 in 1963–65, and for adolescents ages 12 to 17 in 1966–70. A special health and nutrition examination survey directed to persons of Hispanic origin began in 1982. NHANES III is now planned to begin in 1987. Data from NHANES are published in *Vital and Health Statistics* (Series 11) and the *AdvanceData* reports.

> *The National Survey of Personal Health Practices and Consequences* is a one-time study conducted by NCHS to investigate (1) the distribution of preventive health behaviors in an adult population, (2) the stability of these behaviors based on reinterviews with the respondents one year later, and (3) the relationship of these behaviors to health status and mortality. The data were collected in telephone interviews with about 3,000 persons ages 20 to 64, representing a national probability sample. Data are published in *Vital and Health Statistics* (Series 15).

> *The National Ambulatory Medical Care Survey (NAMCS)* provides data on patient visits to office-based physicians in the United States, catalogued by patient and physician characteristics, diagnosis, patients's reason for visit, and service provided. The survey involves an annual sample of about 3,000 office-based physicians. It was conducted

annually from 1973 to 1981 and has been conducted triennially thereafter. Data are published in *Vital and Health Statistics* (Series 13) and the *AdvanceData* reports.

The National Hospital Discharge Survey (NHDS) provides data on patient stays in short-term hospitals, catalogued by patient characteristics, length of stay, diagnoses, and surgical operations based on data from discharge records of patients in a national probability sample of general and special short-stay hospitals. Data collection has been continuous since 1964. Data are published in *Vital and Health Statistics* (Series 13).

The National Natality Survey and National Fatal Mortality Survey obtained data not available on birth and fetal death records, by returning to mothers, physicians, and hospitals for information related to about 10,000 births and 7,000 fetal deaths that occurred in 1980. Similar studies were conducted in the 1960s. Data were published in *Vital and Health Statistics* (series 21) and the *AdvanceData* reports.

The National Survey of Family Growth (NSFG) produces data on factors that influence trends and differentials in fertility, family planning practices, and other variables related to family growth from national probability samples of women of childbearing ages. Surveys have been conducted in 1973–74, 1976, and 1982, with future surveys expected to be conducted at five-year intervals. Data are published in *Vital and Health Statistics* (Series 23) and the *AdvanceData* reports.

The National Vital Registration System provides data on births and deaths based on data provided from the states. Birth data are available catalogued by age of mother, race, parity, and marital status and from many states by number of prenatal visits, timing of first prenatal visit, and educational level of mother. Mortality data are available by age at death, sex, race, and cause of death. Vital event data are available for state and substate levels. Data are published in the *Monthly Vital Statistics Report* and its supplements, in the annual *Vital Statistics of the United States,* and in *Vital and Health Statistics* (Series 20 and 21).

Centers for Disease Control (CDC). This center collects information concerning many reportable diseases, including childhood and infectious diseases. Estimates of these diseases are published in *Morbidity and Mortality Weekly Report.*

The National Institute on Drug Abuse (NIDA). NIDA maintains data bases of special interest to health educators.

The Lifestyles and Values of Youth. This survey collects data from high school seniors each spring, beginning with the class of 1975. Data collection takes place in approximately 125 to 130 public and private high schools selected to provide an accurate cross-section of high school seniors throughout the United States. For eleven separate classes of drugs, data are collected on grade of first use, trends in use at earlier grade levels, intensity of drug use, attitudes and beliefs concerning various types of drug use, and perceptions of certain relevant aspects of the social environment. Data are published in *Drugs in the Class of . . .* (each survey year): *Behaviors, Attitudes and Recent National Trends*

(Series 20). Related publications can be obtained from the Institute for Social Research, Rm. 2030, Box 1248, The University of Michigan, Ann Arbor, MI 48106.

The National Survey on Drug Abuse is one of the most consistent sources of drug use data on youth and young adults. Five separate studies comprise this data base: *Public Attitudes Toward Marijuana* (1971); *Drug Experience, Attitudes and Related Behavior among Adolescents and Adults* (1973); *Public Experience with Psychoactive Substances* (1975); *Nonmedical Use of Psychoactive Substances* (1976); and *National Survey of Drug Abuse* (1977).

The Drug Abuse Warning Network (DAWN) was established in 1972 to monitor the consequences of drug abuse using two indicators: emergency room visits and deaths. DAWN collects its information through episode reports provided by selected hospital emergency rooms, crisis centers, and medical examiners. Reporting facilities are concentrated in 24 Standard Metropolitan Statistical Areas, which are not randomly selected but account for approximately 30% of the population of the U.S. in geographically diverse locations.

Office of Smoking and Health; National Institute of Education. National Surveys on the patterns of cigarette smoking occurred in 1967, 1968, 1970, 1972, 1974, and 1979. The surveys used stratified probability samples that were randomly selected by computer from a telephone data bank. The 1979 survey included 2,639 boys and girls from 12 through 18 years of age. Between 185 and 196 interviews were conducted with boys and girls of each age from 12 to 18. Survey reports are available from the Office of Smoking and Health, Technical Information Center, Park Building, Room 116, 5600 Fishers Lane, Rockville, MD 20857.

The Computer Search

After you realize just how many sources are available to you when conducting a literature search, you might want to conduct a computerized literature search. Most major university and college libraries are equipped with the hardware and software that will enable you to conduct that search. Using the computer search will enhance your ability to check the preliminary sources.

Why Conduct a Computer Search?

A computer search enables you to search the literature by using a computer terminal. This terminal will have access to several databases (stored files) of references to literature. These databases are usually broader and more frequently updated than books or peiodicals. A computer search is certainly faster and more flexible than a manual one. The computer can scan millions of records in seconds and can combine subject terms in a way that is impossible in a manual search. Searches also can be run on phrases or words that appear in the titles of written materials, which enables you to use the most up-to-date, pertinent terminology.

Abstracts also are available via a computer search. This gives the student a more thorough description of the material and can save time in locating unnecessary or unwanted publications. The printouts of the list of citations will devote a full bibliographic entry, and this can save you time in writing the reference on a note card—just paste or tape it on! A final advantage of using a computer search is its relatively low cost, in that a typical search will usually cost between $10 and $20.

Information Available Through Computer Searches

Most university or college libraries subscribe to the large information retrieval services that are available: BRS or DIALOG. These data bases will provide you with needed citations because they both include all of the aforementioned indices including MEDLINE, DISSERTATION ABSTRACTS, ERIC, PSYCINFOR and SSCI. Most libraries use on-line terminals, which enable the investigator to quickly retrieve the citations, in addition to getting other and pertinent information that may lead to new ideas of sources to search. If there is not an on-line terminal available, a search can be run and then mailed to you in about seven days.

How to Conduct a Computer Search

In most colleges and/or universities, you will not be able to actually conduct the search yourself, but rather you will work with a librarian who has special training in using retrieval information systems. The following hints may aid you in conducting your search:

1. **Specify the research problem.** The more precisely your problem statement is written, the more beneficial your computer search will be to you. A generalized statement will garner far too many descriptors that will lead to too many citations. A statement such as "self-efficacy in predicting smoking behavior of junior high school students" will provide a focus for the search because the interest is in *self-efficacy, prediction, smoking behavior,* and *junior high school.* These descriptors will limit the number of citations and be precise enough to home in on the necessary information.

2. **Select the data bases.** As we discussed previously, each university or college will have the software it believes necessary to help its users. With the librarians' help, you can decide which data base or combinations of data bases would be beneficial for your literature search. In the example used above, ERIC (which includes CIJE and RIE) PSYCINFO, and SSCI would be appropriate data bases.

3. **Select the descriptors.** With the advice and consultation of the librarian and the procedure provided by the data base, you should select the descriptors that best describe your research problem. Return to the example used in #1 above; the descriptors might be *self-efficacy, smoking, junior high students*, and *prediction*. Dependent on how the particular data base is set up, the librarian would combine these descriptors with *or* or *and* to limit the number of citations. You will also be asked to set the language limits (English only is most often requested), and to request a year from which to begin the search.

4. **Conduct the search.** Once the librarian (or whoever has access to the on-line terminal) has gotten on-line, you will be asked to enter the descriptors (that coincide with those in the data bases) and determine how many citations are available in each descriptor. At this time, you would probably want to have a printout of approximately ten references to see if you have used appropriate descriptors or their combinations. Once you have decided that you are on the right track, then you can tell the computer to print anywhere from 20 to 200 citations (if available). Some databases also provide abstracts for an additional fee, and you can tell the computer which abstracts you wish to have printed.

5. **Review the citation list.** After you have received the print-out, carefully review it and select those published works that you wish to read. You will probably find additional references in the bibliographies of these citations, which may lead to a second computer search.

Reading and Note Taking

Reading and note taking is perhaps the most important tool in the literature review. Once the materials have been located, the investigator must make notations on each bibliographic entry that is deemed useful and/or important. It is advisable to begin checking the most recent references, because these reports will have been built on earlier research.

After locating the article, you should first read the abstract to determine if the information will prove useful or provide insight into the problem you are studying. If you decide to read the article, use the back of the note card to take notes. Be sure that the bibliographic entry is correct and corresponds to the one directly on the manuscript. Determine an outline you will use for all note taking. A suggestion is in Figure 3.7.

SMOKING AND SEXUAL BEHAVIOR

Zabin, L. (1984). The association between smoking and sexual behavior among teens in US contraceptive clinics. Am. J. Of Pub. Health. 74, 261–263.

Purpose and hypotheses. Relationship of sexual behavior and smoking amongst female teenagers because school-age females are more frequently smokers than males; smoking is particularly hazardous to health when associated with oral contraceptives and smoking may be representative of a cluster of behaviors which are especially problematical.

Methodology. Thirty-two contraceptive clinics in eight US cities participated where 1174 females under age 20, completed a self-administered questionnaire at first consultation. Response rate = 95%; internally consistent instrument.

Results. Strong negative relationship between age of first intercourse and level of smoking. Smoking levels in this group exceed national averages. Girls who prepare in advance for coitus were significantly less likely to smoke. The data exhibited a higher level of smoking among subjects with lower levels of contraceptive usage, or usage of less effective methods.

Conclusions. Designing of initiatives which may be effective in discouraging smoking and unprotected intercourse among young women who demonstrate problem behaviors and who resist preventive behaviors in several health-related areas. Such programs could take place in STD, prenatal, and contraceptive clinics which serve teenagers.

Figure 3.7 Completed note card.

A systematized method for taking notes might include:

1. Use four-by-six-inch or five-by-eight-inch index cards. Keep extra blank cards with you so that you are always prepared to write down a reference or a sudden idea. This is especially valuable when you attend lectures or informal seminars.
2. Read the abstract first to determine if the article is worth reading in its entirety.
3. Read the references in the article, because they may provide valuable leads to other references.
4. File note cards under subtopics or alphabetically, by author. Place the subtopic and bibliographic entry at the top of the note card. If using books, include the call number on the card so that you can easily relocate the reference.
5. Cards should have a single notation—either by subtopic or author. In other words, one card, one subtopic or author.
6. Be prepared never to recopy your note cards. Therefore, write or print carefully at first and you will save time and energy.
7. Try to not carry completed note cards with you, but rather file them in an index card file box. This will eliminate the possibility of losing your cards.
8. Keep your cards for each paper, thesis, or dissertation you may write. You will eventually use these note cards again as you proceed with your career.

Writing the Section on Related Literature

You now have gathered all, or most, of the information necessary to begin writing the review of literature section of a paper, research report, thesis, or dissertation. It is important to note here that you will have already written the Introduction (discussed in detail in Chapter 2), which must be related to the review of literature. In addition, the writer should develop a plan for the review, be sure to have the proper theoretical orientation, and summarize the entire section.

Relating the Review

As we discussed, the purpose of doing the review of literature is to develop an understanding of the background for the study, to delineate very clearly the problem, and to provide an empirical basis for the hypotheses. To present a clear and concise rationale for attempting the study, the information in the literature review should always relate to the introductory material. This will enable the introduction to flow coherently and present an organized approach to theory and research related to your topic. The literature should be related to the purpose of the study, the generated hypotheses, and the population in question.

Development of Plan

We have stressed that being organized is of paramount importance in preparing for the review and in gathering the materials. That organization will help you in writing the review, as you have already established subheadings. Subheadings are usually based on the variables and their relationship to the problem of your study.

To make it easier for the reader, we suggest that each subtopic begin with an introductory sentence to explain the relevance of the section and end with a summarizing section that depicts the conclusions or insights gleaned from this subsection.

Theoretical Orientation

Each literature review in the health sciences must have a theoretical orientation, as discussed in the beginning of this chapter. The theory is usually derived from any of the social sciences and tends to build the theoretical perspectives of the health-related literature. The

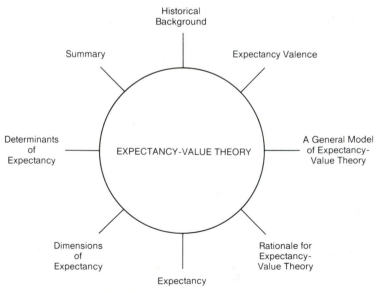

Figure 3.8 Theoretical core and subheadings.

central theme to the review is a theoretical core, from it emanate the subheadings, topics, and even subtheories. During the writing of the review, the theoretical orientation becomes part of the organizing framework, as shown in Figure 3.8.

Summarization

At the conclusion of the review of literature a separate subheading entitled *Summary* should be included. This section recaps the relevant information relating to theory, previous research, new insights, and the stated hypotheses. Generally, one or two paragraphs should suffice, if presented cogently.

Summary

This chapter told you about the tools and information necessary for a review of literature for a paper, research report, proposal, thesis, and/or dissertation. The benefits of the review include being able to limit the problem, develop an understanding and grounding in appropriate theory, review previously used procedures and instruments, originate new ideas, and use the recommendations for further research. A discussion of the steps in the research process included: (1) read the background information, (2) gather the necessary tools, (3) list key words, (4) use preliminary sources, and (5) read and take notes.

A complete listing and annotation of preliminary sources were given to acquaint the reader with the major information sources regarding the health sciences. In addition, a section concerning literature search by computer depicted the relative ease with which one can gather reference materials.

Finally, a strategy for actually writing the review was devised so that you can integrate the literature with the introductory materials discussed in Chapter 2.

Suggested Activities

1. Write a problem statement and prepare a brief topical outline to review the relevant literature.
2. Go to your university library and begin a search using only printed material.
3. After activity 2 above, use a computer index to search for additional sources.

CHAPTER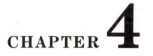

Conducting Experimental Research

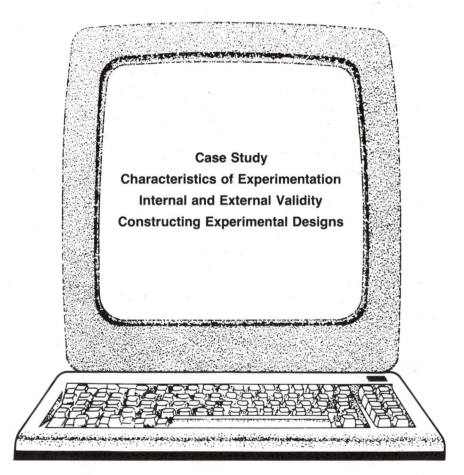

Case Study
Characteristics of Experimentation
Internal and External Validity
Constructing Experimental Designs

Case Study

Jayne was recently hired by the local school board to supervise and coordinate a comprehensive K-12 school health education program. She has had several years experience as a health science teacher and has had the opportunity to review many curricula. While her own philosophy concerning adoption of curricula differs from that of the Board of Education, she is committed to adopt the most suitable program for the district. Her superiors have given her a one-year timetable to adopt the curriculum. Her dilemma: which one should she choose, and how should that selection be made?

Characteristics of Experimentation

The experimental method of conducting research is an attempt to account for a factor in a given situation. It is generally considered to be the most highly regarded research method for hypothesis testing. The experiment carried out by the investigator is really a plan to garner evidence concerning the stated hypotheses. The natural environment is controlled and manipulated so that the researcher can observe and measure the results. When a true experimental situation is determined, the investigator is measuring the relationship between two or more variables in an attempt to discover the effect one variable might have on other variables.

Scientists began experiments with observation of the natural setting, but realized that extraneous events were not being controlled. The next step was to perform experiments in the laboratory where these extraneous factors could be controlled or at least taken into account. Physical and biological scientists used the laboratory method, and in the latter part of the 1800s psychologists began using experiments in the laboratory, and experimental psychology was born. However, experiments are not limited to the laboratory; they are achieved in the classroom, and elsewhere, but with much caution. It is understandable that children in classrooms cannot be randomly assigned to groups and randomly exposed to different teaching styles, because doing so may lead to nonequivalent groups. Although there are some problems inherent in "real-world" research, our behavior takes place in the real world, and thus experimentation should occur in lifelike situations. Behavioral scientists must exercise extreme caution and regard for variables and controls because of these limitations.

An experiment has three characteristics: a manipulated *independent variable,* control of all other variables *(dependent variables),* and the observed effect of the manipulation of the independent variable on the dependent variable. In our case study, if Jayne wanted to examine the effects of a health science curriculum on the gain in knowledge of students, she would manipulate the curriculum (independent variable) to determine the effect on achievement (the dependent variable). As can be deduced from the preceding discussion, the major issue in an experiment is the control of the independent and extraneous variables.

Control in Experiments

Without controlling variables, the experimental method cannot exist. Therefore control is of utmost importance in an investigation. Control allows the scientist to arrange the experiment so that the effect of the variables can be studied. Because health scientists deal with humans outside of the laboratory, not *every* variable can be controlled. However, it is acceptable to attempt to control those variables that might have a significant impact on the experiment. For example, if Jayne wanted to test the effects of a health science curriculum, she would need to have two groups of children who were exactly alike, except that group A would be exposed to the new curriculum, and group B would not receive the treatment (curriculum). These students should be alike in respects that are likely to have an impact on the health science curriculum: reading ability, morale, and motivation. However, other variables such as artistic ability, height, and vocal ability would be variables that could be ignored. Jayne would seek to choose two groups of students who would be most similar in the *significant* variables.

In Jayne's example, the experimenter is attempting to study the relationship between the independent and dependent variables. To do this, Jayne would have to control for *extraneous* variables. An extraneous variable is one that may affect the dependent variable and is not related to the major purpose of the experiment. Here Jayne would have to *control* for the extraneous variable of intelligence, because it would have an influence on the dependent variable. If the students in group A were more intelligent than those in group B, and group A performed better on the health science achievement tests, those gains could not be directly attributed to the new health science curriculum but to the higher intelligence level of the students in group A. In this experiment we have a *confounding* variable. A confounding variable is one in which independent and extraneous variables may each have an affect on the outcome of the experiment, and these effects cannot be separated.

When an experiment is carried out, the investigators must take precautions to be sure that there is as much equivalence as possible among the groups in the study. Several procedures are used to ensure equal groups: random assignment to group, randomized matching, and analysis of covariance.

Random assignment is the assignment of experimental subjects to groups such that every member of the population has an equal chance of being assigned to any of the groups. The investigator numbers all the subjects in the population, and uses a table of random numbers to draw the necessary number of subjects for each group. These groups are then considered to be *equivalent* in a statistical sense. In other words, the groups are so equal that if there is any difference between the groups, then it must be the result of chance alone and not of bias on the part of the investigator. Can Jayne use this method in her study of health science curricula?

Randomized matching occurs when subjects are matched on as many extraneous variables as could possibly effect the dependent variable. Then the matched pairs are assigned to an experimental condition. Variables used for matching usually include sex, age, socioeconomic status, and reading or pretest score. In a school situation where groups preexist (classrooms), investigators match groups on the extraneous variables. The researcher will determine that scores of groups on standardized tests (IQ, reading, pretest scores) are not significantly different in terms of means and standard deviations. Although group matching is not as ideal as individual randomization in certain "real-world" situations, this is the best method left to the investigator.

Analysis of covariance (ANCOVA) can be used to control for differences among the groups in the experiment. ANCOVA is a statistical method that analyzes differences of the experimental groups on the dependent variable only after initial differences on the pretest measures are taken into account. ANCOVA would probably be used in our case study of Jayne, because the method is very useful for intact groups (classrooms). However, ANCOVA only partially controls the extraneous variables that may confound the independent and dependent variables, and attempts at random assignment should be made.

The Hawthorne Effect—Controlling Situations

The experimental situation itself must be controlled to ensure that the differences observed are caused by the dependent variable and not the extraneous situational variables. In the famous Hawthorne experiment it was determined that any attention paid to subjects in the experiments may cause them to behave in a way that they believe is expected of them. At the Hawthorne plant of the Western Electric

Company, a group of investigators wanted to determine the effects of the intensity of light and working hours on the productivity of a group of women factory workers. The workers *increased* their productivity no matter what the experimenters attempted. The study team eventually deduced that the increased productivity was caused by the attention the workers received as subjects in a study.

Investigators involving the use of drugs routinely use a placebo (nonchemical look-alike) so that all subjects believe they are taking the drug. Otherwise, subjects might just react to the fact that they are taking a drug and act as might be expected, which would confound the results of the study. Again, control becomes a large part of the experiment. There are several methods to attempt to control situational variables: (1) hold the variables constant, (2) manipulate the variables systematically, and (3) randomize the situations.

Holding the variables constant is achieved by treating all subjects alike, regardless of group assignment, except for their exposure to the treatment. Ideally, the same teacher should teach the experimental health science curriculum in Jayne's case study. Additionally, all tests, instructions, and general procedures should be as identical as possible for each group.

Manipulating the variables systematically includes controlling the order in which the experiment is given to the subjects. If the subjects were to take a series of achievement tests in relation to the health curriculum, it might be beneficial to split the group in half. One group would receive the knowledge tests first and the second group would receive the decision-making tests first. This is an attempt to separate the groups from the main independent variable.

Randomizing the situational variables can provide a method to deal with the extraneous condition of having the same teacher for each group. The investigator could randomly assign half the experimental group and half the control group to each teacher. In this manner, extraneous conditions are not able to effect the dependent variable.

Advantages and Disadvantages of Experimental Method

It is important to recognize the benefits and pitfalls you might encounter when conducting experimental research. In our case study, Jayne might discuss these issues with her superiors so that they, as well as she, would be aware of the possible effects an experiment might have on the school system. *Advantages* include (1) convenience, (2) replication, (3) adjustment of variables, and (4) establishment of cause-and-effect relationships.

1. **Convenience.** The investigator may decide to carry out the experiment whenever or wherever feasible. Of course, real-world

research puts some limitations on convenience, but nonetheless, the experimenter may choose the time and location.

2. **Replication.** By repeating the experiment or parts of it, the validity of the results increase. This is because the results are based on several observations, rather than just one.

3. **Adjusting variables.** Being able to vary an aspect of the experiment allows the investigator to attempt several steps at a rather rapid pace. As in the previously mentioned Hawthorne experiment, the investigators were able to vary the aspects of the worker's environment in succession.

4. **Establishing cause-and-effect relationships.** This can be accomplished because the experimenter manipulates the independent variables and then observes the effects on the dependent variable. A caution here: make sure your independent variable is valid, because if it is not the effects may not be attributable to that variable.

Disadvantages of the experimental method include (1) cost, (2) inability to generalize, and (3) securing the cooperation of those involved in the project.

1. **Cost** can at times be a hindrance to experimental research. Many times, the training of experimenters and obtaining of equipment is expensive. When this happens, investigators must carry out a bare-bones experiment, or not conduct the study at all.

2. **Inability to generalize** the results of a study usually occurs because the samples used in the project were not representative of the population. In our case study, if Jayne used a group of private school students in her experiment, it would be an inappropriate sample, because the results of the experiment could not be generalized to public schools.

3. **Securing cooperation** from those in the experiment and from significant others (parents, administrators, supervisors) can be a major stumbling block for conducting a study.

Internal and External Validity_____

When designing an experiment the investigator must be certain that the study is technically sound. This is called the *validity* of an experiment. Two types of validity—internal and external—should be dealt with to prevent problems that may cast doubt on the implications derived from the results of the study. This type of validity differs in a way from validity concerning instrumentation.

Internal Validity

Internal validity can be defined as control for all influences between the groups being compared in an experiment, except for the experimental group. In our case study, Jayne would be comparing two methods of teaching the health science curriculum to two groups. The only differences between these two groups would be the teaching method (values clarification or didactic). Figure 4.1 illustrates this concept.

Internal validity is extremely difficult to achieve outside of the laboratory, because there are too many extraneous variables to control. As we attempt to control for internal validity and tighten those controls, external validity (to be discussed later) suffers. As is so often true of the research in the real world, the investigator must compromise! Not all extraneous variables can be eliminated, but the experimenter, in designing a study, should take into consideration the many intervening variables. These extraneous variables, or threats

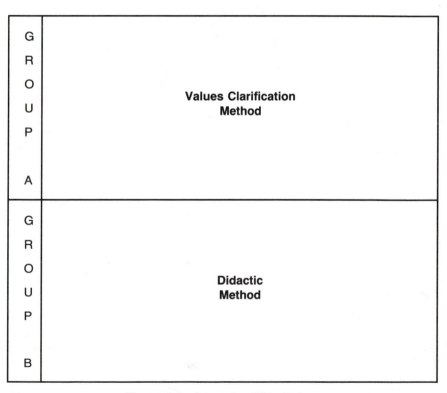

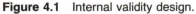

Figure 4.1   Internal validity design.

to the research design, were originally discussed by Campbell and Stanley (1963) and include the following:

Maturation refers to factors that may influence subjects' performance because of the time that has elapsed. The change that has occurred within the participants is the problem, because people normally change over a time regardless of interference (an experiment). This threat is especially apparent in longitudinal studies of young or adolescent children. How can this problem be attenuated? Usually by including a control group in the research design. The members of this additional group should be as comparable to the subjects in the experimental group as possible—they should have similar characteristics in their maturational development.

History is defined as those events that occur at the same time as the study. These external events can interfere with the subjects' performance in the experiment. Sometimes these events are unpredictable, such as a catastrophe in the community (e.g., a tornado). Events such as this make history very difficult to control. In our case study, Jayne has decided to pretest the students on a day when they are having an examination in mathematics. Undoubtedly, the subjects will be under stress, and this may interfere with the performance on the pretest. One way Jayne could attempt to limit the effect on the internal validity of the experiment would be to use a control group, which would be exposed to the same historical experiences during the time of the study. While this may not account for an unexpected event (e.g., a lunchroom fight), it can control for some historical events.

It also should be noted here that the concept of history is within the experiment, including the procedures and materials used to conduct the study. All methods, test instruments, and situations should be the same for every subject in the study, regardless of group assignment.

Testing at the onset of an experiment or actually before it begins, can have an effect on the subjects' performance at the time of the posttest. What is thought to occur is that the subjects practice taking the test and thus are "test-wise." Pretests may even give the subjects information (e.g., about cardiovascular health knowledge instruments), and thus threaten the internal validity of the experiment. This occurs because the investigator does not know if the results of the posttest resulted from the dependent variable (e.g., health science curriculum), or from the practice or knowledge gained from the pretest, or even from a combination of both situations.

To eliminate this test practice threat, two suggestions are offered: (1) use a comparison group that is exposed to the dependent variable but does not receive the pretest, and (2) increase the length of time between the administration of the pretest and posttest. While neither of these plans is absolutely foolproof in reducing the threat to the internal validity of the experiment, they do lessen the chance that the results of the study are suspect to testing practice.

Instrumentation can be a cause for concern in the internal validity of an experiment. The term refers to any changes in the instrument or measuring device used to test the effect of the dependent variable. In addition, changes in those who might be observers or raters in an experiment could change their rating system unknowingly. When considering a written instrument, the posttest should remain the same as the pretest, and procedures for recording the data (e.g., use of scanner sheets) should remain the same each time data are collected.

When observers or interviewers are used to collect data, they must be cognizant that they are fallible to fatigue, boredom, and awareness of the "right" answers. It is advisable that investigators check for intrarater and interrater reliability (Rubinson, Stone, and Mortimer, 1977) of these types of data collectors, to alleviate the possible threat to internal validity.

Statistical regression presents a threat to internal validity when subjects are assigned to a group because of their extreme scores on tests. As an example, students who scored in the highest and lowest quartiles on a nutrition knowledge test were chosen as subjects for the experimental group, and those in the middle 50% were eliminated from the study. At the time of the posttest, the scores of the highest quartile would decrease toward the mean while the scores for the students in the lowest quartile would increase the mean. This condition would produce differences between the groups on the posttest measures regardless of the intervention. So this will not occur, the investigator should make sure that the groups are composed of subjects whose scores represent the full range of possible scores.

Differential selection is actually a bias in selecting individuals for group selection. This usually occurs when participants volunteer for experimental group membership. In this case they usually are more highly motivated, which may cause them to be a biased group. Selection bias also can occur when intact classroom groups are assigned to either an experimental or control group. Here, the students in the seventh hour science class also may be in the advanced algebra class, hence introducing a bias to the study. One of the best ways to avoid this particular threat to internal validity is to randomly assign subjects to each group. However, this usually cannot be facilitated in a school, for obvious reasons. Then the investigators must limit their generalization of findings to the particular sample in the study.

Experimental mortality is the loss of subjects in an experiment (also called *attrition*), especially if there is a differential loss between the experimental and control group. Many times subjects involved in studies in schools will be "lost" due to absence on the day of a test, or they will have moved out of the school district. If this happens equally between the groups, experimentors can select replacement subjects. Other methods to ensure against biased samples resulting from attrition are to choose large groups of subjects and make sure of their representativeness. In addition, it is wise to follow a sample of those who left the study to obtain comparison data.

Selection-maturation interaction occurs when the maturation of subjects becomes the confounding variable. As an example to explain this threat to internal validity, let us use our case study. The seventh grade students selected for the experimental group to test the health science curriculum were from Jayne's school district. The control group of seventh graders was selected from another school district where, because of the different ages of the beginning students, the seventh graders were nine months younger than those in Jayne's school district (the experimental group). If the experiment were to proceed and results indicated that the experimental group's gains in knowledge were not as great as those in the control group, how could we interpret this data? The extraneous variable of maturation has confounded the results of Jayne's experiment. To avoid this situation, investigators must be sure to select groups of comparable maturity levels.

Another threat to internal validity, not discussed by Campbell and Stanley, is that of *contamination*. This bias occurs when the researcher has previous knowledge concerning the subjects in the experiment. The investigator may inadvertently treat the groups differently, or even give the subjects hints as to correct responses on surveys. In medical research, the subjects do not know who receives the experimental medication and who receives a placebo; this is known as a blind study. A double-blind experiment is an even better safeguard against contamination. The person who administers the treatments and records which subjects are in either the placebo or experimental group is not the experimenter, but rather an aide in the study. In our study, Jayne would have to make sure not to involve herself in the teaching and or testing of the curriculum.

External Validity

External validity is concerned with the researcher being able to generalize the findings of an experiment. In an attempt to control threats to internal validity in the behavioral sciences—real-world research—the investigator runs the risk of creating an unreal situation from which generalization to other settings is impossible. Most researchers outside of the laboratory tend to compromise and set up a rigorous experiment in a realistic situation.

Campbell and Stanley (1963) suggested four threats to external validity: the reactive effect of testing; the interaction effects of selection biases and the experimental variable; the reactive effects of experimental arrangements; and multiple-treatment interference. Bracht and Glass (1968) delineated Campbell and Stanley's four factors into a more specific set of threats to external validity. The following discussion is based on their work.

Population validity refers to the extent to which the results of an experiment can be generalized, from the sample used in the study to a larger group of similar people. There are two types of population validity, according to Bracht and Glass. *The extent to which results can be generalized from the experimental sample to a defined population* is the first type. In our case study, if Jayne randomly selected a group of seventh graders to expose to the experimental curriculum and found positive gains in terms of skills in decision making, she would like to generalize these findings to all seventh grade students. However, she can only generalize to those students from whom the sample was drawn: seventh grade students in her school district. This sample is defined as the *experimentally accessible population.* When we read reports of experiments, we sometimes, without thinking, generalize the sample to include all subjects e.g., seventh grade students in all junior high schools in New York. This last group (seventh grade students in all junior high schools) is called the *target population.* When making these generalizations, the researcher must be sure that the two groups are representative of each other. This can be accomplished, although with intact classrooms in schools it is virtually impossible. However, large-scale studies, such as the one conducted by Goodlad (1984) can be generalized to the target population. The schools in this experiment were truly representative of a cross-section of the schools in the United States.

Bracht and Glass wrote about a second type of population validity: *the extent to which personological variables interact with treatment effects.* Personological variables such as ability, sex, anxiety level, extroversion-introversion, and independence can have an effect on students' performance. Hence if the researcher wanted to generalize the findings to another grade level (eighth grade), it would be unwarranted. This phenomenon has gained support as its own branch of research called aptitude-treatment interaction (API) research.

Ecological validity is the second major type of threat to external validity that Bracht and Glass have described. They define ecological validity as the *extent to which the results of an experiment can be generalized from the set of environmental conditions in the experiment to other environmental conditions*. If the results can be obtained only under a very limited set of conditions, those results have low ecological validity. Bracht and Glass described several factors that may contribute to the ecological validity of an experiment:

1. **Explicit description of the experimental treatment.** Researchers must describe the experimental treatment in exact detail, so that it can be replicated by other experimenters.
2. **Multiple-treatment interference.** When it appears that subjects will be exposed to more than one experimental treatment, which may effect the generalizability of the findings of the study, the investigator should choose an experimental design in which one treatment is assigned to each subject.
3. **Hawthorne effect.** This phenomenon was discussed earlier, and can prevent the findings in a study from being generalized because those researchers or other staff personnel are not present in subsequent experimental trials.
4. **Novelty and disruption effects.** An experimental treatment may be effective just because it is different from what the subjects normally receive. This can cause low generalizability, because as novelty wears off so does the effectiveness of the treatment.
5. **Experimenter effect.** This refers to the person who administers the treatment (physician, teacher, nurse practitioner) and their inability to be involved in subsequent investigations. This is also an area of concern for low generalizability.
6. **Pretest sensitization.** As in the case of affecting internal validity, the pretest can act in an adverse way on the posttest performance of subjects. The usual occurrence is that the pretest affects the scores positively on the posttest.
7. **Posttest sensitization.** As in the case of pretest sensitization, at times the posttest can effect the subjects' scores and thus cause concern for generalizability of the experiment.
8. **Measurement of the dependent variable.** When instruments are used to measure the effects of a treatment, they may limit the generalizability of the results to other tests if they are particularly well adapted to the dependent variable.
9. **Interaction of time of measurement and treatment effects.** Experiments may use two or more posttests to measure the effects of an intervention. Usually, the first posttest is administered immediately after the intervention is concluded and then again several weeks or months later to measure the subjects' retention. These second measurements have changed the effects of the intervention and therefore pose a threat to ecological validity.

Investigators must take into account the many threats to internal and external validity when they design an experiment. Because most behavioral scientists work in the real world, some threats must remain, while others can be minimized and even excluded. If the investigator finds that a discrepancy exists between the experimental condition and real-world setting, then she or he should note this in the report as a limitation to the generalizability of the study.

Constructing Experimental Designs To Control Variables

The major purpose in constructing an experimental design is to control as many extraneous variables as possible. Because experimental research in the health sciences is usually conducted outside a laboratory, the investigator must take great pains to ensure that the proper controls are employed. However, in attempting to control for so many variables, real-world research can produce artificial results. This occurs because the environment and/or the subjects are sometimes put into unnatural situations. Snow (1974) has developed an alternative called *representative design,* whereby experiments accurately reflect real-life environments and the natural characteristics of the learners. In our case study, Jayne would then attempt to conduct her experiment in an environment where she could easily generalize the findings of the research.

We shall discuss several experimental designs, which can be divided into the following categories: preexperimental, true experimental, factorial, and quasiexperimental designs. To simplify this process, we will include symbols and terms to describe designs. These symbols are widely used in the literature and include

> *X:* Independent variable that is manipulated.
> *0:* Process of observation or test.
> *R:* Random selection of subjects to groups.
> *X's and 0's across a given row:* Apply to the same people.
> --: Dashed lines between groups indicate no random assignment to groups.

The left-to-right dimension indicates the temporal order, and the *X*'s and *O*'s, when vertical to one another, are given simultaneously.

Preexperimental Designs

The least adequate experimental designs fall into this group; there is no control group, and extraneous variables can cause threats to internal validity. As we progress from these types of experiments to those that do not have such weaknesses, you will be able to build an experiment that will avoid such problems.

The One-Shot Case Study

$$X \quad O$$

In this type of experiment, a treatment is given to one group. Then observations *(O)* are made on the subjects in that group to detect the effects of the treatment. Those observations are made in the form of a posttest. There is no control group, but rather the investigator makes inferences or comparisons of the results based on what the results would have been had the intervention not been given. In our case study, Jayne would introduce a health science lesson to a class of sixth graders and then give a posttest to determine the treatment effects. What might she deduce from this one-shot case-study experiment?

This is the very weakest of experimental designs and should be avoided. As we have discussed, the sources of invalidity in this instance would be history, maturation, selection, and mortality. If Jayne has only one group to use, then it is recommended that at least a pretest be given to the subjects to provide a measure of change.

The One-Group Pretest-Posttest Design

$$O_1 \quad X \quad O_2$$
$$O_1 = \text{pretest}$$
$$O_2 = \text{posttest}$$

Although this design improves the one-shot case study experiment, it is still considered to be weak. The group is administered a pretest to measure the dependent variable and then the treatment is introduced. The same test is readministered at the conclusion of the intervention (posttest). Jayne, in attempting to test the new health science lesson, did give the students a pretest and a posttest. She found that the students increased their knowledge significantly after being exposed to the intervention. Is she correct in believing that the gains in scores resulted from the new lesson? Probably not, because this design does not control for maturation of the students, history, the testing situation, or statistical regression.

The use of the one-group pretest-posttest design is sometimes necessary in school systems that will not allow their students to be treated differently. In other words, a school district insists that a new or experimental program must be made available to all students. In this case, it is necessary for the investigators to make estimates of the gains the subjects would make and then set their experimental significance levels against that standard. Therefore, this type of design can be safely used because most of the extraneous factors that cause threats to validity have been estimated to reach certain levels by the investigators. To test the differences of scores between the pretest and posttest, the usual method of analysis would be to employ the t-test for correlated means, because the same subjects take both tests.

The Static-Group Comparison

$$\frac{X \quad \underline{O}}{O}$$

The static-group comparison experiment includes two treatment groups (experimental and control) where each is given a posttest only. However, the subjects are not randomly assigned to the treatment groups, indicated by the --- lines above. Here selection and mortality interfere with the internal validity of the experiment because the results of the experiment may not be attributable to the intervention but to the differences in the subjects in each group. It is necessary that the groups be equivalent, and because random assignment was not employed, the investigator cannot ensure that the groups are equal.

In our case study, Jayne would select Ms. Evans' class as the control group and Mr. Jackson's class as the experimental group, and each group would be given a posttest after a series of new health science lessons were introduced. She analyzed the data using a t-test of the posttest mean scores and found that Mr. Jackson's class did score significantly higher on the achievement tests than Ms. Evans' class. Does this mean that the new health science lessons are better than the usual science series that Ms. Evans used? Not necessarily so, because Mr. Jackson's students may have had more science knowledge than Ms. Evans' students. They may not have been equivalent at the start of the study, a serious limitation of this type of experimental design.

True Experimental Designs

In these types of real experimental designs, control groups and experimental groups are involved in the study, and subjects have been randomly assigned to each group. These are the strongest types of designs, but Jayne will have difficulty using them because of intact groups, i.e., subjects in classrooms. However, she can assign *classrooms* randomly to groups, and then check students' records for standardized test scores to determine the homogeneity of the classes.

The Posttest-Only Control Group Design

$$
\begin{array}{ccc}
R & X & O_1 \\
R & & O_2
\end{array}
$$

In this true experimental design the experimental group experiences the intervention, but the control group does not. In addition, subjects are randomly assigned to each group and they both receive the same posttest. This is a very powerful design because it controls for all threats to internal validity with the exception of mortality. This is especially useful when the researcher has a large group of subjects because random assignment of the subjects allows for equivalence of the groups.

The pretest is not used in this design, which can be useful in several ways. There is no interaction between the pretest and the independent variable, and therefore the design should be used when there is likelihood that pretest reactivity would occur. In addition, there are cases in which pretests are not appropriate (studies in very young children where learning has not yet happened) or not available. A disadvantage of this design is that you cannot determine if change has occurred. Jayne would have to use a table of random numbers to select subjects to be assigned to experimental and control groups. Sixty students were chosen from an initial pool of 400 seventh graders. The experimental group would receive the new health science curriculum, while the control group would be taught the regular curriculum. All factors would be equated, and at the end of the intervention both groups would be posttested. The data would be analyzed by using a t-test comparison of the mean posttest scores of the groups. If Jayne had used more than two groups, she would use analysis of variance. The results of the statistical scores show that the experimental groups' scores were significantly higher than those of the control group. What can she conclude in regard to the new health science curriculum.?

The Pretest-Posttest Control Group Design

$$
\begin{array}{ccc}
RO_1 & X & O_2 \\
RO_3 & & O_4
\end{array}
$$

This design includes a pretest addition to the previously discussed true experimental design: posttest-only control group design. The subjects in the experimental and control groups are randomly assigned, and each group is given both a pretest and posttest. This design eliminates all threats to validity and thus provides an excellent setting for conducting a study. Randomization of the subjects will ensure that there was no systematic bias in the groups, but in some cases, there *may be* initial differences between groups, as shown on pretest scores. Once again, Jayne randomly selected her subjects, assigned them to groups, administered the pretests, had the appropriate teacher introduce the new health science curriculum, and then posttested each group. She analyzed the data by using analysis of covariance. The posttest mean scores were compared with the pretest scores as a covariate. In this experiment, no significant differences were found on the scores between the groups, but there were some that increased, showing positive changes in the experimental groups' scores. See if you can interpret these results.

The Solomon Four-Group Design

$$
\begin{array}{llll}
R & O_1 & X & O_2 \\
R & O_3 &   & O_4 \\
R &   & X & O_5 \\
R &   &   & O_6
\end{array}
$$

This is a very sophisticated experimental design that takes into account factors associated with external as well as internal validity. The design is set up to determine several factors at once: assess the effect of the treatment in relation to the control group, determine the effect of the pretest, and explain the interaction between the treatment conditions and the pretest. Random assignment of subjects to groups and inclusion of groups that are not pretested add to the significance of the results of the experiment. This results from combination of the previously discussed designs: posttest only and pretest-posttest. The design actually has two experiments going on at once and thus provides replication of the study.

However, there is a major disadvantage to this design: finding enough subjects to complete the four equivalent groups and randomly assigning them to groups. Even if enough subjects can be located, the time to conduct two experiments may not be available to the investigators. Several school health science studies (Rubinson and Stone, 1975; Peterson and Rubinson, 1982; and Bickman, 1978) have been conducted using the Solomon Four-Group Design, therefore Jayne, in our case study, has some frame of reference from which to conduct her investigation.

The analysis for this design is not simple but with today's computers can easily be handled. Campbell and Stanley (1963) suggest disregarding the pretests, except as a treatment, and analyzing the posttest scores with a simple 2 (pretest) x 2 (treatment) analysis of variance design:

	No X	X
Pretested	O_4	O_2
Unpretested	O_6	O_5

From the column means, one estimates the main effect of X, and from the row mean scores, the main effect of pretesting. The cell means provide an estimate of the interaction of testing with X. If the main and interactive effects of pretesting are negligible, an analysis of covariance of O_4 versus O_2, with the pretest scores as the covariate, should be performed.

Factorial Designs

Factorial designs are more complicated than the previously discussed designs where there was a single variable in which one independent variable was manipulated to have an effect on the dependent variable. A factorial design is one in which two or more variables are manipulated simultaneously so as to allow study of the independent effect of each variable on the dependent variable. In addition, the effects caused by the interaction among the several variables are assessed. The effect of each independent variable on the dependent variable is called a *main effect,* while the effect of the interaction of two or more independent variables on the dependent variable is termed an *interaction effect.*

R	O_1	X	Y_1	O_2
R	O_3		Y_1	O_4
R	O_5	X	Y_2	O_6
R	O_7		Y_2	O_8

In the above diagram, an illustration is given of a factorial design where Y is the second variable to be manipulated. In our case study, suppose Jayne were to set up her experiment to determine if a group of randomly assigned sixth graders learned more after being exposed to a new health science curriculum. Two methods of instruction for teachers were used: a three-day workshop and a two-hour orientation session. She set up a Solomon-Four Group Design that looked like Figure 4.2.

The data were analyzed with a two-way analysis of variance using the posttest knowledge scores. The factors considered were training (treatment I, II, or III) and test sequence (pretest or no pretest). Figure 4.3 illustrates the results of the analysis of the mean knowledge

		Pretest	**Curriculum**	**Posttest**
WORKSHOP GROUP	R	O_1	XX	O_{203}
ORIENTATION GROUP	R	O_4	XX	O_{506}
	R	O_7		O_{809}

Figure 4.2 Health science curriculum, Solomon-Four Group Design.

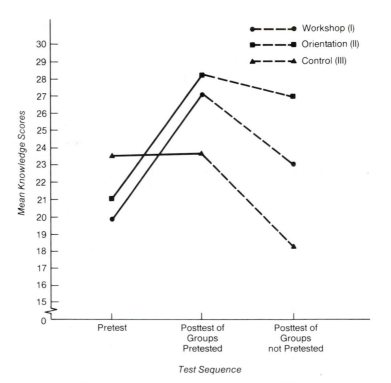

Figure 4.3 Interaction between variables.

scores showing an *interaction* between the variables. The data revealed that there were significant *main effects* and a significant training X sequence *interaction*.

Quasiexperimental Designs

There are times when researchers cannot control all sources of internal and/or external validity. These occasions call for the investigator to use a quasiexperimental design, which although not as strong as the true experimental designs, is certainly preferable to the preexperimental designs. Experiments in this group use designs in which random assignment of subjects to groups has not been accomplished. These experiments are usually carried out where intact groups are available, i.e., schools. In our case study, Jayne would have to use a quasiexperimental design, as she had determined that school officials in her district will not allow students to be reassigned from their original classes.

Campbell and Stanley (1963) originally described thirteen quasiexperimental designs; however, we have decided to explain only those that would have a direct bearing on the health sciences: time-series, nonequivalent control group, and counterbalanced and equivalent time-samples. Each design has strengths and weaknesses that enable investigators to choose the design that would be most appropriate for a particular setting.

Interrupted Time Series Experiment

$$O_1 O_2 O_3 O_4 \qquad X \qquad O_5 O_6 O_7 O_8$$

If Jayne wished to have the entire school system involved in her study, she would want a comparable school district to serve as a control group. Unfortunately, she cannot find one that is both comparable and willing to join in the experiment. Therefore she decides to use the interrupted time series design, as diagrammed above.

As evidenced, there is one experimental group in which observations occur before and after the intervention. Several sources of validity are not threatened when using this design, but the general weakness includes a threat to the effect of history; other influences might have an effect on the dependent variable after it is introduced. This can be controlled by adding a control group, but in our case study this is impossible. Another minor weakness of interrupted time series designs is that of the effect of instrumentation. During the experiment, there are many points at which data are collected, and those who administer the tests may do it differently and even score it improperly. This is especially true of data and record keeping in hospitals, where many different personnel may be involved in this activity.

A caution all researchers should take into consideration when using interrupted time series designs is the cyclical nature of performance and attitudes, which may be attributed to seasonal variations. For example: more hospital admissions occur during the Christmas holidays, and school children will not respond well to serious interventions the day before a vacation. Several other interrupted time series designs may be used. For a thorough discussion of these, refer to Cook and Campbell's *Quasi-Experimentation* (1979).

There are a few limitations associated with interrupted time series designs. They include:

1. Treatments are rapidly implemented, but rather slowly diffused.
2. Effects are not instantaneous.
3. Data observations are too few—50 are recommended.

The statistical analysis for interrupted time series design depends on the number of observations within the experiment. If 50 to 100 observations are available, it is recommended that the autoregressive integrated moving average (ARIMA) models be used. Refer to Box and Jenkins (1976) for a complete description of this technique. However, if fewer than 50 observations occur and the errors are independent, analysis of variance (ANOVA) with repeated measures should be used to analyze the data. If the errors are correlated and the number of observations is small, multiple analysis of variance (MANOVA) is a satisfactory statistical technique.

Equivalent Time Samples

$$X_1O \quad X_0O \quad X_1O \quad X_0O$$

The equivalent time sample design is similar to the time series design; however, the treatment is not introduced once but rather introduced and reintroduced to the subjects. In addition another experience is introduced (X_o) and it too is reintroduced at predetermined intervals. To fully implement this design, the investigator needs large and representative samples and should have a random sample of time periods. In our case study, Jayne would introduce a new health science lesson, using a behavioral approach to 100 sixth-grade students and reintroduce this lesson or an equivalent follow-up. At the same time, another group of 100 sixth graders would be exposed to a different health science lesson that used a values' clarification approach and followed the proper or same intervals.

The equivalent time series design controls for all threats to internal validity, therefore covering the threat of history, which the time-series design does not. In other words, extraneous events should not have an effect on the outcome of the experiment.

Two types of generalizations occur in this type of experiment: (1) across occasions and (2) across subjects. Analysis of the data may be accomplished by comparing the two experiences against a between-occasions-within-experience error term. This provides information about the changes that occur over time.

Nonequivalent Control Group Design

$$O_1 \quad X \quad O_2$$
$$\text{-----}$$
$$O_3 \qquad O_4$$

In this design, both groups are pretested and posttested, no control group is exposed to the intervention, and none of the subjects have been randomly assigned to groups. This design and its many variations (adding non-pretested experimental and control groups) are frequently used in situations such as our case study. As mentioned previously, classrooms are intact, as are other groups: prisoners, some patients in hospitals (dependent on illness), and so on. However, what does become random is the assignment of the intervention. While this design can appear weak, it does become sound in that usually subjects are chosen from a pool of those with somewhat similar characteristics (i.e., age, experience, grade in school). This homogeneity can be tested by comparing scores of the groups on the pretest. The interaction of selection and maturation can be a threat to the validity of the nonequivalent control group design.

To statistically analyze this design, the investigator should use the analysis of covariance (ANCOVA), which would reduce the effects of initial differences between the groups because it makes adjustments to the posttest scores of each group. If you use ANCOVA, remember that only the *measured* variables are used as covariates. There is the possibility that subjects in the groups may differ on other, nonmeasured variables that have not been used in the ANCOVA. The investigator also can use multiple regression to analyze the data from the results of the experiment. This method is advantageous to ANCOVA only because it has less stringent assumptions than ANCOVA. In multiple regression, the posttest scores would be the criterion variable, and the investigator could then decide if the treatment was significant to the prediction.

Counterbalanced Design

	Time$_1$	Time$_2$	Time$_3$	Time$_4$
Group A	X$_1$ O	X$_2$ O	X$_3$ O	X$_4$ O
Group B	X$_2$ O	X$_4$ O	X$_1$ O	X$_3$ O
Group C	X$_3$ O	X$_1$ O	X$_4$ O	X$_2$ O
Group D	X$_4$ O	X$_3$ O	X$_2$ O	X$_1$ O

Counterbalanced designs, also called Latin squares, are usually used when two or more interventions are to be tested. All the subjects will receive all the treatments for a specific time period. The order of administration of treatments is varied between subjects, so that order effects are not confounded with treatment effects. These have been called *rotation experiments*. In our case study, Jayne would use counterbalancing to test the effectiveness of two methods of teaching a health unit to eighth-grade students. The two units, however, must be equal in all aspects—difficulty, age-relatedness, factual information and the like. After each class completed the unit, a cognitive test would be administered to the subjects. This design is especially useful for intact groups and actually is slightly better than the nonequivalent control group design in that it might "rotate out" differences that could exist between groups. In addition, students are matched to themselves, making statistical analysis more discriminatory.

There are some weaknesses in carrying out an experiment like the one just described. A carryover effect from one teaching method to another may effect the scores on the tests. In addition, it is sometimes very difficult to determine that units of study are, in effect, equal in all aspects as prescribed. Also, it could be possible that students would tire of taking as many tests as required in the counterbalanced design.

Summary

This chapter attempted to introduce and explain the very important concept of *control* in conducting experimental research. Good research studies ensure and take into account the advantages and disadvantages of conducting an experiment. While experimentation originally began in the laboratory, it has been successfully conducted in naturalistic settings such as schools, factories, ships, and hospitals. When conducting an experiment, the investigator must be concerned with several threats to internal validity, including variables, history, selection, instrumentation, testing, differential selection, experimental mortality, selection-maturation interaction, and contamination. Another type of validity, external validity, was discussed with specific reference to population validity and ecological validity.

Experimental designs can be classified into four categories: pre-experimental, true experimental, factorial, and quasiexperimental. Ten designs were discussed with respect to controlling extraneous variables. These included the one-shot case study, one-group pretest-posttest, static group comparison, posttest only control group, pretest-posttest control group, Solomon-four group, time series design, equivalent time samples, nonequivalent control group, and the counterbalanced design. Investigators may use each of these designs based on need, availability of subjects, proposed hypotheses, and suitable data analysis capabilities.

Suggested Activities

1. A school decides to implement a health science curriculum for all its seventh-grade students. The investigators predict that the new health science curriculum will increase the subject's knowledge and problem-solving skills in the area of cardiovascular health. Why must a quasiexperimental design be used? Construct the appropriate design.
2. From the following hypotheses, select the independent and dependent variables.
   a. Students exposed to the cardiovascular program will demonstrate superior scores on all scales, as compared to students in the control group.
   b. The percentage of people exposed to the dental screening will increase significantly as compared to those in the control group.
   c. Health knowledge of those teachers attending the in-service training will be greater than the scores of the teachers in the control group.
   d. The treatment group receiving all modes of instruction will achieve a higher score than those subjects in the groups receiving only one mode of instruction.
   e. Students exposed to the human sexuality course will have significantly more liberal attitudes than those students in the control group.
3. Explain the following design

$$R \quad X \quad O_1$$
$$R \qquad\quad O_2$$

4. Choose two research articles that used experimental designs and prepare a symbolic representation of each design.

Bibliography

Bickman, L. (1978) Evaluation plan for Chicago heart health curriculum (unpublished document).

Box, G. and Jenkins, G. (1976) *Time-Series Analysis: Forecasting and Control,* San Francisco: Holden-Day.

Bracht, G. and Glass, G. (1968) The external validity of experiments, *Am. Ed. Res. J.* 5:437–74.

Campbell, D. and Stanley, J. (1963) *Experimental and Quasi-Experimental Designs for Research,* Chicago: Rand McNally and Company.

Cook, T. and Campbell, D. (1979) *Quasi-Experimentation,* Boston: Houghton Mifflin Company.

Goodlad, J. (1984) *A Place Called School,* New York: McGraw Hill.

Peterson, F. and Rubinson, L. (1982) An evaluation of the effects of the American Dental Association's dental health education program on the knowledge, attitudes, and health locus of control of high school students, *J. of School Health* 52(1): 363–69.

Rubinson, L. and Stone, D. (1975) An evaluation of the cositive aspects of the American Dental Association's oral health program, level II, *Proceedings of the National Symposium on Dental Health Education in Schools:* 1–16.

Rubinson, L., Stone, D., and Mortimer, R. (1977) Statistical reliability of NPI administered to a sample of sixth grade children, *Dental Hygiene 51*(3): 109–113.

Snow, R. (1974) Representative and quasi-representative design for research on teaching, *Rev. of Ed. Res.* 44:265–91.

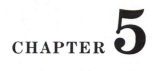

CHAPTER **5**

Survey Research

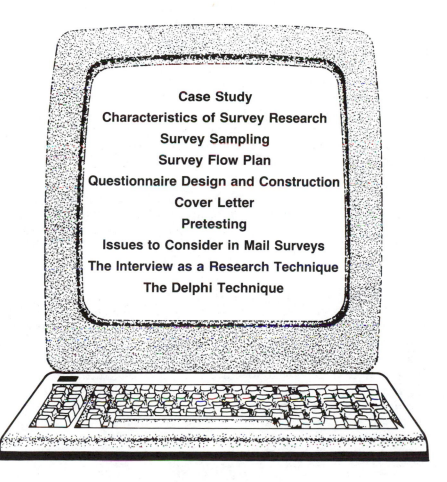

Case Study

Mary was recently hired as community health educator at a bi-county mental health center in rural Illinois. Although some programs had been conducted in the past for the community at large, no one knew of their success or what the populace would really want to see done. Her director, albeit supportive, urged her to develop activities that for the most part would be self-sufficient. Adding to the perplexity of the problem, Mary was unsure as to the best means of advertisement for this rural community. It was obvious that a great deal of research had to be accomplished. The obvious question was, how to go about it?

Characteristics of Survey Research

One kind of research that often appears in the health sciences literature is survey research. For many, this type of descriptive investigation is viewed as unworthy and a misuse of funds. Not unlike other research methods, this perception is correct if the survey is conducted in poor fashion. Trow (1967) observed the following about this form of research:

> The errors and inadequacies of survey research in education appear at many points from the way problems are initially chosen and defined to the choice of the subject population, the selection of the sample, the design of the individual questions and the questionnaire as a whole, and the analysis of the resulting body of data.

To circumvent these dilemmas, the researcher must be cognizant of the salient characteristics involved. First, because observation is the principal means of data collection, population selection must be rigorous and well-defined. Second, one must guard against the introduction of bias. Third, data need to be organized and presented systematically so that valid conclusions can be obtained. In the case study, if Mary were to conduct a survey to determine the opinions of the bicounty residents concerning programs needed, program awareness, financial support, and the best means of advertisement, she would have to keep all three characteristics in mind.

Survey Sampling

Ideally, the researcher would like to observe the entire population to add more weight to the findings. For example, in Mary's situation she may wish to obtain answers from all residents in the bicounty area. However, limitations of resources, time, and money frequently preclude a study of the entire population. This would be even more evident if the study was to survey the State of Illinois or perhaps all midwestern states. Subsequently, a subset of some predetermined size must be selected from the population of interest. The sample or subset should represent the total population so that the data collected from the sample will be as accurate as that from the entire population.

The logic involved is simple. Nonetheless, the importance of this step cannot be overemphasized. As stated by Leedy (1980), "The results of a survey are no more trustworthy than the quality of the population or the representativeness of the sample." A knowledgeable researcher commences with a population and works down to the sample. In other words, the population of interest is designated and then a sample is derived. The neophyte, on the other hand, often works from the bottom up by attempting to ascertain the minimum number of respondents needed for a successful study. The inherent problem with this approach is that it is next to impossible to assess the representativeness of the sample because the entire population has not been identified. Following the example case study, Mary must determine her target population. Is it to be all residents? Or does she just wish to include taxpayers? Her population could be limited to all those who may potentially use the services of the mental health center. Once this decision is made, she may then proceed to the selection of the sample.

The savings in both time and money are obvious reasons to deal with a sample of the population. There are additional advantages, too as described by Bailey (1982). The sample may achieve a greater response rate owing to greater cooperation than might occur in the full population survey. This in itself would tend to make the results more accurate. In health surveys with sensitive items, this point is particularly important. Concomitantly, the researcher can keep a low profile by using a sample. That is, less people may be offended, thereby negating an opportunity for several people to organize a common resistance. In the case of interviewing, a sample reduces the number of interviews and interviewers. This is beneficial in that supervision of an enormous number of interviewers is difficult at best and necessary attention to details such as follow-ups becomes very cumbersome as numbers increase.

There is little doubt that in many instances the use of a sample is much more advantageous than an entire population survey. Yet, the benefits only hold true if the sample is drawn with precision. This involves careful planning and a tremendous amount of work.

The Sampling Frame

The sampling frame is a list of all the persons (objects) from whom the sample is to be drawn. Understandably, the sample cannot be more accurate than the sampling frame from which it is selected. In constructing the sampling frame the researcher lists every person in the population, but only once so as not to increase someone's likelihood of being chosen. If the study is small, it is recommended that the investigator construct the list personally to avoid omissions and repetitions that may be on existing lists. For example, if a student working on a thesis in health sciences desired to survey the heads of health science departments of doctorate-granting universities, it would be relatively simple to construct the sampling frame. In a larger study however, it is much more difficult and perhaps virtually impossible to procure an accurate and complete list. In the case study, it is probable that Mary would not be able to obtain a listing of all residents in the bicounty area. People are born daily, and others die, move, or give incorrect addresses so that they cannot be contacted. As the size of the study increases to include a city, county, state, or nation, the construction of the sampling frame becomes more formidable.

Employment of existing lists, such as telephone directories and county directories, is only a partial answer at best. Both poor people who may not own telephones and wealthy people who may have unlisted numbers will be excluded in the study. Those who have two telephones and multiple listings would have a greater opportunity for selection than those with a single listing. Unless the directory was recently compiled, address changes and people who have left the county would confound the list. If the researcher employs existing lists, an attempt should be made to ascertain the number of persons excluded and whether or not they differ in any systematic way from those on the list. If there is no common bond, that is, the people are excluded randomly from the total population, then little harm will be done.

A possible alternative to the time and monetary demands of listing individuals is to compile residence addresses or households. Residences are relatively stable, and a complete listing could serve as the sampling frame. Further, no groups should be excluded and the risk of bias should be decreased greatly. In attempting to survey the people in the bicounty area, Mary could use this approach and select a sample from the sampling frame of residential addresses.

Types of Sampling

Once the population has been defined and the sampling frame established, the next step in arriving at a target group for research purposes is to select a method of sampling. Basically, there are two types of sampling techniques, which have several different procedures. *Probability samples* are those wherein the probability of selection of each respondent, or address, or even object, is known. In contrast, *nonprobability samples* reflect an unknown probability of selection.

Probability Sampling. Probability sampling techniques include random sampling, systematic sampling, stratifed random sampling, and cluster sampling.

Random Sampling. Simple random sampling is the basic building block of all probability sampling designs. In a random sample, each person (or address or object) in the population has an equal chance of being chosen for the sample. This is accomplished without bias for any personal characteristics. Of course, the underlying necessity is an adequate sampling frame with no one listed more than once and no one excluded. If either of these occurs, then by definition the sampling fails to be random.

An additional point about simple random sampling is that it is sampling without replacement. For example, if the sampling frame comprises 300 people, each person has a 1/300 chance of being selected. After 150 people have been chosen, the remainder will have only a 1/150 chance of being selected. This is considered adequate because the opportunity for selection is equal at any given stage of the sampling process.

While there are many methods for random selection, such as the flip of a coin, a lottery, or the roulette wheel, the usual one used by researchers is the table of random numbers. Each person in the sampling frame is assigned a number to avoid bias through identifiable characteristics (names, age, gender). From the example above, each of the 300 people in the sampling frame would be given one number. The researcher would then employ the table of random numbers to commence selecting the sample.

Examination of a table of random numbers shows that there is no discernible pattern whether one moves up, down, or across the page.

Initially, the researcher selects a predetermined pattern for moving through the table, that is, down columns or across rows. Next, a particular column and row is arbitrarily chosen from which to begin. If the names in the sampling frame are numbered in sequence, the researcher proceeds down the column (or across the row) pulling each name whose number corresponds to the number in the table. Because this is sampling without replacement, a number is simply ignored if encountered more than once. Similarly, if a number is found that is greater than that contained in the sampling frame, it is ignored. This procedure is continued until the desired sample size is obtained.

In the case study, Mary has a sampling frame of 50,000 addresses. Each would be numbered and she would then enter the table of random numbers. At this juncture, she decides to go down columns and arbitrarily choose column one, row three. Since her largest number is 50,000 (five digits), she needs to select five columns of numbers at a time. If the largest number had been 99 (two digits) or less in the sampling frame, she would only need to select two columns of random numbers. She would now proceed to pull out the required number of numbers for her sample size. Each number extracted from the table of random numbers would be matched to the addresses in the sampling frame, and those addresses would be employed in her study.

It can be seen that Mary is just as likely to select a farmer as an industrialist. Moreover, it is highly unlikely that she would obtain all farmers or all industrialists by random sampling. However, it should be noted that her task would indeed be an arduous one unless it were computerized. This may be accomplished with software programs for most personal computers as well as with larger mainframes. If these routes are not feasible, alternative sampling techniques are available.

Systematic Sampling. One alternative to the process of simple random sampling is systematic sampling. As the name implies, it is the selection of specific items in a series according to some predetermined sequence. The origin of the sequence must be controlled by chance. In other words, systematic sampling can be employed only when units in the sampling frame are random. In our case study, the residential addresses would have to be randomly ordered within the sampling frame. If they were not random, then Mary would be unable to use systematic sampling. However, if the items in the sampling frame were randomly listed, the health science investigator could choose $1/k$th of them with k being any constant. If k were two, then the sample would comprise one half of the population. Similarly, if k were five, the sample would be 20 per cent of the entire population. Once again, in the case study, if Mary decided to survey 2 per cent of the population, then k would be set at 50. The number of people in her survey would be 1,000.

Generally, the investigator randomly selects the first item from among the k items in the sampling frame. Next, by definition, a 1/kth sample is established by choosing every kth item in the sampling frame. Subsequently, Mary would randomly select her first address for inclusion in the sample. Needless to say, like Mary, all health science investigators would need to determine sample size before beginning sample selection.

Although simple random sampling is more accurate and does not require the assumption of a randomized sampling frame, systematic sampling involves less work thereby providing more information per dollar. Further, for the inexperienced survey researcher, it may reduce error because it is simpler to perform. In short, the greater the complexity of the method, the greater the opportunity for error. Nonetheless, it must be emphasized that systematic sampling is more dependent on the adequacy of the sampling frame than is simple random sampling. Because any ordering of the sampling frame is retained in systematic sampling, the results can be totally nonrepresentative. If evidence of biased ordering is found in the sampling frame, then steps must be taken to correct it. The most obvious step is to randomize the sampling frame (expensive and time-consuming), or if this is untenable, to return to simple random sampling, or perhaps draw a stratified random sample.

Stratified Random Sampling. At times it is advisable to use stratified random sampling. This means to subdivide the population into smaller homogeneous groups in order to get a more accurate representation or to include parameters of special interest. Herein, the population is broken down into nonoverlapping groups called strata, and then a simple random sample is extracted from each stratum.

The first step in stratified random sampling is to identify the strata (sometimes called stratification parameters). For example, Mary may wish to subdivide the population of the bicounty area into County A and County B. The residential addresses would be split exclusively into the appropriate county and a simple random sample would be taken from each list. Although a simple random sample could have been employed for a listing of combined counties and still have excellent representation, the stratified design could save time and money by requiring a smaller sample size.

If so desired, more than one stratification variable or parameter could be used. That is, the health science researcher can stratify on two or more variables simultaneously. In addition to the county parameter, Mary could stratify on the urban-rural parameter. Now, instead of having two groups, she would have four. Table 5.1 illustrates the four groups or strata. Once the groups have been formed, a simple random sample is taken within each group or stratum.

In proportional stratified sampling, each sample drawn should rep-

TABLE 5.1   Stratified Sampling

	County A	County B
Urban	Cell 1	Cell 3
Rural	Cell 2	Cell 4

resent the population in the proportion in which it exists within the total population. For example, imagine that in County A there were 14,000 addresses in an urban setting and 16,000 in a rural setting for a total of 30,000. Similarly, there are 8,000 urban and 12,000 rural addresses in County B for a total of 20,000. Combined there would be 50,000 addresses that were in the original sampling frame. For Mary to establish a sample size of 1,000, the sample should include approximately the same proportions as the entire population. Table 5.2 illustrates the proportional stratified sampling design.

Each subgroup or cell is drawn randomly in proportion to the total population. Cell 1, comprising 14,000 addresses, makes up 28 per cent of the population and subsequently has a sample size of 280 (28% of 1,000). The remaining cells follow a similar pattern.

In other situations, the researcher may decide to stratify by gender, socioeconomic status, racial origin, education, or religious preference. Obviously, those in the health sciences may wish to stratify by health parameters such as smoking-nonsmoking, hypertensive patients–nonhypertensive patients, pregnancy-nonpregnancy, and many others. The characteristics of the entire population must be considered together with the objectives of the research before the stratified sample design is used. On occasion, stratified random sampling is disproportionate in that a larger proportion of the population is sampled in one stratum than in another. Two reasons for this design are (1) differences in population size, and (2) homogeneity among strata. When the population of a particular stratum is very small, proportionate

TABLE 5.2   Proportional Sample

		County A	County B
Urban	Addresses	14,000	8,000
	Proportion	28%	16%
	Sample Size	280	160
Rural	Addresses	16,000	12,000
	Proportion	32%	24%
	Sample Size	320	240

sampling may leave the researcher with a sample size that is statistically unworkable. Similarly, a larger proportion of the population would have to be sampled in a very heterogeneous stratum. For example, if the health science investigator were to select a stratified sample of nonsmokers, cigarette smokers, and pipe smokers in a company that has 1,000 nonsmokers, 800 cigarette smokers, and 200 pipe smokers, a greater proportion of pipe smokers would have to be sampled than either nonsmokers or cigarette smokers to obtain a sufficient size for sampling adequacy. This delemma will be discussed further in the sample size section of this chapter under disproportionate sampling.

Overall, stratified random sampling is a technique to maintain the same proportionality on stratification parameters in the sample as occurs in the population. The researcher may stratify by demographic characteristics or by health variables. In any case, the characteristics of the entire population must be considered together with the objectives of the research before the stratified sample design is used.

Cluster or Area Sampling. Cluster or area sampling is a variation of the simple random sample and is especially useful when (1) the population to be studied is infinite, (2) a list of members of the population is nonexistent, or (3) the geographic distribution of the population is widely scattered. For example, if an investigator proposed to survey all public school health educators in the United States, a simple random sample would be impractical.

In multistage cluster sampling, the investigator can first randomly sample 20 of the 50 states. In the second stage, from a sampling frame that lists all counties within the 20 states, a random sample of 100 counties could be selected. Then, in the third stage, a random sample of 50 school districts could be drawn from all the school districts within the 100 counties. The fourth stage consists of random selection of 100 school health educators in the 50 school districts. The successive random sampling of states, counties, school districts, and finally health educators is relatively inexpensive and efficient.

Cluster sampling samples among clusters. While it has some advantages over simple random sampling, it does hold the possibility of more error. This is because it is not a single sample but rather two or more, each open to error. Further, there may be sample bias because of the unequal size of some of the subsets or clusters selected. The first stage of sampling may be representative, but the second stage may not be. The researcher must be concerned about sample size and accuracy at every stage of the cluster sample.

In summation, all of the techniques we have discussed, simple random sampling, systematic sampling, stratified random sampling, and cluster sampling may be combined into a single procedure to suit the needs of the researcher. In so doing, the investigator must be familiar with the idiosyncracies of each method.

Nonprobability Sampling. In some instances, the researcher may decide to employ nonprobability sampling. In this method, the probability that a person will be chosen is not known, with the result that a claim for representativeness of the population cannot be made. Concomitantly, sampling error (the degree of departure from representation) is unknown. Subsequently, the researcher's ability to generalize findings beyond the actual sample is greatly limited. This may be a major disadvantage, depending upon the purpose of the study. Nevertheless, nonprobability sampling has an advantage over probability sampling in that it is less expensive, less complicated, and lends itself to spontaneity (spur-of-the-moment investigations). It is particularly useful in small studies or pilot investigations to perfect questionnaires. Nonprobability sampling includes convenience sampling, quota sampling, dimensional sampling, purposive sampling, and snowball sampling.

Convenience Sampling. A common example of convenience sampling is the captive-audience approach such as a classroom full of health science students. While the researcher foregoes representativeness in this case, time and money are saved. It is a simple matter of selecting the closest and most convenient persons.

Quota Sampling. Quota sampling is the nonprobability sampling equivalent of stratified sampling. Initially, the researcher determines which strata are relevant to the investigation and then proceeds to establish a quota for each stratum that is proportionate to its representation in the population. For example, in Mary's study it was found that in County A 28 per cent of the addresses were urban and 32 per cent were rural. In County B, 16 per cent were urban and 24 per cent rural. In selecting her sample Mary would not want all rural residences nor all urban ones. Preferably, the sample would be drawn proportionate to the urban-rural realities of the actual population. Once a quota is set, the sampling merely consists of finding addresses (persons) that fit into the stratum. In Mary's study, a total of 200 residents would mean 56 urban and 64 rural addresses in County A, and there would be 32 urban and 48 rural addresses in County B. Although there is no random selection, at least the strata are in the same proportions as the entire population.

The researcher must make every effort to prevent bias. Bias is most likely to occur when the route of least resistance is chosen, e.g., avoiding houses in questionable neighborhoods or ones that contain unfriendly people. Confining the research to friends and acquaintances is not acceptable.

Dimensional Sampling. Dimensional sampling is principally a multidimensional form of quota sampling wherein the variables (dimensions) of interest in the population are delineated. Each variable and combination thereof must be represented by at least one case. It is a method in which only a small sample is required so that each case selected can be examined in more detail.

Purposive Sampling. This technique falls somewhere between quota sampling, in which various strata are to be filled, and convenience sampling wherein the nearest and most available people are used. In purposive sampling, the researcher employs his or her own discretion to select the respondents who best meet the purposes of the study. This is a great advantage to the experienced researcher who can apply prior knowledge and skill.

Snowball Sampling. There is a multistage technique that literally snowballs. In the first stage of snowball sampling, a person possessing the requisite characteristics is identified and interviewed. This person then identifies others who may be included in the sample. The next stage is to interview these persons who in turn identify still more respondents who can be contacted and interviewed in following stages. As pointed out by Bailey (1982, p. 100), "if one wishes the snowball sample to be probabilistic, one should sample randomly within each stage."

Mixed Sampling Designs. When a population or sample is very large, a mixed model of judgment and probability sampling is frequently used. Discretion procedures are frequently employed in the early stages and probability procedures in the later stages. This combined approach offers a savings in time, money, and effort as well as a sample that can be representative of the entire population.

Sample Size

The determination of sample size usually perplexes beginning researchers because they often have no conception of a minimally adequate sample size. They need to understand that correct sample size is dependent on both the nature of the population and the purpose of the study. Usually, a trade-off is discovered between the desire for a large sample and the feasibility of a small one. An ideal study would have a sample large enough to represent the population so generalization may occur, yet small enough to save time and money as well as to reduce the complexity of data analysis.

General rules are difficult to establish without addressing a specific population. However, Champion (1970) claims that approximately 30 cases seem to be a bare minimum if statistical analysis is to be used. If the researcher intends to subdivide the sample during data analysis; then a minimum of 100 cases may be required to ensure an adequate sample size for analysis in each subdivision. Further, it must be realized that with many surveys the usable cases may vary greatly from the theoretical sample size. This may result from failure to return questionnaires, refusal to be interviewed, items skipped by the respondent, and so on. In all of this confusion, some considerations can be applied in a systematic fashion to assist research efforts.

Considerations in Sample Size. It is a popular misconception that a sample is a small carbon copy of the original population, identical in every way. If this were the case, then the researcher would not have to worry about having a sample size that is representative of the population under study. Needless to say, one can never be certain of representativeness unless the entire population is used. An obvious deduction at this juncture is that the larger the sample, the greater the likelihood of representativeness. This is especially true if the population is quite heterogeneous on the given variable; the greater the heterogeneity, the greater the necessity for a larger sample. For populations in which there is no heterogeneity on a variable (complete homogeneity), a sample size of even one would suffice.

Because use of an entire population total homogeneity are out of the question in most studies, the researcher must have representativeness as the primary consideration. Lack of representativeness is commonly referred to as sampling error. Sampling error is the degree to which the sample means of repeatedly drawn random samples differ from one another and from the population mean. Imagine, for example, that a large number of health science researchers each selected random samples of 50 hypertensive patients from the population of all hypertensive patients in Minnesota. The mean or average blood pressure of each of the random samples would not be identical. Although most of them would tend to cluster around the population mean, some would be relatively high by comparison while others would be relatively low. This variation in sample means is a result of sampling error. It is not a mistake in the sampling process but rather an inevitable variation when a number of randomly selected sample means (herein blood pressure) are compared.

Because means are not identical, it is logical to assume that any one of them differs from the population mean (average blood pressure of all hypertensive patients in Minnesota). A researcher deals with only one sample as a base for generalization about the population, therefore it is necessary to determine whether or not the particular sample is representative. To make this determination the use of statistical techniques and probability theory is required. To put it briefly, the researcher attempts to establish that the sample is representative of the population on critical parameters at an acceptable level of probability. This probability level, called a confidence level, is usually set at 95%, frequently referred to as the .05 level of significance. In lay terms, this means that there is a 95% chance that the sample is distributed in the same way as the population. If he or she deems it appropriate, the researcher may decide to set the level more stringently—at the .01 level, in which there is a 99% chance. Of course, the restrictions could be eased by establishing the level at .10 thereby making a 90% chance that the sample is distributed in the same way as the population. In the past, z critical values of the normal probability table for large samples have been always used; today, t critical values are employed for small samples sizes (fewer than 30 cases). It is suggested that the budding research student consult a text on statistics to learn more about this concept.

Stratified random sampling presents several issues in regard to sample size. As noted in the discussion of sampling types, the sample within each stratum is drawn randomly and as such can be considered an independent sample of the population stratum. Stratified random sampling is such that a very heterogeneous population can be subdivided into several relatively homogeneous strata, each demanding a fairly small sample.

Investigative studies involving a single dichotomous stratification parameter (urban-rural, smokers-nonsmokers, private hospitals–public hospitals) with random sampling in each stratum may employ a formula to determine sample size. The formula considers confidence level and sampling error in calculating a representative sample size.

$$N = (z/e)^2(p)(1-p)$$

where N = sample size
      z = the standard score corresponding to a given confidence level
      e = the proportion of sampling error in a given situation
      p = the estimated proportion or incidence of cases in the population

Confidence level indicates the probability that the sample proportion will reflect the population proportion with a specific degree of accuracy (sampling error designated as e in the formula). With a 95% confidence level $z = 1.96$ whereas with a 99% confidence level $z = 2.58$ and with a 90% confidence level $z = 1.65$.

Suppose that a health researcher decided to investigate patient education programs in public and private hospitals in West Virginia. In ascertaining the sampling frame, it was found that private hospitals accounted for 25% of all hospitals in the state. The proportion of private hospitals in the population of all hospitals would be .25 (p = .25). Employing the usual standard of a 95% (z = 1.96) confidence level and a sampling error of .10, the following calculations apply:

$$N = (1.96/.10)^2(.25)(.75)$$
$$N = (19.6)^2(.25)(.75)$$
$$N = (384.16) \ (.1875)$$
$$N = 72$$

As a point of interpretation, a sample size of 72 private hospitals would give representativeness with no more than a plus or minus .10 sampling error with a confidence limit of 95%.

However, a stratified random sampling is often disproportionate in that a greater proportion is sampled in one stratum than another. The two major reasons for this are (1) differences in population size and (2) differences in homogeneity among strata. As an illustration, an investigation was conducted in West Central Illinois to ascertain the relationship of religion and health habits. The population comprised 1,000 Protestants, 800 Roman Catholics, and 200 Mormons. It is evident that a proportionate sample would leave the Mormons misrepresented or at least without a statistically functioning sample. Further, the decision to work with a sample of 100 from each of the religious strata revealed that the odds of being randomly selected varied tremendously. The Protestants had a 1 in 10 chance of being chosen, Catholics had a 1 in 8 chance, and Mormons had a 1 in 2 chance.

One way around this dilemma is to use weighted sampling. With this procedure the additional problem of combining subsamples (strata) into one overall sample for the purpose of data analysis can be overcome. Weights are assigned to each of the strata. Mormons are given a weight of 2 because they have a 1 in 2 chance of selection. Catholics have a weight of 8 because they have a 1 in 8 chance of selection, and similarly Protestants have a weight of 10. To make calculations more workable, each weight is divided by two to arrive at smaller numbers. This provides weights of 1, 4, and 5 for Mormons, Catholics, and Protestants.

Because it was decided that each religious stratum would comprise 100 individuals, the data for each person were keypunched onto computer cards. As a result, there were 100 cards per stratum (one card per person). To have representative data, each stratum needed to contain data proportional to the population. Therefore 400 cards were required for Roman Catholics and 500 cards for Protestants. To accomplish this feat, the researcher simply duplicated the Roman Catholic cards three times and added them to the original data deck for a total of 400. Similarly, the Protestant cards were duplicated four times and added to the original deck for a sum of 500. The data were then proportional.

To obtain similar results without employing data cards, a researcher can weight the data during analysis using the appropriate weight for each stratum. For example, suppose the following unweighted data shown in Table 5.3 were obtained.

To obtain proportional data, each stratum would be weighted by the appropriate amount. The result would be as seen in Table 5.4.

The figures are changed but the relative values of the data are not altered. Thus, weighting provides adequate and equal representation of all strata. In conclusion, there are several considerations in determining sample size, which are listed below.

1. Select as large a sample size as possible, because the larger the sample, the smaller the sampling error.
2. Cost, in terms of money and time, and subject availability are legitimate concerns in ascertaining sample size.
3. Surveys require a greater sample size than experimental studies because of response failure, item omission, poor interviewing, and so on.
4. When a sample is to be subdivided into smaller groups for data analysis, a large enough sample is required to allow for statistical treatment within each subgroup.
5. Assigning weights is a technique applicable to disproportionate sampling.

As a caveat, however, the researcher should note that more important than sheer size is the selection of the sample. Further, random

TABLE 5.3 Distribution of Smokers by Religion

	Religion		
Smoking	*Mormon*	*Catholic*	*Protestant*
Cigarette	2	25	26
Pipe	10	21	34
Nonsmoker	88	54	40
Total	100	100	100

TABLE 5.4   Distribution of Smokers by Religion

	Religion		
Smoking	*Mormon*	*Catholic*	*Protestant*
Cigarette	2	100	130
Pipe	10	84	170
Nonsmoker	88	216	200
Total	100	400	500

sampling allows for an estimate of sampling error, offering the researcher an idea of the confidence that may be placed in the findings.

Survey Flow Plan

A flow plan is used to outline the design and subsequent implementation of a survey. It begins with the objectives of the survey, lists each step to be taken in the survey, and ends with the final report. In short, the flow plan is an organizational device employed by the researcher to serve as a guide throughout the investigation. The components to be included are

1. **Commencing the survey.** (a) objectives of the survey, (b) amount of time required, (c) money available, and (d) resources available. These should be given in detail.
2. **Survey design.** The design should be according to data needs, sample size requirements, data collection, resources, interviewer selection, data analysis, budget (funds, time, work responsibility), and how the results are to be reported.
3. **Derive from survey design.** From the survey design comes (a) interviewers (when appropriate), (b) questionnaire population, and (c) sample selection.
4. **Pretest.** This is to pretest the questionnaire with a sample that is comparable to the sample that is to be in the full study.
5. **Questionnaire revision.** According to the findings in the pretest, the questionnaire may be revised. If the revisions are heavy, a second prestest should be conducted.
6. **Data collection.** Herein the data are gathered through the appropriate means, e.g., mail, telephone, or personal interview.
7. **Code preparation.** This is the initial step in data reduction. It is the translation of question responses and respondent infor-

mation to specific categories for purposes of analysis. The coding should be consistent and conventional, such as *9* = no answer, *0* = inapplicable. If possible, a precoded questionnaire should be used.

8. **Verification.** This is a very important step particularly with interviewers to check for bias. The answers of respondents from one interviewer can be compared to those of other interviewers to determine whether or not the answers of respondents from the interviewer were leaning in a special direction. Some respondents could be reinterviewed. Also, the researcher could possibly check with some outside criterion, such as whether the respondent really did what he said he would do (e.g., vote).

9. **Editing.** At this point, the answers are checked for consistency. As an illustration, *age* may read *3 years old* and educational level be checked as *college graduate*. The errors should be located and when appropriate the responses sent back to field operations, i.e., interviewers, for correct answers.

10. **Coding.** This is the actual coding of the data that have been received for keypunching. Step number 7 is related to this step.

11. **Keypunching and verification.** The cards are keypunched and verified for possible errors.

12. **Machine cleaning.** A computer program is established to check for inconsistent answers. For example, someone who was supposed to answer a section may have neglected to do so. The purpose is to get "clean" cards.

13. **Tabulation.** Initially, a frequency count should be conducted to ascertain how many answers are in each of the categories for every question.

14. **Analysis.** The analysis will vary according to the purpose of the study but it could include percentages, averages, relational indices, and tests of significance.

15. **Recording and reporting.** All of the previous steps should be outlined in the report with special emphasis on hypotheses, hypothesis testing, reliability of results, and implications of results for the subjects and further survey research.

Employing the flow plan as a guide, in the case study illustration, Mary has decided, as noted previously, to determine the opinions of bicounty residents concerning programs needed, program awareness, financial support, and the best means of advertisement. Her director has allocated a total of $650 for the study not including her own work time. Keeping all the factors in mind for sample size and sampling technique, she has established a sample size of 1,000 (2 per cent) from a sampling frame of 50,000 addresses. To obtain adequate representation Mary employed a proportional stratified random sampling technique with parameters of county (County A, County B) and of setting (urban, rural) as in Table 5.2. The next major task is questionnaire design and construction.

Questionnaire Design and Construction_____

Questionnaire design and construction involve much more than drafting the questionnaire itself. The researcher needs to complete prequestionnaire planning, draft the questionnaire, prepare the final copy, and then pretest it. The following points illustrate the necessary components.

1. **Prequestionnaire planning**
   a. Define the problem and hypothesize solutions.
   b. Speculate the information needed to test the hypothesis.
   c. Review previous research and speak with resource personnel.
   d. Develop preliminary questions.
2. **Drafting the questionnaire**
   a. Considerations for researcher, respondent, and interviewer.
   b. Types of questionnaires.
   c. Types of questions.
   d. First draft of the questionnaire.
3. **Preparing the final questionnaire**
   a. Physical layout.
   b. Reproduction and materials.
   c. Identification of respondents in the questionnaire.
4. **Pretesting**
   a. Value to questionnaire design.
   b. Evaluating the pretest.
   c. Questionnaire revision if necessary (may warrant another pretest).

The emphasis in this section will be on drafting the questionnaire.

Researcher, Respondent, and Interviewer Considerations

Once the hypotheses have been carefully specified and the sample drawn, the next step in the research chain is development of the data collection instrument. Herein the major consideration is questionnaire relevance to the researcher, the respondent, and the interviewer (when appropriate). The researcher must be certain that the questionnaire is relevant to the goals and objectives of the study as set by him or her. No matter how well worded or designed the questionnaire, if it fails to produce the data relevant to the objectives, it is worthless.

Overall, the study and subsequent questionnaire must be relevant to the respondent. This is not always self-evident because research objectives are frequently housed in scientific jargon; therefore they must be clarified and justified in lay terms. This can be accomplished by means of a cover letter. There must be a connection between the respondent and all those questions that apply to the respondent. That is, can the respondents understand the questions? Are they likely to know the answers? Are they willing to respond to the questions? The answer to the last question could be no if the questions are not relevant and thereby offer no motivating force. To make the questions applicable, skips or contingency questions (e.g., *If you answered yes to this question, skip to question 22*) can be used. With this method the respondent only has to read and answer items that are personally relevant.

In drafting the questionnaire that is to be used in an interview schedule, all elements that could lead to interviewer bias must be removed. Questions have to be phrased so as not to be misconstrued. Further, questions should follow a logical order with a smooth transition from topic to topic. Needless to say, all directions to the interviewer and the respondent should be clear and concise.

Types of Questionnaires

Generally, questionnaires forms are closed, open, or a combination of the two. The *restricted* or *closed* form provides fixed-alternative questions that can be answered by a simple "yes" or "no" or by checking an appropriate box. Some of the advantages of this form are (1) ease of completion for the respondent; (2) simplification of coding and analysis, particularly because the questionnaire can be precoded; (3) greater chance that respondents will answer sensitive questions (e.g., about age or income) because they are usually categorized rather than demanding an exact number; and (4) a minimum of irrelevant responses.

On the other hand, some disadvantages of the closed form are (1) given a list of potential answers, the unknowledgeable respondent may guess or randomly select an answer. (2) Variations in answers among respondents may be reduced since only certain categories are available. (3) There may be too many answer categories to be printed simplistically. (4) Frustration may augment since there is no room for a separate, nonprovided opinion. (5) There is the possibility that the respondent may circle the wrong answer, e.g. circle a three when they meant to circle a four.

It is suggested that the categories of "Don't know" and "Other" be included in a closed form questionnaire. In this way, the respondent is not forced to work with just the alternatives provided. Further, it gives the researcher the opportunity to receive more relevant information.

In the *open* or *unrestricted* questionnaire form the response categories are not specified, and the respondent is allowed to answer in his or her own words. Some of the advantages of this type of questionnaire are (1) usable when all the response categories are unknown, (2) preferable for controversial, sensitive and complex issues, and (3) allow for respondent creativity, clarification, and detail. The disadvantages include (1) difficulty in coding and analysis; (2) greater demands on the respondent in terms of time, writing ability, and thought; (3) questions may be too general for the respondent to comprehend or answer; and (4) data collected may not be relevant to the objectives of the study.

Many questionnaires have *combined forms,* including both closed and open items. A questionnaire that is primarily closed should have at least one open-ended item to allow the respondent to express a personal opinion or thought. Each health science researcher must decide which type is more likely to supply the information desired.

Types of Questions

A variety of questions and response category formats are available to the questionnaire builder. In closed form questionnaires the usual types are dichotomous, multiple choice, rating, and ranking. Open form questionnaires generally consist of a blank space in which the answer is to be written. On occasion, sentence completion questions are incorporated into both forms.

To illustrate the different types, suppose that Mary in our case study were to develop a questionnaire with primarily a closed format and a few open-ended items. The basic rule she would follow for writing questions would be to provide all possible answers in as clear a fashion as possible.

In *dichotomous* questions the answer comprises two parts, one of which is to be selected by the respondents. Examples of this type are:

Circle the appropriate number:
1. Gender: Male 1; Female 2
2. Setting: Urban 1; Rural 2

With multiple choice items, each potential answer is listed for the respondent such as:

How far would you be willing to travel for a mental health program of interest to you? (Check One)

One mile or less	[ ]
Two to four miles	[ ]
Five to seven miles	[ ]
Eight to ten miles	[ ]
Eleven or more miles	[ ]

It can be readily noted that this format takes much more space than placing answers side by side; however, the answers are recognized quickly.

Many questionnaires include *rating* questions in which the respondent indicates a particular view about the psychological object. For example:

Several educational services are listed below. Please indicate the importance of each to you.

	Very Important	Some-what Important	Not Important
1. Assertiveness training	————	————	————
2. Marriage enhancement	————	————	————
3. Stress reduction	————	————	————

This format allows several items to be categorized as a series with directions stated only once.

Another fixed-alternative approach is that of *ranking*. Here the respondent simply orders the given answers in rank. For example:

1. The following are some of the mental health problems faced by residents of the county. Please place them in order of greatest problem (rank it 1) to the smallest problem (rank it 5) within the county as you see them.

———— Alcoholism
———— Divorce
———— Drug addiction
———— Incest
———— Unemployment

For the *sentence completion* format, an example item would be:

1. In regard to education, I feel the Mental Health Center should

Frequently, the *open-ended* questions are placed at or near the end of the questionnaire. For example, Mary might ask the following question:

> **1.** In the space below, please write out any particular interests or concerns that you have about attending programs at the Mental Health Center.

It is important that the health science researcher consider the target population when deciding on the type of questionnaire and the types of questions. Further, when writing the questions several pitfalls should be avoided. The following list can serve as a guide:

1. Phrase questions to be comprehended by all those in the target population.
2. Avoid double-barreled questions.
3. Be careful of double negatives.
4. Define terms that could be easily misinterpreted.
5. Underline or boldface a word if special emphasis is demanded.
6. Watch for inadequate alternatives to a question.
7. Do not use adjectives that fail to have an agreed-on meaning.
8. Be sure questions are not leading questions.
9. There should be no ambiguity in the questions.

On completion of the questions, it is necessary to combine them into the final questionnaire in an order that will bring about the greatest response. To assist in this task, some general rules should be followed.

1. Sensitive questions as well as open-ended ones should be near the end of the questionnaire.
2. Place questions in a logical order where possible.
3. Simpler questions should be ahead of more difficult ones.
4. Avoid establishing a response set.
5. Request information needed for subsequent questions first.
6. Vary questions by length and type.
7. Separate reliability-check question pairs, i.e., pairs of questions in which one is stated positively and the other negatively. For example, the Mental Health Center should offer educational classes (agree/disagree) at one point and later state the Mental Health Center should *not* offer educational classes (agree/disagree).

When the questionnaire is complete, a cover letter should be developed.

Cover Letter

Though the instrument constructed is of prime importance, the beginning researcher should realize that an inappropriate cover letter or introductory statement may cause the respondent to discard the questionnaire without even looking at it, or the interviewer may be asked to leave. As a matter of note, the letter should be on an organizational letterhead to indicate the legitimacy of the survey in the case of a mailed questionnaire. When an interview is conducted, the introductory statement serves as a public relations technique.

In regard to content, the cover letter or introductory statement should contain (1) identification of the person or organization conducting the study, (2) the reason the study is being conducted, (3) why it is important for the respondent to complete the survey, (4) assurance of no right or wrong answers, (5) confidentiality of information given, (6) anonymity of the respondent, when applicable, (7) how long it will take to complete, (8) the date of return for a mail survey, and (9) a notice of how to obtain results. (see Figure 5.1).

Scott (1961) reviewed several studies about cover letters and found that a "permissive" letter obtains a greater response than does a "firm" letter. Also, a "short, punchy letter" is better than a longer, logical appeal. Handwriting the address does not seem to increase the response rate. No difference in response rate was found when a true signature or facsimile was used or when the letter was addressed as "Dear Mr. Smith," "Dear Friend," or "Dear Bulletin-User". In short, he concluded that "the content of the letter is very much more important than its trappings."

Pretesting

The constructed questionnaire remains at rough draft stage until a pretest is done to identify flaws and to allow for corrections. Though the sample for the pretest is frequently fellow students, faculty, or coworkers, it is recommended that a subsample of the target population be employed for better results. Further, it should be administered in the same fashion as intended for the actual study; i.e., mail, telephone, or interview.

Those in the pretest sample should complete the questionnaire as directed, and then do a critical analysis of all aspects of the instrument: sensitivity of issues, question wording and order, response categories, reliability checks, physical layout, length of time for answer-

February 8, 1989

Dear (Respondent):

The Bi-Counties Community Mental Health Center, a nonprofit organization responsible for mental health services in your area, is conducting a survey to determine how people feel about mental health education programs.

Enclosed is a questionnaire that we are asking you to complete as part of this survey. The questions are very easy to answer and should not take any more than 20 minutes of your time. There are no right or wrong answers. You have our assurance that the information that you provide in this survey will be kept anonymous. Your answers will help us to plan mental health education services throughout the bi-county area and to promote better health for all our residents.

Since a limited number of these questionnaires are being sent out to select residents of the bi-county area, your individual opinion is highly important to the success of this undertaking. We therefore request that you please complete and return this questionnaire in the enclosed, self-addressed, stamped envelope no later than March 3, 1989. If you have any questions about this survey or want to have a copy of the results, please contact Mary _____ at 555-9115.

Thank you for your cooperation.

Sincerely,

John Doe, Executive Director
Bi-Counties Community Mental Health Center

Figure 5.1 Cover letter.

ing, instructions. Any comments given in the margins or elsewhere should receive special attention particularly if several respondents hold the same view. In addition, the researcher should seek indicators of other problems by calculating the "no response" or "don't know" answers. Pattern of response should be observed for set responses.

Only when the corrections have been made should the questionnaire be used in the research project. If several alterations were required, another pretest should be conducted. All of this takes time and should be built into the time frame for the entire study. Omission of this step could prove to be a grievous error if the final data fail to correspond to the objectives.

Issues To Consider in Mail Surveys

Whether to use a mail survey or an interview technique should be determined before sample selection and questionnaire design and construction are done. Subsequently, Mary should have made this decision some time ago in her survey of two counties. This section will deal with some of the advantages, disadvantages, and factors involved with mail surveys. For a complete discussion of mailed questionnaires, it is suggested that *Methods of Social Research* by Bailey (1982) be consulted.

Advantages of Mail Surveys

Briefly, some of the advantages of a mailed questionnaire are (1) a savings of money and time, especially as compared with the interview technique, (2) no interviewer bias, (3) greater assurance of anonymity, (4) completion by the respondent at his or her convenience, (5) accessibility to a wide geographic region, (6) accurate information because the respondent can consult records before answering, and (7) identical wording for all respondents. In short, there are some definite pluses for using the mail survey technique. On the other hand, drawbacks do exist.

Disadvantages of Mail Surveys

While a mailed questionnaire may have appeal to Mary, she should consider the disadvantages of (1) lack of flexibility, (2) likelihood of unanswered questions, (3) low response rate as compared to interviewing, (4) inability to record spontaneous reactions and/or nonverbal responses, (5) lack of control over the order in which questions are answered and over the immediate environment, (6) no guarantee of return by the deadline date, and (7) inability to use a complex questionnaire format.

Factors Influencing Mail Surveys

Further consideration of whether or not to do a mail survey should include seven variables enumerated by Sellitz et al. (1959). that affect the adequacy of data and the number of questionnaires returned.

One factor is sponsorship of the questionnaire. The organization or individuals involved may enhance or detract from the legitimacy of the study, thereby influencing questionnaire completion. A second variable is questionnaire format and color. It appears that color makes little or no difference in the rate of return. In regard to questionnaire length, it seems that a less cluttered questionnaire, although longer, will bring a higher return rate than a shorter version. Ease of completion and return serves as a fourth factor. It is suggested that directions be explicit and that a stamped, self-addressed envelope be supplied. Incentives, which can range from money to a copy of the survey results, usually increase the response rate. Monetary incentives should be seen as a goodwill gesture and not payment for time—unless of course you are enclosing a large sum of money! Moreover, incentives should be sent on the first mailing. The nature of the respondents also affects the number of questionnaires returned and the adequacy of data collected. If a highly select group is used, such as Directors of Mental Health Centers, responses tend to be more favorable than if mailed to the general public. Sellitz et al. also noted that the cover letter, discussed previously, is of great importance.

The time and type of mailing as well as the nature of the follow-up also play a role in mail surveys. As may be expected, first-class mail provides a greater return than any other class of mail. Concomitantly, a hand-stamped envelope may increase the return slightly over a business-reply envelope. This difference seems to be shrinking, however, and with rising postal rates the researcher should seriously consider the use of business-reply envelopes to save money.

Mailings must be well-timed. Obviously major holidays should be avoided. Surveys received during the latter part of the week are more likely to receive quick response than those received early in the week. The months of February and April offer the lowest rate of return and March the highest, although for school surveys September may be the best month.

As a final note on factors influencing mailed questionnaires, follow-up letters or telephone calls should be employed. This should be standard procedure. The literature reveals that an increase of 20 per cent can be expected with one follow-up or more. Frequently the researcher may send out a reminder letter, followed by an additional questionnaire and letter, and then either another letter or a phone call.

A reasonable rate of return is a highly questionable topic because so many factors affect it. Some researchers hold that a 90 per cent return rate is needed, others claim that 50 to 60 per cent is permissible, and still others believe that a lower rate is acceptable depending on the target population. Whatever the response rate, it is important that there be a demonstrated lack of response bias. Of course, the greater the return, the less opportunity for response bias. The amount of time and money available to the researcher will dictate response rate too.

In summary, the mail survey is a technique with much potential and several advantages. Nonetheless, drawbacks do exist and many factors influence the rate of return and adequacy of response. The decision to use or not use a mail survey must be couched within the framework of the entire study and in particular the objectives of that study.

The Interview as a Research Technique

Traditionally, interviews have dealt with an individual on a face-to-face basis. It may be the principal method of investigation in some studies, but in others it is more of an exploratory tool to acquire more information, e.g., a pilot study to develop a more extensive questionnaire. Less traditional is the group interview. While not appropriate for all occasions, it may be an excellent technique if the researcher is concerned with a behavior that takes place in a group interaction setting. The advantages of the group technique over the individual approach are (1) greater efficiency in time and money, (2) observation of group interaction patterns, (3) reflection of group behavior in results, and (4) productivity of others can be stimulated. On the other hand, the group approach (1) may intimidate and suppress responses, (2) promote conformity, (3) polarize opinions, and (4) be susceptible to manipulation by an influential group member (Issac & Michael, 1981).

Advantages of Individual Interview Studies

Some of the major advantages of the individual interview study are (1) personalization of the study to the participant; (2) flexibility so that further probing may occur or questions can be repeated; (3) a response rate that is usually higher than a comparable mail survey; (4) observation of both verbal and nonverbal behavior; (5) control over question order that cannot be accomplished by a mail questionnaire; (6) spontaneity and "no help from others," as contrasted with either the mail survey or the group interview technique, (8) recording of the time of the interview—this may be important if events affecting the object under study have occurred; and (9) ability to use more involved and complex questionnaires.

Disadvantages of Individual Interview Studies

As with all research methodologies, the interview study has some inherent disadvantages. Some of these are (1) cost in terms of money and time (including training period and travel allowance); (2) openness to manipulation or interviewer bias; (3) vulnerability to personality clashes; (4) lack of anonymity; (5) inconvenience to the respondent as well as lack of opportunity to consult records, e.g., medical records for immunization or booster shots; (6) lack of standardization in questions because probing or question repetition may bring about a rewording that produces different responses for different respondents; (7) lack of access to respondents because of distance or other factors that may make the mail survey appear more desirable; and (8) difficulty in summarizing the findings.

Factors Influencing Interview Studies

As in the mail survey, several factors may influence the quality of the data received through the interview technique. The principal one, of course, is the effect of interviewer characteristics.

Both race and ethnicity were found to have an effect on responses according to Hyman (1954), Dohrenwend (1968), and Bradburn and Sudman (1979). These studies revealed that differences in race or ethnicity between the respondent and the interviewer may bring forth biased results.

Research by Hyman (1954) and Benney (1956) have shown that the gender of the interviewer can affect the respondent's reaction. Similarly, social status (Katz, 1942) and social distance (Dohrenwend 1968) have been discovered to bias results. Further, Bradburn and Sudman (1979) found that interviewers with the most education made the fewest errors in question asking.

Benney et al. (1956) had inconclusive results in studying the effects of the age of the interviewer and respondent. However, with age and gender combined, young female interviewers tended to attribute a higher honesty ranking to young male respondents than to older male respondents.

Finally, in regard to clothing and grooming, little research has been completed. However, it is generally thought that both are important because appearance is the first thing a respondent notices. According to Bailey (1982), three important points are (1) dress to look like an interviewer, (2) dress neutrally in a fashion similar to that of the people to be interviewed, and (3) dress unobtrusively so the emphasis is on the interview.

Interview Structure

Several interview structures may be employed by the researcher, all of which may be placed into one (or more) of three categories. All three will be presented briefly. The researcher should note that reliability increases with objectivity.

Unstructured interviews offer broad freedom to the respondent in terms of both response and time. This type of interview is usually reserved for obtaining information that is very personal or potentially threatening. As to be expected, this format is the most susceptible to subjective bias or error.

The middle road is the *semistructured* interview, which contains a core of structured questions from which the interviewer may move in related directions for in-depth probing. This allows accurate information on certain questions with a built-in opportunity for exploration. Training is important so that the interviewer knows when and how to probe as well as how to avoid the introduction of interviewer bias.

In the *structured* interview, a well-defined pattern is followed, similar to a questionnaire. The interviewer only strays from the pattern to clarify questions or allow for elaboration. The type of information sought through this technique must be factual and specific. The interview itself is usually brief.

Telephone Interviewing

The use of the telephone in interviewing has increased greatly over the past few years. The chief advantage over face-to-face interviewing is cost. One study by Graves and Kahn (1979) estimates a savings of 50 per cent by telephone while another purports a reduction of 75 to 80 per cent (Klecka & Tuchfarber, 1978).

A second advantage is that telephone interviewing is much faster than either a mail survey or interview study. Third, the researcher can select subjects from a much broader area because travel is not involved. Fourth, the respondent remains more anonymous in a telephone interview. Fifth, monitoring of interviews and quality control is much easier in telephone interviews because all calls can be made from a central location. Sixth, if no one is home, frequent callbacks can be made with little expense, as contrasted to an interviewer returning to the household or business. Seventh, the researcher has access to security buildings and dangerous neighborhoods with the telephone interview. Finally, it has been shown by Bradburn & Subman (1981) that the telephone interview may be better than the face-to-face interview for collecting sensitive data.

However, the telephone interview does have some drawbacks. Generally, respondents are less motivated and often may see the interview as a hoax or a cover for some ulterior motive. Of course the use of checklists and visual aids is eliminated, as compared with the interview study. Further, the telephone interviewer has very little control over the situation; all the respondent has to do is hang up the telephone. Although, Graves and Kahn (1979) in their study found that, while a 74 per cent response was obtained in personal interviews, a 70 per cent response was received through the telephone interview. Because the same questionnaire was employed for each method, the results could be compared easily. It was discovered that the results were very similar over a wide range of topics.

The major problem with telephone interviews is that not all people have a telephone. Tull and Albaum, (1977) and Kviz (1978) found that in those homes with no telephone, the head of the household is likely to be black, under 40 years of age, and not married, to have a low income and little education, and to reside in a rural area. The head of a household with a telephone generally is a white male who earns a higher than average income, has a higher education level, and is married. According to the figures of Klecka and Tuchfarber (1978), 92.8 per cent of U.S. households had a telephone and by the mid-1980s that figure may be expanded to 98 per cent. Consequently, for most studies the number of people without a telephone would be very small and thereby not introduce a significant bias in the research effort.

A related problem is that of unlisted numbers. The advent of random digit dialing (RDD), however, has allowed the researcher to circumvent this dilemma. The researcher simply selects four digit numbers from a table of random numbers and adjoins them to the prefix (first three numbers) and then dials that number. This makes unlisted numbers available.

Microcomputer Revolution in Telephone Interviewing. Before the increase in telephone accessibility and random digit dialing, the telephone interview was a poor technique for gathering adequate data. Now, accessibility, RDD, and widespread usage of WATS (Wide Area Telephone Service) lines, the telephone interview has come of age.

To help the growth of telephone interviewing, the microcomputer can be used to assist in data collection. Computer-assisted telephone interviewing, referred to as CATI, can virtually eliminate the recording of data in the wrong place and the incorrect asking of questions. For example, if the question "Do you smoke?" arises in a health interview and the answer is affirmative, the interviewer may be required to turn two pages to a set of questions about smoking, e.g., about inhaling or frequency. If the interviewer failed to do this that data may be lost and/or the respondent may be asked other questions that could be embarrassing and shorten the interview. The microcomputer can be programmed so that an answer automatically moves the interviewer to the next, appropriate question. Response accuracy is increased, especially because the interviewer does not even see the questions that do not have to be asked.

Groves, Berry, and Mathiowetz (1980), Nicholls, (1980) and Borg and Gall (1983) suggest several advantages of CATI over regular telephone interviewing.

1. CATI requires a well-thought-out questionnaire and a logical progression throughout.
2. Question branching is done methodically and easily, eliminating a type of interview error.
3. Codes that do not have any meaning (wild codes) can be readily detected during the interview and resolved by having the computer direct questions to either the respondent or interviewer.
4. CATI allows close supervision and an opportunity for checking inconsistencies and estimating interrater reliabililty. These can be accomplished by having an additional interviewer simultaneously code the interview and then check the recording of each interviewer.
5. CATI can produce error-free data ready for analysis.

In order to achieve these advantages, the researcher needs to have a computer that will perform RDD, store and retrieve telephone lists, dial automatically, present questions, check codes, input to a dataset, and perform interviewing management. Initially CATI required a large computer, but today even 16-bit memory microcomputers are capable of completing such research.

The Delphi Technique_____

The Delphi technique designed by Helmer (1967) is a method of reaching group consensus on any psychological object. It was originated to circumvent the traditional round table approach of group consensus with the inherent problems of power by individuals to sway the group, the bandwagon effect of majority opinion, manipulation of group dynamics, and the unwillingness of individuals to alter publicly stated positions.

While the Delphi technique is not new (Dalkey & Helmer, 1967), it is relatively recent to health science research. Two examples are those of Weller (1977) and Frazer et al.(1984). The technique was used by Weller to ascertain the knowledge competencies needed by secondary school health educators. Frazer et al. employed a modified technique to identify the most important research questions in health education. There is little doubt that the Delphi technique will be used more as the health education profession continues to grow.

Generally, group members are identified who will generate the consensus position and each member interacts individually to provide collective feedback. Individuals then reconsider their initial positions in light of group trends and can make adjustments accordingly. Eventually, this leads to an informed consensus isolated from the forces of the traditional approach.

Specifically, the sequence of events are as follows:

1. Identify the group members whose consensus opinions are sought. If they are representatives of a group (e.g., heads of departments of health sciences in universities) the sampling technique must be appropriate.
2. First questionnaire: Each member of the group generates a list of concerns, goals, or issues toward which consensus opinions are desired (e.g., knowledge competencies for health educators or research issues confronting health education). The combined lists are edited, randomized, and placed in a format acceptable for a second questionnaire.
3. Second questionnaire: Each member rates or ranks the items derived from the initial questionnaire.
4. Third questionnaire: The results of the second questionnaire are present, revealing the preliminary level of group consensus to each item as well as repeating each member's previous response. The individual group member then rates or ranks each item a second time. If the member differs greatly from the group trend, a brief explanation should be given.

5. Fourth questionnaire: At this juncture the group trend becomes quite evident, as the results of the third questionnaire are presented for each item as well as the member's latest ranking or rating. Along with this is a listing by item of the major reasons for dissent from the group trend. In this questionnaire each member ranks or rates each item for a third and last time, keeping the group's emerging pattern in mind.

6. The results of the fourth questionnaire are calculated and presented as the final statement of group consensus.

If this technique is employed, it is necessary to have all the knowledge and skill required for survey design as well as questionnaire construction and design.

Summary

This chapter discussed survey research commencing with the characteristics of such research. It was seen to be a more complicated matter than frequently perceived. One of the major issues is survey sampling and the development of the sampling frame, which is a list of all the persons or addresses from which the sample is to be drawn. Probability sampling techniques discussed included random sampling, systematic sampling, stratified random sampling, and cluster sampling. Convenience sampling, quota sampling, dimensional sampling, purposive sampling, and snowball sampling were reviewed as nonprobability techniques.

Factors determining sample size were presented, particularly representativeness. A formula was discussed to take confidence level, sampling error, and representativeness into account when dealing with single dichotomous stratification parameters. Disproportionate sampling was seen as a viable route when differences in population size and differences in homogenity among strata existed in stratified random sampling.

The survey flow plan consisted of fifteen steps that outline the overall approach to doing a survey. Four necessary components were presented for questionnaire design and construction: (1) prequestionnaire planning, (2) drafting the questionnaire, (3) preparing the final questionnaire, and (4) pretesting. Emphasis was given to drafting the questionnaire with attention to researcher, respondent, interviewer considerations, types of questionnaires (open or closed), types of questions (dichotomous, multiple-choice, rating, ranking, sentence completion, and open-ended). A checklist of nine pitfalls in question writing was presented as well as seven general rules in arranging the final draft.

The importance of the cover letter accompanying the instrument was discussed in addition to the necessary content and trappings. Pretesting was viewed as a critical analysis so that further modification may be made of the questionnaire.

The mail survey was looked at specifically because it is a time-honored technique of health scientists. This discussion included advantages, disadvantages, and many factors that influence the rate of return and the adequacy of data received. The latter included sponsorship, time and type of mailing, questionnaire length, color and format, ease of completion and return, incentives, nature of respondents, and follow-up procedures. There is little consensus as to what is an appropriate minimum number of returns.

The interview study was discussed including advantages and disadvantages of both the one-on-one interview and the group interview. The effects of interviewer characteristics—race, ethnicity, gender, social status and distance, age, clothing, and grooming—were presented and seen to have an effect on the interview process and results. Unstructured, semistructured, and structured interviews were perceived according to reliabililty and ease of use.

The telephone interview was seen to have several advantages over the face-to-face interview methodology despite some drawbacks. The increase in accessibility and the use of RDD combined with CATI has made the telephone interview more popular as a research technique.

As a final note, the Delphi technique was reviewed in some detail, with reference given to two health science studies. This unique group consensus approach appears to be one that is of great benefit to a still-growing profession.

Suggested Activities

1. You are interested in finding out about the attitudes of hospital administrators toward patient education, especially the need for it. Construct three sequential interview questions.
2. You are going to interview 60 health education teachers in a system of 200 health education teachers. In this system there are 100 elementary teachers—20 men and 80 women; 50 junior high school teachers—20 men and 30 women; 50 high school teachers—30 men and 20 women. How many teachers in each of the six categories would you include in your sample of 60?
3. As a school health educator, you are interested in surveying the parents, administrators, and teachers within your school district to ascertain their

opinions about mandated school health education. To do so, what could you use as a sampling frame for each group? How would you go about selecting a sample of parents, administrators, and teachers? What would be the sample size for each group? What sampling technique should be employed? Would it be different for each group?

In designing the questionnaire, what types of questions should be asked and in what format? Construct a cover letter for this type of survey. Would you have it mailed or completed by interview? Why? Who could you use to pretest the questionnaire?

Use the survey flow plan to get started and include a time frame.

4. Your employer, the head of the Dental Section in the State Department of Public Health, has requested that you conduct a survey of a local community with regard to their feelings about flouridation. There is a strong contingent of people residing therein who have voiced opposition to flouridation, and this has come to your employer's attention. He foresees possible court action and would like some data from the community. Outline all the steps necessary to conduct such an assessment.

Bibliography _____

Bailey, K. (1982) *Methods of Social Research,* New York: MacMillan.

Benney, M., Riesman, D., and Star, S. (1956) Age and sex in the interview, *American Journal of Sociology* 62:143–52.

Borg, W. R. and Gall, M. D. (1983) *Educational Research,* 4th ed., New York: Longman.

Bradburn, N. M. and Sudman, S. (1979) *Improving Interview Method and Questionnaire Design,* San Francisco: Jossey-Bass.

Bradburn, N. M. and Sudman, S. (1981) *Improving Interview Method and Questionnaire Design,* San Francisco: Jossey-Bass.

Champion, D. (1970) *Basic Statistics for Social Research,* Scranton, PA: Chandler.

Dalkey, N. and Helmer, O. (1963) An experimental application of the Delphi Method to the use of experts, *Management Science* 3:458.

Dohrenwend, B. S., Colombotos, J., and Dohrenwend, B. P. (1968) Social distance and interview effects, *Public Opinion Quarterly* 32:410–22.

Frazer, G., Kush, R., and Richardson, C. (1984) Research questions in health education: a professional evaluation, *Journal of School Health* 54(5):188–92.

Graves, R. M. and Kahn, R. L. (1978) *Surveys by Telephone: A National Comparison with Personal Interviews,* New York: Academic Press.

Groves, R. M., Berry, M., and Mathiowetz, N. (1980) Some impacts of computer assisted telephone interviewing on survey methods, *Proceedings of the Section on Survey Research Methods, Houston, 11-14 August, 1980.* Washington, D.C.: American Statistical Association.

Helmer, O. 1967. *Analysis of the Future: The Delphi Technique,* Santa Monica, CA: Rand Corporation.

Hyman, H. (1954) *Interviewing in Social Research,* Chicago: University of Chicago Press.

Issac, S. and Michael, W. (1981) *Handbook in Research and Evaluation,* 2nd ed., San Diego: Edits Publishers.

Katz, D. (1942) "Do interviewers bias polls?" *Public Opinion Quarterly* 6:248–68.

Klecka, W. R. and Tuchfarber, A. J. (1978) Random digit dialing: a comparison to personal surveys, *Public Opinion Quarterly* 42:105–14.

Kviz, F. J. (1978) Random digit dialing and sample bias, *Public Opinion Quarterly* 42:544–46.

Leedy, P. (1980) *Practical Research: Planning and Design,* New York: MacMillan Publishing Company.

Nicholls, W. (1980) Computer assisted telephone interviewing, *Computer Center Newsletter* 3:1.

Scott, C. (1961) Research on mail surveys, *Journal of the Royal Statistical Society* 124(A):143–95.

Sellitz, C., Jahoda, M., Deutsch, M., and Cook, S. (1959) *Research Methods in Social Relations,* New York: Holt, Rinehart, Winston.

Trow, M. (1967) Education and survey research, In Clock, C. (ed.), *Survey Research in the Social Sciences,* New York: Russell Sage.

Tull, D. S. and Albaum, G. S. (1977) Bias in random digit dialed surveys, *Public Opinion Quarterly* 41:389–95.

Weller, R. (1977) Identification and evaluation of knowledge compentencies in health education. Unpublished doctoral dissertation, University of Illinois.

CHAPTER 6

Qualitative Research

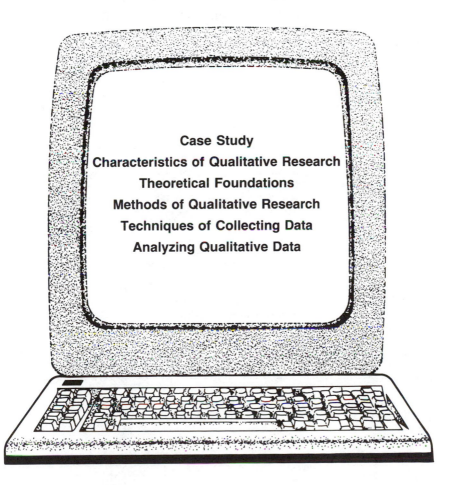

Case Study
Characteristics of Qualitative Research
Theoretical Foundations
Methods of Qualitative Research
Techniques of Collecting Data
Analyzing Qualitative Data

Case Study

Health Data Analysts, a research consortium, has been awarded a contract to examine the efficacy of a hospital's Wellness Center. Steven has been named the project director of this study, and he will head a team comprised of several staff people who are all trained and educated to gather and interpret data for the layperson. The consortium devised a methodology to use qualitative research in order to best reach the goals and objectives of the project.

Some of the previous chapters of this textbook have dealt with collecting and reporting data in a quantifiable manner. This chapter discusses another method of gathering data that is different to experimental and survey research in that it is *qualitative*. As an introduction to this chapter Table 6.1 compares the two approaches of qualitative and quantitative research. After you review the chart, you will be able to see that the need, setting, and type of problem to be studied will eventually determine the research approach you will use.

TABLE 6.1 Comparisons Between Qualitative and Quantitative

Qualitative		Quantitative	
Phrases associated with the methodology		*Phrases associated with the methodology*	
Case study	Naturalistic	Empirical	Positivist
Documentary	Observation	Experimental	Social facts
Ecological	Participant	Hard data	Statistical
Ethnographic	Phenomenological		
Field work	Soft data		
Life history	Symbolic interaction		
Key concepts associated with the methodology		*Key concepts associated with the methodology*	
Common sense	Negotiated orders	Hypothesis	Statistically significant
Definition of situation	Process	Operationalize	Validity
Everyday life	Social construction	Reliability	Variable
Practical purposes	Understanding	Replication	
Meaning			
Academic affliation (beginnings)		*Academic affiliation* (beginnings)	
Anthropology		Economics	
History		Political science	
Sociology		Psychology	
		Sociology	

TABLE 6.1 (continued)   Comparisons Between Qualitative and Quantitative

Qualitative	Quantitative
Goals	*Goals*
Describe multiple realities	Establish the facts
Develop sensitizing concepts	Prediction
Develop understanding	Show relationships between variables
Grounded theory	Statistical description
	Theory testing
Relationship with subjects	*Relationship with subjects*
Empathy	Circumscribed
Emphasis entrust	Distant
Equalitorian	Short-term
Intense contact	Stay detached
Instruments and tools	*Instruments and tools*
Tape recorder	Computers
Transcriber	Indexes
	Inventories
	Questionnaires
	Scales
	Test scores
Data analysis	*Data analysis*
Analytical induction	Deductive
Constant comparative method	Occurs at end of data collection
Inductive	Statistical
Models, themes, concepts	
Ongoing	
Problems in using the approach	*Problems in using the approach*
Data reduction difficult	Controlling extraneous variables
Difficult to study large populations	Obtrusiveness
Procedures are not standardized	Validity
Reliability	
Time consuming	
Design	*Design*
Design is a hunch as to how to proceed	Design is a detailed plan of operation
Flexible, evolving	Specific
General	Structured
Data	*Data*
Descriptive	Counts, measures
Field notes	Operationalized variables

Continued

TABLE 6.1 (continued)   Comparisons Between Qualitative and Quantitative

Qualitative	Quantitative
Data (cont'd)	*Data (cont'd)*
Offical statistics	Quantifiable coding
Personal documents	Quantitative
Photographs	Statistical
Subjects' own words	
Sample	*Sample*
Nonrepresentative	Control for extraneous variables
Small	Control groups
Theoretical	Large
	Precise
	Random selection
	Stratified
Methods	*Methods*
Observation	Experiments
Open-ended interviewing	Data sets
Participant observation	Quasiexperiments
Reviewing documents	Structural interviewing
	Structured observation
	Survey research

Source: Adapted from Bogdan, R. and Biklin, S. *Qualitative Research in Education.* Boston: Allyn and Bacon, 1982, p. 45–48.

Characteristics of Qualitative Research

What is different about qualitative research? The following characteristics, adapted from Bodgan and Biklin (1982), help to describe some traits about this methodology:

1. *Qualitative data has the natural setting as the direct source of data and the research is the key instrument.* The data is collected at the location of the study. Steven, in our case study, will go directly to the Wellness Center to study the actual goings-on firsthand. The researcher is really the instrument most readily used. Even if tape recorders or other equipment are employed, the researcher has the insight into where he or she should be and exactly how to collect the necessary data. The reason that qualitative researchers go to the location under study is that they are concerned with context and feel that situations can best be understood when they are directly observed. The setting has to be understood in the history context of the

institution of which it is a part. When the data with which qualitative researchers are concerned are produced by subjects, as in the case of official records, they want to know where, how, and under what circumstances the data came into being. Of what historical circumstances and movements are the records a part? Qualitative researchers believe that behavior is influenced by the setting and therefore always go to that location to collect the necessary data.

2. *Qualitative research is descriptive.* Numbers are not used to collect data, but rather words and pictures form the basic methods of data collection. The data include transcripts of in-depth interviews, field notes, photographs, tapes, memos, personal documents, and other official records. In our case study, Steven might ask the director of the Wellness Center for files pertaining to the goals and objectives stated when the center first opened.

Quotations are very often used in collecting qualitative data. In addition, a record is made of everything that occurs in certain situations. For example, when observing a conversation between two people, the researcher would probably describe the initiator, the person who did most of the talking and listening, the immediate surroundings (e.g., near a drinking fountain), and so on. The researcher is attempting to get a very comprehensive and deep understanding of the situation being studied. Therefore every detail must be described, and this is a very laborious task!

3. *Qualitative researchers are concerned with process rather than with outcomes or products.* The researcher is concerned with the natural history of the situation being studied. Questions related to how decisions are made in the context under study, and what becomes "common sense," are areas of concern. Qualitative studies tend to decipher exactly what goes on in an institution so that the expected outcomes are fulfilled. That is the *process* leading to the outcomes. In quantitative research, subjects are given tests (pretest and posttest) to determine the effectiveness of a program. The qualitative process discerns activities that would occur between the pretest and posttest and analyze those events, with no concern for the outcome.

4. *Qualitative researchers tend to analyze their data inductively.* Qualitative investigators do not collect data to prove or disprove a prior hypothesis, but rather they collect the data first and then group them together. Glaser and Strauss (1967) describe a type of theory that builds from the bottom up as *grounded theory.* The qualitative investigator puts together a theory after the data have been collected and after much time has been spent at the location with the subjects. Part of this process is to find out what the concerns are, as opposed to quantitative research in which investigators come into a situation with predetermined questions.

5. *"Meaning"* *is of essential concern to the qualitative approach.* Qualitative researchers are concerned with how different people live their lives and make sense of it; this is called *participant perspective.* For example, investigators might ask what people in a certain situation take for granted.? In our case study, Steven may ask Wellness Center personnel for their perspectives on the efficacy of the center. He would ask other personnel in the hospital the same question. In other words, he would attempt to get the participants' perceptions about the Wellness Center and relate those to the perspectives of other people, looking for common ground.

Many situations in which qualitative research is conducted will not include all of the characteristics we have discussed, but they should include a majority. Investigators using this research method must have time and patience, as the study will undoubtedly demand much painstaking effort.

Theoretical Foundations

For any researcher to adequately collect and analyze data, he or she should be aware of and have an understanding of the theoretical base on which the research is based. The theoretical foundations of qualitative research are similar to those in anthropology and sociology, in which paridigms are used to guide research. A *paradigm* is a research perspective that hold views about how research is to be conducted and has its own assumptions about how the world works and what is important in that world. Most qualitative researchers use a phenomenological perspective, which is the basis for most research in this area.

Phenomenological Perspective

Max Weber was the leading proponent of the phenomemological approach to research. The phenomenologist is concerned with attempting to understand human behavior through the eyes of the subjects in the study. This has been called *verstehen,* which is the interpretive understanding of human interaction. The phenomenological approach is used throughout most qualitative studies because of the importance of interviewing the subjects in a program or institution. Here the investigator has not made any presumptions about how the subjects view something, and goes about an informal interview without any structure. This perspective is ever present as a theoretical framework for qualitative researchers.

Symbolic Interaction

Symbolic interaction originated with George Herbert Mead in his book *Mind, Self and Society* (1934). He viewed communication as the key to understanding the connection between intelligence (mind), self-consciousness (self), and the community (society). Gestures (verbal or not), made by people are symbols, taken to mean acts that stand for something else. Another aspect of Mead's work dealt with the fact that humans have a self-conscious awareness of themselves. Interaction between people depends on the degree to which it possesses a self-conscious quality. How others intepret the interactions depends on experience and history. In other words, symbolic interaction theory asserts that people's self-concepts are influenced by the way others respond to them.

People act not on the basis of predetermined responses but as interpreting, defining, symbolic animals whose behavior the researcher can only understand by entering the defining process (Bogdan and Biklen, 1982). This is accomplished with a type of qualitative research called participant observation, which will be discussed later in this chapter. Defining is a shared event, and the people involved usually developed congruent definitions of interpretations. As people see a need, they may change their definition of an interpretation, and this is where the qualitative investigator steps in to determine how definitions develop.

Culture

Cultural anthropologists study other cultures, sometimes from a phenomenological perspective. *Ethnography* is the term used for the description of a particular culture. All anthropologists use the theoretical framework of culture in their research studies and this organizes the ethnographic work. The ethnographer has few if any hypotheses and there is no structured instrument with which to collect the data. The goal of the ethnographer is to describe in as much detail as possible the customs, religious ceremonies, mores, language, and other pertinent variables of a subculture or group. The best way to do this is for the investigator to become a participant observer and in so doing attempts to put aside her or his own culture.

Ethnomethodology

Harold Garfinkel (1967) coined the term *ethnomethodology* to refer to the study of how individuals create and understand life. It is the study of everyday, commonplace, routine social activity. Ethnomethodologists attempt to understand how people make order out of the complex world in which they live. A more complete discussion of ethnomethodology will appear later in this chapter, because it is a type of qualitative research that has taken on importance in the last 20 years.

Methods of Qualitative Research

Qualitative methodologies are research procedures that enable the investigator to produce data. The methods that will be discussed include observation and participant observation, ethnomethodology, and document study. Although in-depth interviewing is also a qualitative research method, we chose to discuss it in Chapter 5, "Survey Methods."

Observation

One of the primary methods of qualitative research is observation. It is a scientific technique if conducted under the proper circumstances. Observation must (1) serve a research purpose, (2) be planned systematically, (3) be recorded systematically, and (4) be subjected to checks and controls on validity and reliability (Bickman, 1976). The following section will describe the value and purposes of the observation, what to observe, methods of observation, and the training of observers.

Value and Purposes of Observation. Observational data are collected in a naturalistic setting in that the researcher does not manipulate or control people or other significant things related to the study. It is a discovery-oriented approach carried out in the field. Because the investigator is in the field, he or she can become very close to the situation and better understand the context within the program and its various complexities. Therefore, the value of observational data is that it enables those who asked for the information (the users) to understand the entire program through detailed and very descriptive information that is provided through the collection of observational data.

The purposes of observational data include: (1) descriptions of the behaviors; (2) situational behavior may be recorded; and (3) the topic lends itself to this method. First, providing detailed descriptions of the behavior patterns of people is one of the purposes of health science research. The observational method of data collection enables researchers to accomplish this task. When observational data is recorded, it is done at the time a behavior pattern is occurring. This allows investigators to get a true sense of individual and group behavior under real and accurate circumstances.

A second purpose for using observational data is that behavior can be recorded as it actually occurs. In our case study, Steven will use observation so that he and his staff can directly observe behaviors as they happen. In this manner they will be able to observe how Wellness Center personnel interact with each other under varied circumstances and in several situations.

The remaining purpose of observational methods is that there are certain circumstances under which they are the *only* feasible method to collect the appropriate data. Infants and toddlers cannot be interviewed or given a survey to complete; hence, observation becomes the method to use to collect data concerning these types of subjects. Another example would be a study of people with severe diseases (terminal cancer, autism, schizophrenia), which is not possible except through observation.

There are several values or advantages of direct observation. Patton (1980) has best described the advantages of direct, personal observations

1. By directly observing program observations and activities, the investigator is able to understand the *context* within which the program operates.
2. The firsthand experience with a program enables the experimenter to use the inductive approach.
3. The study personnel can observe things that are routine to those in the program.
4. The investigator can learn things about the program that cannot or will not be revealed in an interview or through completing a questionnaire.
5. The observers are able to present a comprehensive view of the program because they can move beyond the perception of the participants.
6. The investigator uses her or his knowledge and experience in terms of feelings, reflection, and introspection about a program.

Methods of Observation. There are two major types of methods of observation: relatively unstructured and structured. In the former method, the investigator attempts to get directly involved in the situation and to describe it as nonselectively as possible. In structured methodologies, the investigator codes or categorizes the observed behaviors of the program participants.

Unstructured methods may involve filming or videotaping an occurrence, being involved as a participant observer, using specimen records, and recording anecdotes. Because participant observer methods will be discussed later in this chapter, we will focus here on the other unstructured methods.

By using *film or videotape* one could ideally get a complete and accurate view of a program. However, is this really the goal of observation? Or is it to summarize, systematize, and simplify the event, rather than depict an exact replication? (Bickman, 1976) Even if one does use film to record the program, the film really is not an exact reproduction because of biases caused by the presence of the camera and microphone.

Specimen records are descriptions of behavior over a brief continuous time period. It allows for extrapolations of one event to several or a series of events. Behaviors are noted with painstaking care and the interventions of those observed are recorded so as to define a standing pattern of behavior. If these patterns of behavior can be observed under various environmental settings, a behavioral consistency can be determined. This is the major advantage of using specimen records.

Anecdotes are used very widely by many people attempting to observe behavior. The observer selects places and particular events to observe before actually completing the anecdote. This is not true of specimen records or films. Anecdotal records are objective and usually written after the incident has occurred. This type of record can test hypotheses if proper sampling is used. In the previously mentioned methods, hypotheses are generated *after* the observations are made. Anecdotal records should not be interpretive, but merely descriptive and accurate.

Generally, unstructured methods lead to problems of reliability, observer bias, and memory distortion. Because these problems can damage any study, we suggest that unstructured methods be used to generate rather than to test hypotheses.

Structured methods are more formal methods used to observe behavior and to set up or test hypotheses. The investigator is able to select activities to observe before they occur and can plan a systematic recording of observations. There are several ways to record this type of information: duration, continuous, frequency-count, and interval.

Duration recording is used when the observer wishes to record the elapsed time during which the behavior occurs. In our case study, if Steven wanted to find out how long the coordinator of the Wellness Center talked during a staff meeting, he could use a stop watch to accomplish this task.

Continuous recording occurs when the observer records all the behaviors of the subjects and thereby creates a *protocol*. A protocol is a narrative in chronological order or everything that occurred in a given setting, such as the Wellness Center staff meeting. This is a very comprehensive method in that the observer must use a content analysis system to classify the observed behavior.*

When using *frequency count recording,* an observer simply counts the number of times a particular behavior occurs. This is especially useful when behaviors occur at low frequency and observers can count several different behaviors at the same time.

Interval recording is used to study the sequence of behaviors of subjects. The observer records a specific behavior at specific intervals, e.g., every ten seconds. If Steven were to record, at intervals, when the coordinator of the Wellness Center asked a rhetorical question, Steven could get an idea of the sequence of that behavior. In addition, if Steven had a frequency count of rhetorical questions and multiplied it by the interval, he could get the duration of that behavior, which could prove to be very important in diagnosing possible personnel problems.

What should we observe? Many program aspects should be observed to get a comprehensive view of that program. We will discuss (a) program setting, (b) activities and participant behaviors, (c) informal interactions and unplanned activities, (d) nonverbal communication, and (e) unobtrusive measures. Much of the following has been abstracted from Patton's *Qualitative Evaluative Methods.* These occasions can help an observer to organize a methodology that will emphasize certain kinds of observations. These are called *sensitizing concepts,* and they provide a framework to enhance the importance of behaviors and events.

The program setting is the physical environment in which the research takes place. When the reader can visualize the setting through a complete and detailed description provided by the investigator, then the program setting is helpful. The researcher should avoid using interpretive words such as "very," "wonderful," and "lovely."Rather, words that actually describe the setting—colors, dimensions of space, or quotations of participants—should be used.

Program activities and participant behaviors involve asking questions such as, What do the participants do? What is it like to be a participant? What do the observers see while the program is in progress? Units of activity are generally regarded as organizers for the researcher. These units may include staff meetings, formal sessions, patient-client sessions, and the like. The investigator must focus the

---

*For a more complete discussion of content analysis see *Miles and Huberman's,* (1984) Qualitative Data Analysis.*

sequence of events in a chronological order: when did the activity begin, who introduced it, who is in charge of the activity?

Gradually, the researcher attempts to observe each activity by asking questions that deal with statements made by staff and participants during the event. How did behaviors change over the duration of the activity? How did it feel to be engaged in that activity? At the end of the activity, the observer asks, what signals that the event has ended, what is said by whom, and what is the relationship of this particular activity to the other parts of the program?

Observation of *informal interactions and unplanned activities* is just as valuable as viewing formal activities in a program. Investigators should ensure that time is allotted for this activity. It can occur during breaks or meals, before and after formal working hours, and during the workday. The researcher will probably overhear conversations or conduct face-to-face or small group interviews. The way people interact or do not interact after a meeting or part of a program should also be observed. The fact that people do not interact is a part of the data and should be noted.

Nonverbal communication has received much attention by behavioral scientists, who of course include health scientists. When observing groups, noticing how people sit, what they do in their seats, how they dress, and how they space themselves in discussion groups (e.g., who sits next to whom and how often) enriches description of the process of a program. Investigators should describe the nonverbal cues of others, as well as their own reactions to those cues. And by watching for behavior patterns, they can learn about significant nonverbal behaviors.

Unobtrusive measures are helpful in obtaining data without the participants realizing that they are part of the study. Examples of this type of data collection include analyzing contents of wastepaper baskets, counting cigarette butts before and after meetings, and noting what is written on a blackboard or memo pad. These unobstrusive measures are very helpful, because once people know that they are in a study, their reactions may become self-conscious and inhibited. Unobstrusive measures should not contaminate the way people respond. Additional ways to collect unobstrusive data include looking through directories, calendar diaries, and other such documents.

In our case study, Steven could observe reactions of people leaving a conference room, witness daily calendars to see the meetings scheduled, and look at internal memos. These would be unobstrusive measures and could possibly reinforce the results of other, reactive data-gathering methodologies, such as surveys and interviews. The more varied the data-gathering techniques, the more congruence should

TABLE 6.2 Observation Form

1. *Check each question asked by the Wellness Center coordinator into one of the categories.*

	Frequency	Total
a. Asks personnel for direct input	x x x	3
b. Asks personnel to answer specific questions	x x x x	4
c. Asks for general questions	x x x x x	5
d. Other	x x x x x x x	7
	Grand Total	19

Adapted from Borg, W. and Gall, M. (1983) *Educational Research*, N.Y.: Longman.

appear among the results. This provides a more true and accurate picture of the program being observed.

The Observation Form. There are so many types of observations and situations in which they take place, that we encourage all investigators to prepare their own forms. Each time an observation takes place, a new form is required. Researchers should attempt to plan their observations, so they can devise appropriate forms. Table 6.2 is an example of a form that Steven might utilize when observing a staff meeting of the Wellness Center.

As is evident, observation forms can be easily devised and when utilized properly can provide necessary and valuable information for the study.

Observer Training. Many reviews on observer training (Hartman and Wood, 1982; Haynes, 1978; and Wildman and Erickson, 1977) provide helpful information on the training of observers. You should refer to these references for a more complete review. We will discuss the observation manual, training for the observational setting, and training in the observational setting.

The observational manual becomes the bible for all observers. Steven will have worked on this manual before contacting his staff. The manual should clearly define all code categories, and positive and negative examples should be included to more explicitly depict the coding techniques. Researchers in Health, the research consortium that Steven is employed by, would have a well-developed manual for use in most of the research projects the consortium conducts.

The manual should discuss and explain ethical issues, dress codes, courtesy protocols, and all other matters that pertain to the collection of data by the observational method.

Observer orientation occurs when observers have been selected by the project director to be oriented to the purpose of the study, and where the observational method fits into the specific research project. All observers must be encouraged to follow the coding system exactly, and not allow other information to interfere with completion of the forms. The observers should not be told any hypotheses, if any exist, because this knowledge might bias them when they are completing the necessary observation forms.

During orientation the observers must be informed about subjects' rights and the confidentiality of the study. Observers should not discuss their reactions with each other until the observations are complete.

Training for the observational setting includes having observers memorize the manual, especially the coding rules and definitions. This will eliminate confusion and disorganization when the actual observations occur. It might be worthwhile for Steven to ensure his staff's knowledge of the manual by having them practice and then demonstrate mastery on a test regarding the manual. Observers should be exposed to and trained in using the actual forms and any other equipment (videotape or audiotape recorders, etc.).

One way for training to take place is to place the trainees in settings that require them to use the materials that will be used in the actual study. This can be accomplished by having trainees watch videotapes and listen to tape recordings, called analogue tapes. These are made by experienced observers. They enable the trainees to proceed from the simple to complex tasks, approximating an actual situation.

While the trainees are using the analogue tapes, they should receive constant, consistent, and constructive feedback as to the accuracy of their responses. This can be done by comparing trainees' responses to experienced observers' responses and discussing the discrepancies. In addition, this method can be useful to reconstruct forms and/or categories of behavior on the forms.

After the analogue tape training is completed and the trainees have demonstrated almost perfect accuracy in their response to the tapes, they should begin *training in the observational setting*. This is the final phase of the training and is conducted under supervision. Steven would take one of his staff to a very straightforward observational setting (behind a one-way mirror in a person's office) and encourage the staff member to begin making observational recordings. Afterwards, Steven would review the staff member's forms to check for accuracy. Each staff member would go through the same type of procedure before attending larger, more complicated observational situations.

Participant Observation

Participant observation involves the collection of data in the field that combines document analysis, interviewing of respondents and informants, and direct participation, observation, and introspection (Denzin, 1978). The field of anthropology is best known for using participant observation, but more recently, sociology, education, and health science researchers have used this method of qualitative data collection. The aforementioned disciplines have used participant observation in natural setting such as schools, hospitals, and clinics. Our case study would lend itself to participant observation as a methodology.

The observer becomes part of the setting and "goes native." The observation may take serval forms and may vary as to the degree of the researcher's participation, how much is disclosed to the subjects in the study, and the degree to which the activities and subjects are directly observed by the investigators (Walizer and Wienir, 1978). Researchers can become totally involved in the setting (e.g., a staff member of the Wellness Center in our case study), or be a partial participant in a tribe or religious group without becoming an actual member of that group. When an observer goes native, he or she wants to understand the values and experiences of that group. The participant observer must disregard her or his own values, because they might interfere with the ability of the participant observer to become emotionally involved with the group. This becomes a difficult dilemma for the participant observer. He or she must share experiences of the group, but cannot become totally involved, because some sort of detachment must be retained to accurately report the observations.

How much is told to the subjects can vary from everything to nothing at all. At times it is necessary to conceal the fact that there is a study being conducted. This may result in some ethical problems. However, compromises are usually achieved by using partial disclosure. Here, only a few select people are informed about the participant observer. Junker (1960, pp. 35–38) has described four types of participant-observation situations

1. *Complete participant.* In this role, the observer's activities are entirely concealed. The observer is a complete member of an in-group, thus sharing secret information guarded from outsiders. The observer's freedom to observe outside the in-group system of relationships is severely limited, and in such a role tends to block perception of the workings of the reciprocal relations between the in-group and the larger social system, nor is it easy to switch from this to another role permitting observation of the details of the larger group.

2. *Participant as observer.* Here, the observer's activities are *not* entirely concealed, but are "kept under wraps," or subordinated to activities as participant. This role may limit access to some kinds of information, perhaps especially at the secret level.
3. *Observer as participant.* This is the situation in which the observer's activities as such are made publicly known at the outset, are more or less publicly sponsored by people in the situation studied, and are not "kept under wraps." This role may provide access to a wide range of information and even secrets may be given to the participant observer.
4. *Complete observer.* This describes a range of roles where, at one extreme, the observer is behind a one-way mirror, and at the other extreme, her/his activities are completely public.

Participant observation must involve direct observation and is usually supplemented by other data collection methodologies. One of the most common complementary sources of data collection is the use of informants. *Informants* are a group members who are in a position to reveal worthwhile information or who are wholly representative of the group under study.

Advantages and Disadvantages of Participant Observation. The first advantage of participant observation is the ability of the process to *explore* a theory or a type of measurement. In addition, it allows for hypothesis formation whereas it is impossible to formulate hypotheses before the beginning of the study. A further point of exploration lies in the investigator being able to research a new area as a participant observer.

A second advantage to participant observation is that investigators can gain *access* to subjects or to data, where it might not otherwise be feasible. Organizations that might feel threatened, such as in our case study, would be prime candidates for participant observation. This methodology would enable a researcher to gain valuable data as an insider of the organization. A further consideration is that in some instances subjects are unable to recall events or may not view events as important, thereby not giving the investigator accurate, reportable information. Additionally, participant observation becomes advantageous when subjects cannot self-report data, as in the case of very young children, impaired people in hospitals, or those who are afraid to self-report data (prisoners, gang members, etc.)

The third major advantage to participant observation is the possibility of gathering *richness* of data. While other methods provide hard data in terms of numbers and statistics, participant observation enables the researcher to see variables within the context of the natural setting. Subjects are off guard and the descriptions garnered are accurate as to what exactly occurred.

As with any methodology there are both pros and cons; there are several disadvantages with participant observation. The most serious of these is the ethical element, especially when no one under study is apprised of the investigation. The problem then is one of deception and of the reaction of subjects who were, in effect, duped.

Another disadvantage of participant observation is the possibility that the participant observer will become too emotionally involved, lose objectivity in reporting, and then later provide interpretation to the data.

A third disadvantage lies in the reliance on the participant observer's memory to recall all aspects of the events that occurred. This can be a slow and arduous process, because the observer must covertly write or dictate notes whenever feasible.

Being a Participant Observer. Many of the considerations previously discussed concerning validity, reliability, sampling, and subject selection must be adhered to in participant observation. However, as Walizer and Wienir (1978) discuss, some special concerns pertain to participant observation.

Problem selection is a consideration for participant observation. Investigators may have relied on previous research to pose the problem, or even have used participant observation to find the problem. There are some major things to look for when observing a particular group that guide the problem selection. The following has been adopted from Walizer and Wienir (1978, p. 338):

1. How is the institution or program organized?
2. What is the nature of the social relationships that exist within the program?
3. What types of technology are utilized to make the work environment plausible?
4. What are the relationships between management and staff?
5. What activities do employees do together? Apart?

These questions are just a few examples of how participant observers begin a framework for their study. These questions naturally lead to others and thus can readily focus the problem to be studied. There are times when participant observers are given the problem before embarking upon the research.

A second consideration is *choosing the setting* for participant observation. If the problem has previously been delineated, then the participant observer must choose an appropriate site that would contain that problem. For example, if one wanted to study the relationship between secretaries and middle managers, the chosen site must include both these characters and both must have expressed the desire to participate in the study. Another aspect to consider in choosing the setting is to ensure that the participant observer will be comfortable in the setting. If you were asked to be a participant observer in a nuclear power plant and did not feel at ease in that situation, the study would not benefit from your participation.

Another consideration is *establishing social relationships* with the subjects. This is the most important part of the design, because the entire concept of participant observation relies on acceptance of the observer by group subjects. Before the study commences, it would be wise to obtain the necessary entree from high-level employers, presidents of corporations, chieftains of tribes, etc. In our case study, Steven would get permission from the hospital director and clinic president if he wanted to conduct part of the research by using participant observation.

Once the study is in progress and the necessary permissions have been granted, the participant observer should begin to become associated and acclimated to the program. In this regard the observer should attempt to remain in the background and not attract attention. This prohibits people from being too curious about the "new person on the block."

A fourth consideration in attempting to become a participant observer is *finding informants*. These persons are used to observe for the participant observer and to suggest to and inform the participant observer about the program and its problem or problems to be studied. The observer must make sure that the informant is reliable and is relaying truths about what he or she sees and hears. The informant should be tested by the participant observer to verify her or his comments and perceptions.

A further consideration for the participant observer is to *establish rapport* with the subjects. The goal of the investigator is to blend in with the program, and act as natural as possible. Bogdan and Taylor (1975) have delineated ways in which a participant observer can establish rapport.

1. Attempt to be yourself.
2. Dress in a manner that is both comfortable for you and is appropriate to the setting.
3. Begin to establish relationships very slowly.
4. Establish common interests with the subjects.
5. Participate in activities and events with subjects, if they are of interest to you.

6. Do not disrupt the subject's routines.
7. Do not assume that hostile subjects will remain hostile as the study progress.

Participant observation is absolutely demanding and can take a great deal of time, patience, and effort. While the observer is spending the day with the subjects in a group, the other waking hours are spent recording, collating, and analyzing data. Hence, participant observation can be a very time-consuming activity, especially if it endures long periods of time. However, the rewards are great in that participant observation, a qualitative research methods, gives the richness and completeness needed for obtaining information and drawing conclusions concerning some research problems.

Ethnomethodology

Ethnomethodology is the study of methods used in everyday, commonplace, and routine social activities. Garfinkel (1967) believes ethnomethodology is an organizational study of a person's knowledge of his or her ordinary affairs, of his or her own organized enterprises, where that knowledge is treated by investigators as part of the same setting that it also makes orderable. It should be made clear here that ethnomethodology is not an alternative methodology aimed at a more effective solution of traditionally formulated problems. Focusing upon the complicated character of action scenes, ethnomethodology necessarily develops a style of research responsive to its subject matter (Turner, 1974). In other words, ethnomethodology is *not* a research method per se, but rather it is a method to attempt to find out how people make sense out of ordinary situations in which they live. Ethnomethodologists, then, examine common sense in an attempt to understand how people see, describe, and explain order in the world in which they live.

As an example, Wieder (1974) explored how narcotic addicts in a halfway house used a "convict code" ("do not snitch," "help other residents") to explain and account for their behavior. He illustrated the way in which residents "tell the code," apply maxims to specific situations, when they are called upon to account for their behavior. He wrote: "the code, then, is much more a method of moral persuasion and justification than it is a substantive account of an organized way of life. It is a way, or set of ways, of causing activities to be seen as morally, repetitively, and constrainedly organized" (p. 158). This is an example of how ethnomethodologists suspend their own common-sense assumptions to study how common sense is used in everyday life.

Advantages and Disadvantages of Ethnomethodology. The *advantages* of ethnomethodology are many. The first is that it studies nonverbal as well as verbal behavior. Second, it is longitudinal because it is ongoing and changes in behavior can be viewed over a long period of time. Third, this type of study can provide insight into what and why people think about commonsenese activities and behaviors, enabling health scientists to make better order of why people behave the way they do in areas of health.

One of the *disadvantages* of ethnomethodology in relation to the health sciences, is that this type of study involves investigating the *process* of how something occurs, rather than the product of that occurrence. As an example, in our case study Steven would not use ethnomethodology to ascertain the attitudes of Wellness Center personnel toward centralized management, but would use ethnomethodology to study the process of how those attitudes were formed. Another disadvantage is that enthnomethodology does not lend itself to large-scale studies, but is better for process-oriented, smaller investigations.

An interesting point to include here is that ethnomethodology actually studies all the previously discussed methods as a means to garner knowledge about the process of how people make sense of their commonplace lives. In this manner, researchers can gain valuable insight into questionnaire construction and coding of other survey materials.

Indexical Expressions. Indexicals are situation-specific words and/or phrases whose meaning changes from situation to situation and may depend upon who is uttering the word or to whom the remarks are directed. Garfinkel and Sacks (1970) listed the following indexical words: *she, we, he, you, here, there, now, this, that, it, I, then, soon, today,* and *tomorrow.* These words have varying meanings, dependent upon the context. The indexicals have to be interpreted by an individual who is participating in the interaction before the meaning of the words is clear. The ethnomethodologist does not want to convert these indexical expressions into objective, nonindexical expressions, as a traditional researcher might approach this situation. Instead, the ethnomethodologist wants to study the rules people set to make sense of these indexicals in everyday conversation. This can be a very important aspect of a research project: the interpretation of important words.

Another aspect of ethnomethodology is that conversation and interaction are regulated by rules or norms. Ethnomethodologists discover how sense is made out of the structuring and ordering of indexicals. Ethnomethodologists can put meaning to indexicals that are made clear through a situationally specific process in which the context may be problematic and differ from place to place or time to time. However, the rules by which meaning is explicated remain objective, constant, and nonproblematic (Baily, 1982). Topics that are usually studied by ethnomethodologists are

1. Formulating: the process by which one conversationalist interprets or explains a part of the conversation.
2. Sequencing of a conversation.
3. The termination of conversations.

All of these and many other topics provide invaluable information to the health scientist, especially when conducting a qualitative research study. Experimental and survey research results may tell us what the subject knows or thinks, but ethnomethodology takes it one step further in an attempt to find out why the respondent answers in particular ways. Ethnomethodologists are indeed interested in human behavior in that they seek to find the rules that govern behavior.

Document Study

We shall discuss the study of documents with specific reference to nonpersonal documents. Personal documents will be discussed in a later section of this chapter, under Techniques Utilized in Data Collection, and in Chapter 8. A very valuable source of information is retained in a program's or institution's records and documents. The investigator will have a better understanding and increased knowledge about a program once he or she reads its documents. At the outset of the project in our case study, Steven should negotiate receiving at least the following types of documents: routine client records, correspondence from and to staff, financial charts, and official or unofficial documents generated by or for the program (Patton, 1980). These documents can avail the investigator of basic sources of information regarding the activities and processes of the organization, and they can enable to researcher to view other questions not previously considered to follow up on observations, participant observation, or ethnomethodological research.

Types of Documents. There are many official documents that the researcher should attempt to obtain: minutes of meetings, memos, newsletters, policy documents, code of ethics, philosophy statements, etc. The qualitative researcher is looking for how the organization or program is defined by those who are involved in that program. Therefore, a review of these documents will prove beneficial.

Internal documents include memos and other communications that abound in any organization. In a hospital, such as the one where our Wellness Center is located, the amount of paper that flows from the top to the bottom is immense. Of course, some flows in the opposite direction as well. These documents can reveal the true chain of command, the interoffice fighting and subsequent negotiation, and rules and regulations. In addition, leadership styles might emerge from these documents. It is advised, as we stated in the beginning of this section, that the researcher ensure that he or she will have access to this information before the project actually commences.

External communication includes those materials that are circulated outside the organization. This would include newsletters, public philosophic statements, news releases, marketing advertisements, and public access programs (health fairs, open houses). These documents can provide official points of view and administrative hierarchy. Many organizations, especially hospitals, such as that in which our Wellness Center is located, have hired public relations firms. This makes it a little difficult to ascertain who wrote what. In any case, the researcher should obtain the necessary information regarding the public relations organization, such as whether all external documents get reviewed in-house previous to publication. These documents are readily accessible because they are produced for outside consumption. In many instances, files will be kept of these types of documents, so they will be very easy for the researcher to obtain.

Personnel records can provide valuable information about hiring and firing practices, promotion and reward systems, and administrative policies regarding personnel. In addition, these files also can provide information about the people (personnel managers, supervisors) who add paper to the file. Access to these files may be granted, if researchers agree not to identify people but use a coding system to describe the content of the files.

Document study can provide a well-rounded view of the organization or program that the researcher is studying. The aforementioned methods of qualitative research—observation, participant observation, ethnomethodology, and document study—all enhance the researcher's ability to gain an understanding of the events and activities of a particular program or an organization. A good qualitative study would most likely put to use most of these methods, beause they will prove to be beneficial. The next part of this chapter will discuss how, using various techniques, Steven may actually collect the necessary data concerning the efficacy of the hospital's Wellness Center.

Techniques of Collecting Qualitative Data_____

There are several techniques to use when you are collecting qualitative data. These include: fieldnotes, subjects' written words, photography, and official statistics. The following sections briefly describe these techniques.

Fieldnotes

Fieldnotes are the most important part of collecting data in qualitative research. They are used in *all* methodologies: observation, participant observation, ethnomethodology, and document study. Fieldnotes contain everything and anything that the observer feels is worth noting. Any information that will enable the observer to gain a better understanding of the program must be written down immediately. If one leaves observation to memory, one is leaving much to chance.

Descriptions are the basics of fieldnotes. Basic information as to who was there, what was happening, and where the observation took place should be included in the notes. In addition, a description of the event, what took place, and the interactions between people should be recorded. Fieldnotes also should contain quotations of what people said. In addition, the notes should reflect the observer's feelings and reactions to the experience, as well as the meaning and significance of the event. Furthermore, the notes should contain the observer's insights, interpretations, beginning anaylses, and working hypotheses regarding the situation (Patton, 1980). These comments are noted by using observer's comments (OC).

Lofland (1971) has some suggestions for those writing fieldnotes:

1. Record the notes as quickly as possible after the observation.
2. Discipline yourself to write notes quickly and reconcile yourself to the fact that recording of the notes can be expected to take as long as is spent in actual observation.
3. Dictating rather than writing is acceptable, but writing may have the advantage of stimulating thought.
4. Typing fieldnotes is preferable to handwriting because it is faster and easier to read.
5. Make at least two copies of the fieldnotes. One original copy is retained for reference, and other copies can be used as rough drafts to be cut up, rewritten, and reorganized.

Content of Fieldnotes. Two types of materials are included in the fieldnotes: descriptive and reflective (of the observer's ideas and concerns). The *descriptive* part of the fieldnotes include the following (Bogdan and Biklin, 1982):

1. *Portrait of the subjects.* Include their physical appearance, dress, style of talking, and mannerisms.
2. *Reconstruction of dialogue.* The conversations between subjects, as well as what subjects might say to the observer are recorded. Use direct quotations, especially when they are unique to the setting.
3. *Description of the physical setting.* The observer should draw this with spacing furniture arrangements and where people are sitting. Note blackboard writing, what may be on bulletin boards.
4. *Accounts of particular events.* Note who was involved in the event, in what manner and the nature of the action.
5. *Depiction of activities.* Include detailed descriptions of behaviors.

As we discussed previously, the reflective part of the fieldnotes should be recorded as well as descriptions of events, activities, and behaviors. These notes are designated by "OC." Bogdan and Biklin (1982) offer the following comments in relation to the reflective part of the fieldnotes:

1. *Reflections on analysis.* Speculate about what the observer is learning, emerging themes, patterns and adding ideas.
2. *Reflections on method.* Include comments on the study design, accomplishments, plan what to do next.
3. *Reflection on observer's frame of mind.* Observers may have preconceived notions about the subjects. When these are changed or reinforced, they should be noted.
4. *Points of clarification.* Make additional notes to add or clarify a previous notation.

Fieldnote Form. Observers should adopt a standard form for their fieldnotes. They should include at least the following:

1. *A title page:* Date, time, place of observation as well as when the notes were recorded. Title of the event may also be included here.
2. *Diagram of setting:* As mentioned previously, a diagram of the activity or event should be included at the beginning of the notes.

3. *Wide margins*: Necessary because the observer or someone else might want to make appropriate comments.
4. *Paragraphs*: Should be formed very frequently to correspond with each new person speaking, or every change in the setting occurs.
5. *Quotation marks*: Should be used as often as possible. Even though the observer may not quote exactly, if it's very close to an exact replica, enter the quotation marks.

Fieldnote Techniques. There are various ways to record field-notes, but the observer must find the technique that is most comfort-able for herself or himself. Most people use pen and paper on site and then use a typewriter, dictating machine, or word processor to rewrite and embellish the notes later on. Another on-site method that is used is a tape recorder. If an observer wishes to use a tape recorder or other equipment (silent typewriter, portable word processor, etc.), then the observer must make sure that the equipment does not inter-fere with the natural workings of the group of subjects within the group. In other words, the equipment must be unobstrusive.

Another mechanism is available for recording fieldnotes called the Stenomask. It is a sound-shielded microphone attached to a portable tape recorder that is worn on a shoulder strap (Patton, 1980). The handle contains the microphone switch and allows the observer to talk into the recorder during an activity without the subjects being able to hear the dictation. Of course, this can be distracting to the group, and therefore should be used with caution.

Fieldnotes provide the basis from which qualitative data is re-corded and then analyzed. It is a tedious task that requires patience and long hours after the observations have been completed. It is nec-essary that notes be organized and clear so that all involved in the project may benefit from the effort.

Personal Documents

Much information can be obtained from studying people's personal effects. This may include their clothing and the furnishings in their home or office. What may be of greater significance to qualitative re-searchers is examination of documents that indicate how people lead their everyday lives. These include calendars, diaries, letters (per-sonal and business), autobiographies, scrapbooks, books read, and po-etry written. Thomas (1923) was an early proponent of utilizing per-sonal documents to make inferences about people's lives. He believed that autobiographies, letters, etc., were an important source of data because they were capable of presenting life as a connected whole and of showing the·interplay of influences on individuals. Thomas' research focused upon immigrants at the beginning, and later analyzed their diaries, letters, and other personal documents. From these analyses he was able to depict some central themes of these people: individualization, demoralization, and deregulation.

The use of personal documents usually does not allow for a large sample size, although the Thomas study, as just described, must be considered an exception. This enables the qualitative researcher to make a generalization about a subject, and then use excerpts from personal documents to illustrate them. In our case study, if Steven believed that the coordinator of the Wellness Center was autocratic, he would search the personal documents of that coordinator to look for a sense of autocratic personality.

How to Obtain Personal Documents. Obtaining personal documents such as diaries, autobiographies, and letters is not an easy task. One way that was used by Thomas and Znaniecki (1927) was to advertise in a newspaper to find the appropriate materials. Some people might be willing to share diaries and letters. Organizational files would be very helpful in our case study. These personnel files should contain references to people in the organization, indicating how people define themselves in their respective positions.

The written words of subjects can be of invaluable assistance to the qualitative researcher who is attempting to gain an understanding of how and why a system works. Although obtaining these personnel documents may be difficult, it allows the investigator to exercise her or his imagination.

Photography

Qualitative research can be greatly enhanced by photography. The following section is taken from Bogdan and Biklin's (1982) excellent work on the benefits of photography in relationship to collecting qualitative data.

Social scientists have used photography since the nineteenth century to depict social documentaries on how people live (Thomson and Smith, 1877; Riis, 1890; Stott, 1973). The adage: "a picture is worth a thousand words" has been adhered to by recent social scientists utilizing photography (Becker, 1978 and Wagner, 1979). The advent of photography has enabled researchers to study aspects of life that cannot be researched through other approaches: images are more telling than words. There are two categories of photographs that qualitative researchers may use: found photographs (pictures others have taken) and those that the researcher has produced.

Found Photographs. Many organizations have archives of photographs depicting ground-breaking ceremonies, outings, and other events germane to that organization. Newspapers usually have photo libraries as well as book libraries. In addition, county offices will have aerial photographs of land.

Photographs can reveal factual information that may shed light onto organizational structure. Parties may have been photographed, depicting who was there, seating arrangement, mistress or master of ceremonies, and the general ambiance of the party.

A photograph is like all other forms of qualitative data: to use it, the investigator should place it within the proper context and understand what it is capable of telling. Photographs can represent the photographer's point of view, a superior's orders, or even the subject's demands. This can present valuable information in that when photographs are studied, clues are ascertained as to what people value by the images they prefer. These add to the evidence that the other qualitative techniques have enabled the investigator to gather.

Photographs may present anomalies, images that do not fit the theoretical constructs that the investigator has been forming. This can enhance the researcher's analysis and insights and even alter preconceived notions about the subject. Researchers may utilize photographs to discern how people define their world: what people take for granted, what they assume is unquestionable, and organizational assumptions.

Researcher-produced Photographs. Investigators can collect factual information by using photographs to depict utilization of facilities. The technique requires the use of hidden cameras, but it is a technique that is acceptable. Participant observers take photographs in the course of the study, so they can more accurately recall events, activities, people, what they were wearing, seating arrangements, etc.

There are the usual advantages, disadvantages, and cautions when researchers are about to use photography as a data collection technique. In certain instances, picture taking may inhibit the establishment of rapport (the researcher appears to be an outsider), and there are other occasions when it is advantageous to rapport (other cultures may feel a sense of pride at being asked to pose—this serves as a discussion tool). We recommend that you do not take pictures at the very beginning of a project, but wait to establish rapport and you might even wait until subjects start snapping—thus giving you a chance to join in the photography session.

Photographs, whether found or taken by the investigator can serve as a tool for enabling the researcher to better understand the values and inner workings of the organization or program being studied. Photography can be a researcher's tool as well as a cultural product and a product of culture.

Official Statistics

Quantitative data that have already been collected can serve to help qualitative researchers in that the data may suggest trends (e.g., the Wellness Center has had five coordinators in four years) and also provides descriptive statistics (e.g., age, sex, race, socioeconomic status of Wellness Center staff). In addition, hypotheses may be broadened and/or delineated dependent upon what the official statistics delineate.

Qualitative researchers tend to be critical of quantitative statistics because they are asking questions that cannot easily be answered with numbers. "Rather than relying upon quantitative data as an avenue to accurately describe reality, qualitative researchers are concerned with how enumeration is used by subjects in constructing reality. They are interested in how statistics reveal subjects' commonsense understandings" (Bogdan and Biklin, 1982, p. 113).

Types of Official Statistics. There are several different kinds of official documents that provide statistics for researchers. They include census documents; health statistics provided by insurance companies; statistics provided by voluntary health organizations; and personality inventories provided hospitals, schools, clinics, personnel departments and social service agenices. For the purpose of brevity, we will discuss census documents and other directories that can provide data for the qualitative research.

Census surveys are conducted every ten years in the United States. They supposedly enumerate every person living in the country. (The first modern United States census was taken in 1790.) These massive undertakings are computed so that apportionment of government representatives remains accurate and truly representative, and to provide data for a wide variety of research interests. The census asks general questions regarding age, sex, socioeconomic standing, number of people living in a household, etc. It should be noted here that not all households are asked the same questions, because the census, at times, uses sampling to gather some of their information.

Directories are another source of vital statistics that can be valuable to the investigator. Telephone directories and city directories usually have information that is needed and useful when conducting a study. City directories usually list the name, address, and occupation of a person, but these are not representative of the population, because people have to agree to be listed in the directory. There are also professional directories, such as the *American Association of Sex Educators, Counselors, and Therapists Directory*. These are compendiums that may include brief biographies, which will be helpful to the researcher.

Occupational directories, such as the *Dental Association Directory*, can provide information that allows construction of indexes to compare cities. This has been especially useful in depicting utilization and placement of physicians. There are also a vast array of *Who's Who* directories, many with regional and professional classifications. In addition, county and state governments keep records that provide information concerning financial transactions. These include automobile registration, pet ownership, collected fines, and residential taxes. Abrahamson (1980) put these kinds of records to use by analyzing a sample of winners of a state lottery and the effect winning tickets had on these people's lives.

Problems in Using Statistical Records. There are several problems inherent in amassing voluminous amounts of data that the qualitative researcher should take into account:

1. *Data collection methods.* Reporting of deaths in a region is created locally and may not mean the same thing to the entire universe. Undercounting is another problem inherent in data collection.
2. *Ambiguous terms.* Categorical definitions that are used by governmental agencies are not always used in the same way as other nongovernmental agencies. Boundaries of districts and regions may change as the population changes. In addition, technical definitions (the United States census defines an urban area as a town of at least 2,500 people) do not always coincide with common useage of these terms.
3. *Bias.* Lists for directories are not assembled for research purposes, and are not usually completed with the care of accuracy necessary for a research project. Professional directories might be incomplete because a fee was charged for inclusion, which causes a bias in the reporting.

Official records and statistics can be an invaluable aid for the qualitative researcher. Easy access to a great deal of information may enable an investigator to get a good picture or sense of an organization or of the place where that organization exists. As with any compilation of large amounts of data, cautions must be observed in the use of these compendiums. While we have reported on only a few

types of census-like compilations, the United States government gar-
ners many special subtopic reports from the census and other mass
surveys.*

Analyzing Qualitative Data _____

After collecting reams of data, most of it containing voluminous
words, the researcher asks, How can I make sense of this mess? What
needs to be done then is make coherent sense out of these many pages
of words. The qualitative investigator will look in the data for themes
and patterns that might help construct and/or support hypotheses.

Recognizing Themes and Constructing Hypotheses

Bogdan and Taylor (1975) offer the following suggestions for constructing hypotheses and recognizing themes:

1. *Read the notes carefully*: Read everything, even minor incidents
   very carefully. Write margin notes recording possible patterns
   and trends leading to themes and hypotheses.
2. *Code important conversation topics*: Code those conversation topics that keep recurring. (Coding will be discusses later in this
   chapter).
3. *Construct typologies*: These are classification schemes and can be
   useful when formulating hypotheses. This is accomplished by de-
   noting how your subjects classify people and behavior and the
   differences between and among subjects that allow them be to
   be classified.
4. *Read the relevant literature*: Consult the professional literature
   to compare the literature findings with what is beginning to appear in the data. In addition, utilize the concepts, models, and
   paradigms of others.

It is very important that the researcher be able to determine common threads and themes through analysis of the data. This process
then leads to hypothesis formulation and support for those hypotheses. To accomplish what at times seems like an insurmountable
task, the investigator must develop a coding mechanism by which to
organize and assemble the data.

---

*Information about these reports may be obtained from the Department of Com-
merce, Bureau of Commerce, Washington, D.C.

TABLE 6.3 Section of a Coding Sheet

Administrative Hierarchy	AH (DUR) (END)	2.1
AH: Style	AH - ST	2.1.2
AH: Role	AH - RO	2.1.3
AH: Demeanor	AH - DR	2.1.4
AH: Subject use	AH - SU	2.1.5

Coding the Data. Once the notes have been reread, typologies constructed, and literature reviewed, an elaborate coding system must be devised. This system will serve to organize and assemble the mounds of data that have been collected. When the review of the notes commences, the investigator makes notes and begins to code as described in the previous section. There are several type codes that include (1) descriptive and (2) explanatory. *Descriptive* codes do not require interpretation but indicate a class of phenomenon in the notes. As as example, in our case study, Steven would note in the margin *PERS* to denote "personality" wherever appropriate. This will enable him to quickly note where all relevant personality notes appear in the text.

Explanatory codes indicate where patterns or themes have emerged. Steven could use pattern or theme (PAT or TH) to indicate an administrative style that he has seen as evident in the data. Codes, no matter which kind, tend to pull the data together and make sense of the fieldnotes.

Creating the Code. There are several methods to help the investigator create the code. Miles and Huberman (1984) suggest devising *start lists* previous to doing fieldwork. The list develops from the conceptual framework, list of research questions, problem areas, and key variables that were determined at the beginning of the study. Usually, a master code is developed. For example, in our case study, *ADM ST* might mean "administrative style," and *AUT* ("autocratic") might be a subcode under *ADM ST*. This list may have as many as 90 codes and should be kept on one piece of paper for easy reference. Table 6.3 is an example of a section of a code sheet. The first column denotes a descriptive level for the general categories, the second column indicates the code, and the third column keys the code to the research question from which it derives.

Bogdan and Biklen (1982) suggest another mechanism for determining coding subsections:

1. *Setting/context*: information on surroundings;
2. *Definition of the situation*: how people define the setting;

3. *Perspectives of subjects*: ways of thinking, orientation;
4. *Ways of thinking about people and objects*: subject's understanding of each other, of outsiders, and objects that are included in their world;
5. *Process*: categorizing events, changes over time, and flow.
6. *Activities*: regularly occuring kinds of behavior;
7. *Events*: specific activities;
8. *Strategies*: tactics, methods, techniques, plays and other conscious ways subjects accomplish things;
9. *Relationship and social structure*: behaviors not officially defined by the organization;
10. *Methods*: material pertinent to research-related issues.

These coding patterns can enable the investigator to think about the categories for which codes are to be developed. This method has its advantages and disadvantages over the start list. However, it is recommended that the researcher find the coding method that is easiest to work with and will provide the most complete listing of codes to organize the data.

Data Organization. Now that the investigator has developed a coding system, the mechanics of actually going through the data and organizing it becomes the main task. The first step is to number all the pages of data numerically so that the location of sources is easily accessible. Numbering the data in chronological order of their occurrence is a good way to sequence the data. A second step is to begin coding the data using any of the methods previously discussed, or even one that the investigator may construct on his or her own. After the coding categories have been designed, the third step is to go through the data and mark each paragraph (or sentence) using the appropriate coding category. The fourth step is to sort the data.

Sorting the Data. Bogdan and Biklin (1982, p. 166) have several recommendations for sorting data and encouraging researchers to utilize the method that is best suited to them and the data.

1. *Cut-Up and Put-in Folders*: Utilizing manila folders for each coding category, the fieldnotes are cut up and file into the appropriate folder. Go through all the notes, placing a number next to each coded unit of data which corresponds to the number of the page it is on. It is less confusing if you circle that number or in some way mark it so you do not confuse the coding numbers with the page numbers. The page numbers enable you to refer back to the master copy if confusion arises concerning the original context.
2. *The File Card*: To utilize this method, the paper on which the origi-

nal fieldnotes were typed have to have each line on the page numbered consecutively. In addition, a stack of notecards with the code number and corresponding phrase and word written on the top. Record on each card on what page in the data and on what lines on that page, data relevant to the category can be found.

3. *Information Retrieval Cards*: These cards are available at most college book stores and two brands are McBee and Indecks. Each card contains a large space where data is typed according to each paragraph or sentence. Each card comes with the same numbered holes around the rim. After each paragraph or sentence is typed on the card, cut off all those holes except those that correspond to the number of the coding categories to which the sentence or paragraph pertains. After all data has been transferred to the cards, they are placed in the box that originally held them. The box is the same dimensions as the face of the card and thus holes with the same numbers line up perfectly. A long, needle-like instrument, that comes with the cards and box, is used to pull cards out of the box. Line up the cards and pass the needle through the hole that corresponds to the category and pull on the handle. The cards not wanted fall off and the others are available for study.

Each method of sorting the data has advantages and disadvantages that should be obvious. A researcher may try all three of the methods discussed, at different times, to find out which is most appropriate.

The analysis of qualitative data can be a taxing and tedious task, and at the same time the most rewarding. Hypothesis construction and the recognition of themes are the primary reasons for analyzing the data. Coding of the data enables the researcher to organize the substantial amount of data collected. Once the data have been coded, it then has to be sorted, so that themes, patterns, categories and trends can become evident.

Summary

Qualitative research is an approach utilized to collect data and report the findings. It differs from quantifiable methods by having as its main goals the description of multiple realities, development of sensitizing concepts, and understanding of a particular program, organization, or setting. The designs utilized are generally flexible and they evolve as the study progresses. Data come in different forms; fieldnotes, official statistics, personal documents, photographs, and subjects' written words. Methodologies used are observation, participant observation, ethnomethodology, and document study. The samples utilized are usually nonrepresentative and small. Analysis of the data is very time consuming because it is done by hand, without the aid of mechanical devices (computers).

There are several problems in utilizing qualitative research methodologies. These include (1) the data reduction is difficult, (2) large populations are not easily studied using this approach, (3) the procedures are not stabilized, (4) reliability is subjective, and (5) the method is very time consuming. However, qualitative approaches are very useful when a researcher wants to study naturalistic settings, such as schools, hospitals, organizations, and the like. In our case study, the consortium, *Researchers in Health*, decided quite appropriately to utilize qualitative methods to study the efficacy of the hospital's Wellness Center.

Suggested Activities

1. Devise a list of topics that could be studied utilizing the qualitative approach.
2. Conduct a literature search on one of the topics in your answer to Activity 1 and attempt to set up a coding system for those citations.
3. Describe, in detail, a situation wherein you could be a participant observer. What are the steps you would take from the conception of the idea to the completion of the data analysis.

Bibliography

Abrahamson, M. (1980) Sudden wealth, gratification and attainment, *American Sociological Review* 45:49–57.

Bailey, K. (1982) *Methods of Social Research,* New York: Free Press.

Becker, H. (1978) Do photographs tell the truth? *After Image* 5:9–13.

Bickman, L. (1976) Observational methods. In Selitz, C., Wrightsman, L., and Cook, S. (eds.), *Research Methods in Social Relations,* New York: Holt, Rinehart and Winston.

Bogdan, R. and Biklin, S. (1982) *Qualitative Research for Education,* Boston: Allyn and Bacon.

Bogdan, R. and Taylor, S. (1975) *Introduction to Qualitative Research Methods,* New York: Wiley.

Borg, W. and Gall, M. (1983) *Educational Research,* New York: Longman.

Denzin, N. (1978) The logic of naturalistic inquiry. In Denzin, N. (ed.), *Sociological Methods: A Sourcebook,* New York: Appleton-Century-Crofts.

Glaser, B. and Strauss, A. (1967) *The Discovery of Grounded Theory: Strategies for Qualitative Research,* Chicago: Aldine Press.

Hartman, D. and Wood, D. (1982) Observational methods. In Bellack, A., Hersen, M. and Kazdin, A. (eds.), *International Handbook of Behavior Modification,* New York: Plenum.

Haynes, S. (1978) *Principles of Behavioral Assessment,* New York: Gardner.

Junker, B. (1960) *Field Work: An Introduction to the Social Sciences,* Chicago: University of Chicago Press.

Lofland, J. (1971) *Analyzing Social Settings,* Beverly Hills: Sage Publications.

Patton, M. (1980) *Qualitative Evaluation Methods,* Beverly Hills: Sage Publications.

Riis, J. (1980) *How the Other Half Lives,* New York: C. Scribner's Sons.

Stott, W. (1973) *Documentary Expression and Thirties America,* New York: Oxford University Press.

Thomas, W. (1923) *The Unadjusted Girl,* New York: Harper and Row.

Thomas, W. and Znaniecki, F. (1927) *The Polish Peasant in Europe and America,* New York: Alfred A. Knopf.

Thomson, J. and Smith, A. (1877) *Street Life in London,* London: Sampson Low, Murston, Searle and Rurington.

Turner, R. (1974) *Ethnomethodology,* Baltimore: Penguin.

Wagner, J. (Ed.) (1979) *Image of Information,* Beverly Hills: Sage.

Walizer, M. and Wienir, P. (1978) *Research Methods and Analysis,* New York: Harper and Row.

Wieder, D. (1974) Telling the code. In Turner, R. (ed.), *Ethnomethodology,* Baltimore: Penguin.

Wildman, B. and Erickson, M. (1977) Methodological problems in behavioral observation. In Cone, J. and Hawkins, R. (eds.), *Behavioral Assessment: New Directions in Clinical Psychology,* New York: Burnner/Mazel.

CHAPTER 7

Evaluation Research

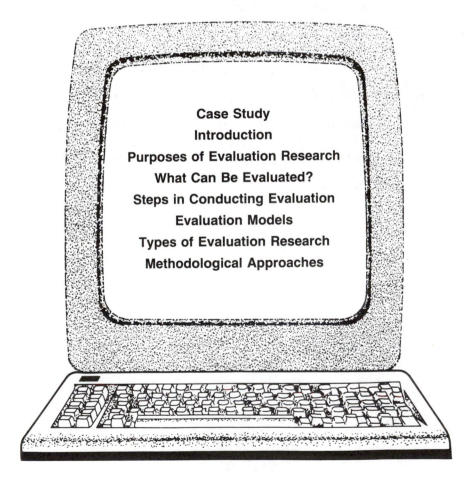

Case Study

The Homewood School district has had a health science program for the gifted in their high school for 2 years. A new superintendent is searching for cost-cutting measures and has asked for an evaluation of the health science program. The Homewood Board of Education agreed to the superintendent's request, and sought proposals from agencies, universities, and other groups. They eventually awarded the evaluation contract to the Department of Health Behavior of the University of Anset. The department's evaluation team was headed by Sarah, a professor with varied experiences in education evaluations.

Introduction

Evaluation research is yet another type of research that health scientists utilize for a myriad of reasons. Usually in evaluation research, scientists seek to determine if a program's goals and objectives have been achieved. Evaluation research has been defined as

1. The application of scientific principles, methods, theories to identify, describe, conceptualize, measure, predict, change, and control those factors or variables important to the development of effective human service delivery systems (Struening and Brewer, 1983, p. 211);
2. The systematic application of social research procedures in assessing the conceptualization and design, implementation, and utility of social intervention programs (Rossi and Freeman, 1982, p. 20);
3. A judgment regarding the degree to which desired outcomes of a program have been achieved or can be achieved (Caro, 1977, p. 3).

These definitions give us a sense of what evaluation research is about: *a process of determining the effectiveness of a program.* We emphasize *process* as opposed to product. Once the process is completed, decisions are then made about the program being evaluated. For instance, in our case study Sarah may provide information about the health science program concerning its length, duration, and cost benefits, which can provide valuable information to the superintendent of schools. The superintendent may decide to improve the program's weaknesses, terminate the gifted program, or add more funds to the program.

Purposes of Evaluation Research_____

As we have stated, there may be many and varied reasons for a research evaluation project to be undertaken. We can look at the purposes for evaluation research from different vantage points: (1) the program evaluator, (2) the administrator, (3) the consumer or public, and (4) the organization, or in our case study, the school district.

Sarah's team of evaluators from Anset University may wish to contribute to the knowledge and the discipline of evaluation research. In addition, the team may view this as a means for advancement in their area of expertise. An altruistic purpose for Sarah's group may be a belief they can help the discipline of health science by conducting this evaluation.

The superintendent (administrator) of the Homewood school district may have other purposes for the evaluation, including (1) gaining control over the program, (2) bringing attention to the health science curriculum for the gifted, or (3) bringing the program to the attention of the Board of Education (Shortell, 1978).

The Homewood Board of Education may want to be able to justify the money it spends on the program. Additionally, they may want to determine that the program is indeed worth the expenditures, and plan for its expansion. The citizens who pay taxes in the Homewood school district may want the evaluation to ensure their tax dollars are well spent. Furthermore, special interest groups, such as health science teachers, may have gotten community support for the program, and therefore need to prove its worthiness.

Chelimsky (1978) describes the following purposes for evaluation research; e.g., management and administrative reasons, assessment of the appropriateness of program changes, identification of ways to improve the delivery of interventions, or accountability to funding agencies. In addition, evaluations may be completed for planning and policy purposes, to test innovative ideas, to decide if programs should be curtailed or expanded, or to support one program in lieu of another.

Whatever the purpose that underlies evaluation research, those involved in the process must be sure to accomplish the task by utilizing appropriate methodologies, processes, and analyses. In other words, the research project must be able to be replicated by other evaluation groups.

What Can Be Evaluated?_____

Almost anything can be evaluated, and it usually is in some manner or form. Listed here are some examples of things that have been or could be evaluated:

- Curricula
- Drugs
- Health
- Data bases (for computers)
- Life-styles (singlehood, married, etc.)
- Software programs
- Teaching styles
- Workshops
- Staff and personnel
- Management systems
- Organizations
- Needs-assessment strategies

Even evaluation models and schemes can be evaluated, and some have been so scrutinized. The next section will discuss some evaluation models and attempt to critique them.

Steps in Conducting Evaluation_____

Once Sarah was appointed to conduct an evaluation of the health science program for gifted students, she had to determine a plan of action. We will use this portion of the chapter to describe step-by-step the process of setting up an evaluation of a program. Two major sources were utilized in the writing of this chapter: Rutman's *Evaluation Research Methods* (1984) and Shortell and Richardson's *Health Program Evaluation* (1978). Figure 7.1 depicts the process of evaluation. From the inception of the project to the final report, there must be interaction between the evaluator(s) and the person or group for whom the evaluation will effect: the decision makers. Although we have depicted the steps as separate entities, in reality some may be working at the same time. In other words, they are interactive.

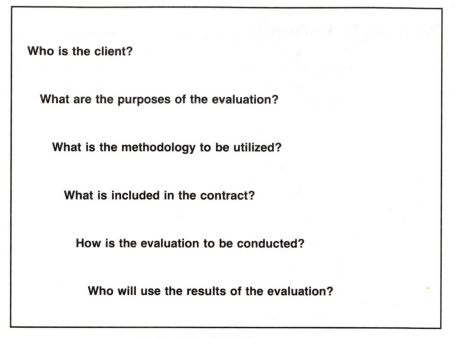

Who is the client?

What are the purposes of the evaluation?

What is the methodology to be utilized?

What is included in the contract?

How is the evaluation to be conducted?

Who will use the results of the evaluation?

Figure 7.1 Evaluation process.

Who Is the Client?

In our case study, Sarah has been hired by the seven-member Homewood Board of Education. Are all these people the primary client? Sarah must determine the power structure of the Board of Education and those persons who will be instrumental in making decisions with the added information provided by Sarah's evaluation group. She might interview the Board members, or ask the superintendent of schools or informed teachers and parents, to ascertain who the decision makers are in Homewood. This can become a cumbersome and complicated process, but one that is very worthwhile. If it does appear that the entire seven-member Board is the actual client, then the evaluation group must take this into consideration at every phase of the evaluation process.

What Are the Purposes of the Evaluation?

Sarah should determine the exact purposes for which the evaluation is to be undertaken. If possible, she should ascertain the covert as well as the overt reasons for conducting the study. Earlier in this chapter we discussed the major purposes of conducting an evaluation and refer you to that section for a brief review. In our case study, let us assume that the members of the Board of Education and the superintendent of schools disagree about their evaluation plans. They want to know if the health science program is cost-effective and if they should they keep it in lieu of other programs. Knowing the main purpose of the evaluation, the team will have the necessary insight as to what specific methodologies and techniques should be utilized to conduct the study.

What Is the Methodology to Be Utilized?

When determining the methodology to be used, the evaluator must be familiar with the purposes of the evaluation as we have discussed. We will discuss the various methods to use later on in this chapter. However, briefly, they are experimental and quasiexperimental, correlation, surveys, personnel assessment, expert judgment, and testimony. Once the methodology is determined it is then necessary to consider the feasibility of implementing that method. The following characteristics must be considered when determining the feasibility of the method: available funds, time schedule, availability of data, and the legal, political, ethical and administrative constraints that usually occur when conducting an evaluation.

What Is Included in the Contract?

When the Homewood Board of Education sent their request for proposals (RFPs) across the nation, they specified funding levels time frames, purpose of the study, and other information. Once they contracted with the University of Anset to perform the evaluation, Sarah had to develop a more inclusive contract between the Board of Education and the evaluation team. The contract that they will develop should determine responsibilities of the evaluation team and should include

1. A line-item budget.
2. The entire scope of the evaluation.
3. Details concerning the research design and data collection procedures.
4. Levels of cooperation of the Board of Education.
5. Controls to ensure adherence to the evaluation plan.
6. Determinations as to the publicity of the final report.

How Is the Evaluation to Be Conducted?

As Rutman (1984) has so adequately explained, conducting a program evaluation entails three tasks: (1) measurement, (2) use of a particular research design; and (3) analysis of the data. Each of these areas must receive the necessary attention so that the evaluation process will produce usable results.

Measurement. The evaluation team decides on the type and amount of information that is necessary to answer the questions posed at the beginning of the study. Evaluations may obtain four categories of information: (1) program, (2) objectives and effects, (3) antecedent conditions, and (4) intervening conditions.

Program information is collected on how the program is run. Information on the process of the program can determine how the program was implemented; if it was implemented as designed; how the implementation process affected the results of the program; and whether the program was cost-effective.

Objectives and effects are the central point of evaluating programs. The extent to which a program reaches its goals and objectives can be measured in addition to the effects it has produced.

Antecedent conditions refer to the context within which the program operates, the characteristics of the client, and the background of program personnel. Antecedent information helps to interpret the findings, which enables the evaluator to determine what is most beneficial to the client, what type of personnel benefit the program best, and whether the context in which the program operates is best so that the program's objectives are met.

Intervening conditions are occurrences not planned during the program's activities. For example, in our case study, the head teacher of the gifted health science program may leave that program, thus causing a disruption to the organization. Measurement of the impact of these intervening conditions can enable the evaluators to determine which factors help the program reach its objectives.

Another consideration is to determine the methods by which the information will be collected. Data may be collected through questionnaires, interviews, observations, program documents, and official statistics. These methodologies have been discussed in detail elsewhere in this text; therefore we will not discuss them here. Validity and reliability of instruments become important considerations. *Validity* refers to the extent to which a procedure measures what it is supposed to measure. There are several types of validity:

1. *Face validity:* On the face of it, it is obvious that the instrument measures what it purports to measure.
2. *Content validity:* The instrument will produce a reasonable sample of all possible responses, attitudes, and behaviors.
3. *Construct validity:* The extent to which scores on a proposed instrument permit inferences about underlying traits, attitudes, and behaviors.
4. *Predictive validity:* The instrument can accurately predict a future occurrence.

Reliability refers to the stability of the instrument. In other words, the same results will be consistently reproduced in subsequent administrations of the instrument. To avoid unreliability, evaluators must ensure that instruments are properly worded and administered in a consistent manner.

Research Design. Evaluation research treats research design as other types of research do; very importantly. A good research design enables researchers to ask the pertinent questions and determine the answers to those questions. In this regard Cook and Campbell (1976) state the importance of *attribution* and *generalizability* in the choice of a research design. Designs concerned about attribution (the program has produced the measured results) use several measurements, pretests and posttests, control groups, and random assignment to groups.

To ensure generalizability, the sample must be comprised of people who are representative of the population. In addition, the experiment should be replicable by other investigators. These issues have been discussed, in detail, in Chapter 4.

Data Analysis. The final task in conducting a program evaluation is concerned with analyzing the data. For inferences to be made about the program, the correct statistical techniques need to be employed. Statistical methodologies are usually determined by the hypotheses (questions asked) and the research design. Conclusions and recommendations about the program are based on the data analysis; therefore, inappropriate techniques can lead to false or erroneous statements concerning the program.

Who Will Use the Results of the Study?

At the beginning of this section we described the importance of determining who the decision maker(s) will be or who the client is. The decision makers will utilize the study's findings for a multiplicity of reasons. Therefore, it is imperative that the decision makers are involved in the evaluation so they will feel a commitment to utilize the findings of the project. It is anticipated that if the many groups that have a stake in the program (in our case study, members of the Board of Education, the superintendent of schools, teachers and students of the gifted health science program, the parents, and administrators) receive information about the process and outcome of the program, then more appropriate decisions can be made concerning the program.

The steps in conducting an evaluation have been discussed with the idea that they are interactive with each other. The evaluation team should determine, in advance, a well-conceived plan of action to carry out the evaluation. Communication with pertinent personnel is of utmost importance when these procedures are drawn up. Planning is imperative, no matter the type of evaluation research.

Evaluation Models

Evaluation research dates as far back as 2200 BC when the Chinese emperor insisted that all of his public officials pass proficiency tests. Would that be possible today? Testing seems to have stimulated the evaluation movement in that Alfred Binet was asked by France's public instruction minister to devise a test to screen for mentally deficient children in the classrooms. This test became the basis for the IQ tests currently in use in the United States. With time, evaluation and measurement took a firm foothold in science. Individual differences were characterized by evaluation studies, and toward the middle of the twentieth century evaluation strategies began to concentrate on groups, organizations, and curricula.

The following discussion depicts several evaluation models and explains advantages and disadvantages of each model.

The Behavioral Objectives Model

The behavioral objectives model, advanced by Tyler (1950), Mayer (1961), Bloom (1956), Suchman (1967), and Popham (1975) starts with a program's goals and collects data to determine if these goals were met. The program's success is measured by the outcomes of the program in relationship to the stated goals. The field of education has had much to do with this model because Tyler defined educational goals in terms of student behaviors. These student behaviors were then assessed to determine if modifications or refinements in the curriculum were needed. The *behavioral objective* approach, as proposed by Tyler (1949), included the following:

1. Derive a pool of candidates by examining learner studies and by soliciting suggestions from content specialists.
2. Pass the pool of candidates through a series of three screens: philosophical, psychological, and experimential.
3. The candidates who survive the screening process are put into a matrix whose rows depict the content areas and whose columns depict the student behaviors expected in relation to the content areas. The individual matrix cells represent individual objectives.
4. Identify situations where students can express the behaviors mentioned in the objectives.
5. Develop instruments that can test each objective.
6. Apply the instrument, in pretest and posttest paradigms, so that behavioral changes assigned to the curriculum can be measured.
7. Examine the results to determine the strengths and weaknesses of the curriculum.
8. Develop the hypotheses that account for the pattern of the strengths and weaknesses.
9. Modify the curriculum and begin the process once more.

Tyler's approach led the way for program and organizational evaluations, in addition to the individual evaluations that were being conducted before Tyler came upon the evaluation research scene. In the health sciences, this model has been used in the area of dental health by the American Dental Association. More recently, his model has taken on additional refinements in the form of criterion-referenced tests, where objectives are first set, and then the test is based on that set of objectives. In addition, competency testing has become popular in many states. Here, objectives that are the basis for a test serve as the minimal objectives for a particular grade level. In other words, students must pass the competency test to go on to the next level or grade.

Education is not the only field in which the behavioral objective model has been used. Businesses and other organizations have utilized the management-by-objectives (MBO) approach whereby personnel determine their own objectives, and then are evaluated on the basis of how well they met those predetermined objectives. In the public health arena, Suchman (1967) wrote a book using a goal-based approach in which he identified goal activity and put it into operation. The reader was to assess the effect of the goal operation, form a value about that goal, set the goals and objectives, and finally measure those goals. Suchman said, "The most identifying feature of evaluative research is the presence of some goal or objective whose measure of attainment constitutes the main focus of the research problem" (p. 37).

This model has its *weaknesses* in that questions usually arise concerning who sets the goals and objectives, whose interests they represent, whether the goals really are a complete set of the desired behaviors, how these goals can be measured, and whether important outcomes are reflected by the respecification of objectives (House, 1980). These questions or inherent problems of this approach must be carefully thought out before one embarks upon a behavioral objectives model toward evaluation.

A *strength* of the behavioral objectives approach is that it provides validity. As we discussed in Chapter 4, *validity* means that the program, or instrument, does what it claims to do. By applying this model, the objectives should be directly linked to the measured outcomes of the program. A second advantage is that this model enables the evaluator to have a set plan of action by predetermined steps to be taken.

The Systems Analysis Model

The systems analysis model had its roots in the Department of Defense and in what was then called the Department of Health, Education, and Welfare, now called the Department of Health and Human Services. In this model, a few output measures are determined and then the differences in programs or their policies are measured as they vary against the predetermined indicators.

When the U.S. government began utilizing this model it was to evaluate Title I, a program that provides funds for disadvantaged youth. There were 30,000 projects to be evaluated by using test scores as the measure of success. The results were to be reported in a normal curve and aggregated at the state and national levels. These evaluations led the government to act concerning certain programs. What developed was a systems approach to a cost-benefit analysis that would compare programs.

Cost-benefit analysis is a distinct and difficult methodology to undertake, even for a governmental organization. The goals are predetermined and then the outcomes of the program are measured. Once the outcomes have been measured, the programs then must be compared on a cost level, which should determine the best outcome for the least amount of money.

Systems analysis can be used for evaluating management and planning procedures, policy structure, and budget procedures. Rossi et al. (1979) ask the following questions when preparing an evaluation:

1. Does the intervention reach the target population?
2. Is the intervention implemented in the manner specified?
3. Is the intervention effective?
4. How much does the intervention cost?
5. What are the intervention's costs relative to its effectiveness?

These types of evaluations must be very objective and leave no room for the commonsense–type of qualitative research discussed previously. It is obvious that the social scientist's method of conducting this type of evaluation is relied upon very heavily. These evaluations usually can produce realistic evidence, which should be able to be duplicable by other researchers. A comprehensive evaluation can illuminate facts about program planning, program monitoring, impact assessment, and economic efficiency (House, 1980).

This model has been used with great success by many economists, especially within the governmental sector of our nation. Evaluators utilizing the systems analysis model have a preconceived notion as to the function of the program under scrutiny. The role and function of that program have been well delineated by the government, thus enabling the evaluative researcher to answer concrete questions relative to that program. This model has recently begun to be utilized in the health science area. Investigators attempt to determine the cost-effectiveness of a program, such as in hospitals where patient-education programs are utilized. In our case study, Sarah would most certainly choose this method as one of many to evaluate the program.

The major *disadvantage* of this model is that, because it is utilized so often by governmental agencies, it excludes the interest and concerns of the program participants. In an excellent critique of this model, House (1980) claims:

> At its worst, the systems analysis approach leads to scientism—the view that the only way to the truth is through certain methodologies. Objectivity is equated with reliability, with producing information from only certain types of instruments. Impartiality and validity are sacrificed. In reducing everything to a few indicators so that one can demonstrate reliability, do cost-benefit analysis, and discover the most efficient programs (thus maximize utilities), the outcomes of complex social programs are narrowed to a few quantitative measures. (pp. 226–227)

At times, the systems analysis model takes an almost hard, cold approach to evaluation, and seems to not consider the human, social context of the program or organization.

There are *advantages* to this model, especially when the evaluator is looking for simple cause-and-effect relationships. In this case, a few indicators may indeed be enough to determine those relationships. For example, the systems analysis approach may be utilized to determine physician shortages in certain areas of the country. A simple count would suffice, here using one indicator. However, the evaluators must ensure not to extrapolate a possible shortage of physicians to indicate insufficient health care delivery.

The Decision-Making Model

Evaluation research made perhaps one of its largest contributions in the field of decision making. Evaluators believed that they could enable decision makers (program leaders, administrators) to make more informed decisions based on the data they collected. Stufflebeam (1971) developed the CIPP model to enable evaluation to contribute to the decision-making process in program development. CIPP is an acronym for four types of educational evaluation processes in the model: context, input, process, and product. The model also includes three settings where decisions are made: homeostasis, incrementalism, and neomobolism. There are additionally four types of decisions that can be made: planning, structuring, implementing, and recycling. Stufflebeam also delineated three steps in the process of evaluation: delineating, obtaining, and providing.

We have chosen to discuss the types of evaluation Stufflebeam described, because they have wide implications for health science evaluation research. *Content evaluation* involves analyzing problems and needs (a discrepancy between a desired condition and an existing one) of a program. In our case study, Sarah might find there are 85 gifted students in the science program but has determined that there is a need, by consensus, to reduce that number to 50. Hence a *need* has emerged. Once the needs have been determined, program objectives that will alleviate that need are proposed or determined.

Input evaluation considers the resources and strategies of the program. The data that are collected during this stage of the research project enable the evaluator to make decisions regarding equipment or resources that might be too expensive, if a particular strategy could be effective in achieving the program's goals, whether strategies are legally or morally acceptable, and how to best utilize staff as resources.

Process evaluation begins once the program is underway. For example, Sarah will begin to observe and collect data relative to the gifted health science program. If she were to find that students did not attend the special sessions and had higher absentee rates than other students, the program decision makers may take some action based upon this information. They might encourage students to attend classes or have teachers attend special in-service programs geared for educators of the gifted. In addition, process evaluation methods serve to keep records of the events that occur during the program. These records should be kept over a relatively long time period, so that peaks and valleys can be ascertained.

Product evaluation determines the extent to which the program's goals and objectives have been achieved. The evaluators develop measures of the goals and then administer them to the proper audiences. The results enable program administrators to make decisions concerning modifying or ending the program.

There is another approach to the decision-making model as suggested by Patton (1978). He suggests that for evaluations to be successful and relevant, the decision makers must be identified so that the gathered information gets to the people who can implement change. A second step in conducting this type of evaluation is to identify and focus the relevant questions. The program administrators also may specify how they would use the answers to questions, and thus provide much-needed input into the research study.

Decision-making approaches primarily use survey methods such as questionnaires, face-to-face interviews, and small group discussions. The evaluator goes to the setting, such as Sarah going to the Homewood school district, and does not necessarily set up an experiment. The program administrator, or decision makers play a very important role in this type of evaluation model.

The major *advantage* of this model is that the methodology selects the information that would be most useful to the evaluator. Criterion measures are predetermined, so that the evaluation is actually focused for the evaluation team. In our case study, Sarah would meet with the administrator of the gifted health science program to help determine the questions to be asked during the evaluation process. At this point, some might believe that the decision maker (the administrator) may have too much to say concerning the evaluation, and thus not be objective to the approach.

This leads to some *disadvantages* of the decision-making model: the administrator is preferentially treated, the evaluator becomes very close to the managers of the program, and the evaluation can become undemocratic and unfair. In addition, the identification and specification of important decisions is a difficult task for the evaluator. Who should be included in this process? How should these people be utilized before, during and after the evaluation?

The Goal-Free Model

The goal-free model was developed by Scriven (1973) when he was employed as one of a group of advisors to the Educational Testing Service to screen candidates for a list of innovations and developments that had been funded by the federal government, and whose evaluations proved that they were worth giving to schools. During this experience he delineated intended and unintended effects, or side effects, of a particular program. If one knew the goals of a program, this might serve as a contaminating effect. Therefore, Scriven decided that evaluations should be goal free, and the organizational framework of the process becomes the effects of the program, rather than the goals.

Goal-free evaluation is not widely utilized because of two factors: (1) Scriven has not given much guidance as to the procedures of the model, and (2) evaluators cannot easily find criteria to judge the program if they are not to use the administrators or the developers' goals and objectives. It is apparent that social science areas may find it difficult to utilize this model, but one good example of its use is by Consumers' Union. This group typically evaluates all sorts of products using what the members believe are criteria that consumers would prefer. Goal-free evaluation uses the reference group of the consumer of programs, rather than the producers or administrators.

Scriven has developed the concept of a consumer's need to be analyzed and does so through needs assessments of a particular group of people. He has insisted upon a bias-free approach when conducting the research, so the evaluator can remain as objective as possible. The techniques that are utilized include double-blind experiments, in which neither the subject nor the evaluator knows which is the treatment and which is not. Scriven describes goal-free evaluation as a triple-blind experiment where neither of the treatments is known.

The goal-free model, though not utilized very frequently does serve to point evaluators to the important aspect of the unintended or side effects a program may offer. Evaluators have become sensitized to the not-so-evident effect, and therefore have added a richness to the field of evaluation research.

Scriven's goal-free model is implicit in reducing bias in the evaluation. Because the evaluator has no contact with program personnel and does not have an inkling as to the goals of the program, a supposedly unbiased evaluation can occur. Unfortunately, there have not been many goal-free evaluations, assumedly because of the unwillingness of administrators to allow strangers to act as investigators, or hunters. The major *disadvantages* of the goal-free model include (1) a lack of a clear methodology as to how to approach this model and (2) the lack of social interaction between normally social people: evaluators and administrators of human service programs.

The *advantages* of the goal-free model lie in its ability to be completely bias-free from stated or predetermined goals. Consumers' Union does evaluate products in this manner. However, we must remember that products are not processes and it is process that concerns most evaluations in the health sciences. It appears that goal-free evaluations, in combination with other models, make a contribution to program or organizational evaluations.

The Connoisseurship Model

Connoisseurship is the art of perception that makes the appreciation of complex educational practices possible (Eisner, 1979). In this model, a judge is used to determine the effects of a program, curriculum, or educational system, Just as an art critic might write about a painting, so will the connoisseur of program evaluations. Connoisseurship consists of recognizing and appreciating the qualities of a program, and the connoisseur writes about that program; in other words "renders" a critique or criticism of that particular program. Sarah, in our case study, would be the connoisseur in this study.

The connoisseur, or critic, must be an experienced evaluator who will point out the significant aspects of a program through writing about his or her feelings about the program. With such an approach there are many methodological considerations to take into account: How can one know whether a critic is to be trusted? How can one be sure that the critic is not imagining the events? How can one know what confidence to place in the critic's description, interpretation, and evaluation of a program?

Eisner (1979) does suggest that to obtain validity for this model, one should look for instances of structural corroboration where separate pieces of evidence validate each other if they fit together to form a coherent, persuasive whole. Another way to validate the critic's findings is to ensure that the language used is referentially adequate by having other critics view the program through analysis of videotapes and audiotapes to assess if the critic's rendition of the material did really exist.

The critic must be experienced and trained in utilizing the connoisseurship model. The evaluator becomes totally involved in the program and becomes as familiar with it as is possible. The criticism that comes about through this model will usually lead the program to improve the standards and probably perform better than previous to the criticism. Although this model is not in the traditional mode of collecting and analyzing data, it does serve to supplement other approaches and to provide additional insight to what is being evaluated.

This model, because it is very closely aligned with art criticism, provides a very impressive and expressive idea for completing an evaluation. Because this type of method has worked very well in the arts (drama, music, painting, etc.) it should prove valuable to the science of evaluation. Connoisseurship has the *advantage* of adding another way to accomplish and augment an evaluation. It provides an expert review that, although biased, can detect weaknesses, flaws, and strengths of programs and/or organizations.

However, as with all of our evaluation models, there are *disadvantages* in utilizing the model. The connoisseur, really an expert, must decide on criteria in making judgments about programs. How does the evaluator decide on these criteria, and how are these criteria justified to the administrator of the program? A second disadvantage is that Eisner (1979), the creator of the connoisseurship model, maintains that the evidence for the criticism is the teachers of programs being evaluated. If this is so, can, or will teachers readily accept the criticisms? Have they?

The Case Study Model

In this model, the *process* of a program or an organization is the focus of the study. The evaluator attempts to depict the program to those involved in the program by presenting a case study. This is usually accomplished through interviews that serve the same purpose as those that ethnomethodologists conduct. You will often hear the term *naturalistic* applied to these methodologies. The major proponent of the case study model has been Stake (1978), who stated:

> [C]ase studies will often be the preferred method of research because they may be epistemologically in harmony with the reader's experience and thus to that person a natural basis for generalization. . . . If the readers of our reports are the persons who populate our houses, schools, governments, and industries; and if we are to help them understand social problems and social programs, we must perceive and communicate in a way that accommodates their present understandings. Those people have arrived at their understandings mostly through direct and vicarious experience (p. 5).

It is evident that the case study model enables people to gain an understanding of their world through complex descriptions of that world. The methodologies utilized to collect the data are interviews, as we stated previously. However, the writing becomes very informal, with illustrations and allusions. This evaluation model has led Stake (1975) to develop and implement responsive evaluation, which will be discussed later in this chapter.

The case study model comes from the qualitative research methodologies in which participant observation, interviews, document study, fieldnotes, and subjects' own words are utilized to collect and record the data. Because this has been discussed in depth in Chapter 6, we refer you to that chapter for reiteration of these methodologies. Although the case study model is similar to the connoisseurship model there is a difference in that the case study evaluator determines the perceptions of other people in addition to his or her own, whereas the connoisseur relies on only his or her own experience and values. Sarah would utilize these methodologies and act as the sole case study evaluator.

The case study model is a subjective approach to evaluation and has met with criticism as compared to the more scientific methods of evaluation. Because of the nature of the methodology of the case study, different observers will emphasize different parts of a program. This leads to the *disadvantage* of inconsistency. Another disadvantage is the interpretation made by the evaluator. The evaluator must observe all parts of a program, and then draw conclusions. Whose values are the basis of these conclusions?

There are many *advantages* to the case study model. As House (1980) has stated, these include (1) rich and persuasive information based on program participants and other people removed from the program, (2) representation of diverse points of view and different interests, and (3) potential for being persuasive, accurate and coherent.

Accurately depicting a case study and trying to avoid becoming personally involved can be a difficult task for any evaluator. Although this model has many advantages, it suffers from the same weakness that other models do: not having written methods and procedures.

The Accreditation Model

Many professional associations conduct evaluations of their respective professional training programs. In the area of health science, one of these accrediting bodies is the Council for Education in Public Health (CEPH), which accredits schools of public health and community health programs outside schools of public health. Other examples of professional reviews involve lawyers, physicians, educators, social workers, and speech and hearing therapists.

The CEPH accrediting process is similar to that of many professional organizations, so we have chosen to use it as an example. Typically, the accrediting body sets up criteria that are organized into several sections concerned with the professional training program. The approach that CEPH utilizes involves a self-study evaluation of the program. The program personnel have several months to prepare an in-depth analysis of the program and submit it to the CEPH staff.

A subcommittee of CEPH is appointed as the visiting, on-site group, and they review the self-study report previous to the on-campus visit. Once on the site, the committee interviews staff, faculty, and students associated with the program being evaluated. The committee prepares a brief report and gives their findings, informally, to

TABLE 7.1 Evaluation models

Model	Audience or Reference Group	Methodology	Outcome	Typical Questions
Behavioral objectives	Managers, social scientists	Behavioral objectives Achievement tests	Productivity Accountability	Is the program achieving the objectives? Is the program producing?
Systems analysis	Economists, managers	Cost-benefit analysis Planned variation	Efficiency	Are the expected effects achieved? Can the effects be achieved more economically? What are the *most* efficient programs?
Decision-making	Administrators	Surveys, interviews	Effectiveness, Quality control	Is the program effective? What parts of the program are effective?
Goal-free	Consumers	Bias control	Consumer choice Social utility	What are *all* the effects?
Connoisseurship	Consumers, connoisseurs	Critical review	Improved standards Heightened awareness	Would a critic approve this program? Is the audience's appreciation increased?
Case study	Client, practitioners	Case studies, interviews, observations	Understanding Diversity	What does the program look like to different people?
Accreditation	Professionals, public	Self-study review by panel	Professional acceptance	How would professionals rate this program?

Adapted from House, E. (1980) *Evaluating with Validity*, Beverly Hills: Sage.

the program director. Typically a few months later, a formal report is forwarded to the director with comments regarding the strengths and weaknesses of the program. The program director is then given an opportunity to correct any perceived weaknesses or devise a plan to do so. Program representatives are then invited to a meeting of the full council for a final disposition. The results of this process are then communicated to the appropriate program personnel.

Accreditations are useful in that they provide a mechanism for self-evaluation, as well as simultaneous peer evaluation. Programs that have been accredited are believed to have met criteria and standards set by the profession.

The accreditation model has grown as professional groups come under increased pressure to evaluate their own programs. The *advantages* of this model include (1) the self-evaluation mechanism, (2) setting of criteria and standards for a profession, (3) a continual effort at evaluation, and (4) accountability to the public. Although these advantages place a great burden on the profession in question, it seems apparent that a review of methods and procedures of professions can only help to improve that profession.

The accreditation model also has its *disadvantages* in that the public has challenged the model and the process, and thus it can bring about disharmony within the profession itself. A second limitation is the procedure that professional organizations utilize in their evaluations. The accrediting teams may not always have fair and competent people and each team may vary when conducting a site visit. This can lead to uneven evaluations among member programs and create a system of review that does not promote equality.

Table 7.1 summarizes the evaluation models we have discussed.

The models we have discussed can be utilized alone or in any combination. We have attempted to give a clear description of each model with a sense of their advantages and disadvantages so that evaluators may be able to decide which model is best suited for each evaluation situation. In our case study, Sarah might appropriately choose a combination of the decision-making and case study models. Can you suggest another model that Sarah could utilize to evaluate the health science program for the gifted?

Types of Evaluation Research

There are several types of evaluation research, some of which have developed from or have been precursors to the models previously discussed. We have chosen to discuss four types of evaluation research:

(1) needs assessment; (2) formative, (3) summative, and (4) responsive. These types of evaluation research can be utilized in the health sciences because they have broad application in the social sciences.

Needs Assessment

Usually, a needs assessment occurs when someone at the decision-making level feels there is a discrepancy between an acceptable condition and the existent condition. In our case study, the needs assessment would have been conducted *previous* to the implementation of the health science program for gifted students. Often, needs assessments are conducted at the community level: hospitals begin wellness centers, voluntary associations set up screening programs, and public health departments determine the *need* for free services.

Public support of a program should be demonstrated before that program becomes an actuality. Recently we have seen strong support for child abuse education programs, both in schools and other community groups. This has resulted because of the exposure of several child abuse cases involving adults who were in charge of preschools, parents abusing their own children, and abuse of elementary school children. Even though there appears to be widespread support for child abuse education programs, it is best to carry out a needs assessment to determine if a *specific group* would support such a program.

Needs assessment has been called front-end analysis (Harless, 1973), in which the assessment of the needs of a program, evaluation of the program's conception, a cost estimate, determination of feasibility, and projections of demand and support are researched before the programs commence. Two factors that might determine if a program is needed are frequency and intensity. If many people have a need for a program (frequency) then public support can be elicited, as in the case of the child abuse education program. In addition, if the need is seen as intense or grave, the program will receive support as well. There are some questions that researchers should consider when they are about to undertake a needs assessment (Anderson and Ball, 1978, p. 20):

1. What made us think that there were needs requiring investigation?
2. Whose needs are we talking about?
3. How can we find out whether the needs are frequent or intense enough to justify intervention?
4. How much frequency or intensity is sufficient—how much discrepancy between acceptable state and observed state is undesirable?

Once researchers have determined to undertake a needs assessment it becomes a fairly straightforward matter. The need has been determined; there is a discrepancy between an acceptable condition and one that is underway. Let us assume that our case study began at the needs assessment stage. Sarah was asked to determine if a health science program for gifted students would be accepted in the Homewood School District. The major design would be to survey the important figures (as previously mentioned) and perhaps interview a smaller, select group. The survey would be designed so that as many issues relevant to the gifted program would be discerned to elicit an analysis, which would compare the status of the current program with the desired program.

The final report that Sarah submits to the Board of Education should enable the decision makers to be better informed about the gifted health science program. Many specific objectives and goals of the program can be determined by the outcome of the analysis of the results.

Formative Evaluation

Scriven (1967) distinguished between two forms of evaluation: formative and summative. Formative evaluation occurs when data are being collected. This process provides information so that revisions and improvements can be made for the program. Formative evaluation can occur when instructional programs or curricula are to be evaluated. The gifted health science program would have been a good target for formative evaluation. Industry also utilizes this type of evaluation when evaluating products during particular stages of development.

Baker (1974) describes four areas of concern where an evaluation of a new program (formative evaluation) is undertaken:

1. Determine the results of the program.
2. Diagnose the weak areas.
3. Limit the number of subjects exposed to the new, unproven program.
4. Limit the costs of the program.

Keeping these guiding principles in mind, the evaluator should then decide on what kinds of data are to be collected. Outcome data is the first category of data collection. Here, the researcher is concerned with how the program affects those people directly involved in the program. A second type of data that is to be collected is that about the implementation the program. How does the program operate? Is the sequence adequate? What about the format in its presentation? At this stage, weaknesses of the program may be enlightened, and thus serve as targets for revision. So the revisions will have a high probability of success, it is suggested that the data collected on program effects should be correlated with that concerning its implementation. The data collected are usually in the form of observations, questionnaries, and interviews.

Formative evaluations are usually conducted by an "in-house" or internal evaluator. Formative evaluators are concerned with several important questions when conducting the review (Baker, 1974). The first to consider is, *Are the instructional materials accurate?* This leads evaluators to examine the curriculum materials, instructional guides, plans, and activities to ensure that the concepts are properly presented and are accurate. For example, in our gifted health science program, all the materials and subsequent examples would be scrutinized.

A second major concern is, *Does the content reflect an appropriate range?* The researchers would look for a broad range of materials, rather than a set of materials that represents only one point of view. For example, in our case study, it would be inappropriate for the materials to contain an overabundance of information about microbiology, if that took away from a well-rounded program.

A third consideration is, *Is the product well designed instructionally?* The evaluation team has to determine if the prescribed goals and objectives of the program are being met. In addition, if the program planners had designed the program to utilize a certain learning theory, were the principles of that theory ascribed to in the delivery process of the program?

A fourth question to be asked is, *Does instruction account for all planned outcomes?* In this situation, the evaluator is faced with determining whether the outcomes, or goals, as stated by the program developers have been accomplished. In health science, we must ensure that all domains—cognitive, affective, behavioral, skills, and decision-making—are taken into account when developing and evaluating a program.

A fifth consideration is, *What is the instruction's level of quality?* Here, the program activities are judged to see if they are effective. An evaluator can determine, by assessing the participants' level of activity and consequent outcome, if learning opportunities meet their objectives.

A final question in the internal review of a program is, *Do things fit together?* The evaluator must ask when reading through a program, do references match, are page numbers accurate, are the objectives clearly met, and there typographical errors, and can the program be easily utilized by the intended user? Once the internal review has been completed and is communicated to the program planners, it is up to them to institute the changes or make revisions.

Preliminary Field Test. After the internal review process has been completed, the program is tried out on a small sample of potential program participants. Two areas of concern are of importance here: the *effects* of the program on the participants and the *implementation process* of the program. At this phase of the evaluation, questionnaires, observations, and tests are used to collect the data.

Participant tests are utilized to determine the outcomes of the program. These can be used in a pretest-posttest manner, or any other experimental design that is appropriate. The use of standardized tests is not recommended here, because those tests would not necessarily reflect the anticipated outcomes of a particular program. Tests also can be in the form of observation of behavior and attitudes, or observing skill in decision making. These are conducted by the evaluation team in various ways, as mentioned in Chapter 6.

To obtain data concerning the implementation process of the program, the evaluator can collect items completed by the participants during the program. These materials can be in the form of assignments, memos, letters, field work situations, etc. The data can be related to the participant's postprogram scores to determine any weaknesses in the program, or areas necessary for revision. Observational data become very useful at this stage because the evaluator can pinpoint when certain activities work, are helpful, provide enrichment, and the like. The data collected during the preliminary field test enable the evaluator to gather information regarding the program participants' reactions, and to detect unplanned outcomes of the program (Baker, 1974). The evaluators then prepare a report for the program planners so that they can debug the program and get it ready for an operational field test. In this context, the program is then placed in the situation for which it was intended. At this stage, the evaluation is not as concerned with meeting program goals and objectives, but attention is directed toward issues of program utility, integration, and access. In our case study, Sarah must ask if the gifted health science program fits in well with the other science programs? Here, administrators and teachers would become actively involved in the evaluation process.

Summative Evaluation

Once the program has been evaluated in the formative manner, summative evaluation can take place. The purpose of this type of evaluation is to access the overall effectiveness of a program and the extent to which the program is worthwhile in comparison to other, similar programs. The results of the evaluation assists decision makers in terms of whether or not to adopt a particular program, utilize a product, or implement a procedure. An external evaluator usually is employed to conduct the summative evaluation. This person should be as impartial as possible and have no connection to the program whatsoever. In our case study, Sarah is conducting a summative evaluation in that she is concerned with evaluation of the gifted health science program after it has been in effect for 2 years. Once Sarah completes the evaluation process, administrators and the Homewood Board of Education will be able to determine if the health science program for the gifted is worthwhile and whether it is cost-effective for the school district. Thus, summative evaluation can provide the consumer with an independent assessment of a program.

Summative evaluation is concerned with the impact of a program, and because of this, the researcher has to ask, impact with respect to what? Many evaluators set about conducting a summative evaluation with a behavioral objectives approach, and yet others advocate employing a goal-free approach. Once the criteria against which the program's effectiveness will be measured are chosen, the evaluator then chooses measures that reflect the chosen criteria. The researcher also is concerned with the target population, sampling, and the study design. An evaluation report usually is rendered to those who called for the evaluation. This report should indicate the successes and weaknesses of the program and should be able to point to those program features that influence successes or failures (Anderson, Ball, Murphy, et al., 1975).

Planning Summative Evaluations. There have been many summative evaluations in the health sciences, especially in the area of curriculum evaluation. There also have been summative evaluations in the medical field in which a product or procedure has been evaluated for its effectiveness. No matter the context of the evaluation, planning is a very important and vital aspect in summative evaluation. Because external evaluators are utilized, the process can be costly and very time consuming.

Purposes of Summative Evaluation. Anderson and Ball (1978) have delineated the various purposes of summative evaluation that include the *monitoring of the continuing needs for program*. At times, the program has met its original intent, and should be disbanded. This is true in some health maintenance programs, where hypertension is under control, smoking has ceased, or weight loss has been achieved. This purpose can be achieved through collecting survey data, conducting personal assessments of the participants, and gathering expert judgments about the program.

A second purpose for summative evaluation is the *assessment of the cost-effectiveness of the program*. Sometimes it appears that it may be impossible to evaluate human effectiveness in terms of costs, e.g., if a medical procedure saves one life at a huge cost, is this cost-effective? An example is the use of artificial heart implants in very ill people. If the evaluator were to ask the recipients' family about the cost-effectiveness, and then survey the general public, disagreement about the outcome would certainly become apparent. In terms of our case study, the evaluators of the gifted health science program would address one of the following decisions:

1. Determine the least-expensive means of achieving a specified level of performance.
2. Determine the greatest level of performance that can be obtained for a specified cost.

In cost-effectiveness analysis it is easier to determine the cost-effectiveness of a program when it is evaluated against another, similar program than it would be to evaluate a program as an absolute. Sarah will have to determine which approach to take when determining the cost-effectiveness of the health science program. Methods to utilize in determining these factors include surveys and correlational status studies.

A third purpose of summative evaluation is to determine the *global effectiveness of the program in meeting the goals and objectives of that program*. Most programs have predetermined goals and objectives and, as discussed previously, criteria and measures by which to determine the success of the program. Factors such as long- and short-term effects also should be considered. If a program was instituted as a precursor to a more advanced program (e.g., Health Science I before Health Science II), the effects of that program should be evaluated at the end of the program. On the other hand, if one of the aims of the Health Science I program was intended to teach students to utilize health maintenance programs, this cannot be evaluated until the students have a chance to choose their type of health care delivery. Long-term effects are much more difficult to evaluate because of the impracticality of following subjects over a long period of time. Methodologies that are utilized for this purpose include experimental and quasiexperimental studies.

The fourth purpose of summative evaluation involves *determining the possible side effects of a program*. Although program objectives may have been clearly delineated at the outset, other positive and negative effects may occur because of that program. For example, the gifted health science program may have had a positive effect in keeping students from high rates of absenteeism because of their interest in the program. On the other hand, a negative, and unintended, side effect may be that some students enrolled in the program resented it because of the time commitment they were supposed to give to the program. Side effects can be determined by using the case study, experimental, or quasiexperimental approaches.

Responsive Evaluation

Responsive evaluation research focuses on the issues and concerns of the persons who have a stake in the evaluation; hence the term *stakeholder*. The evaluator *responds* to what different audiences wish to know. Stake (1975) was the first to use the term *responsive evaluation* and says the following:

> An educational evaluation is responsive evaluation if it orients more directly to program activities than to program intents; responds to audience requirements for information; and if the different value perspectives present are referred to in reporting the success and failure of the program. To do a responsive evaluation, the evaluator conceives of a plan of observations and negotiations. He arranges for various persons to observe the program, and with their help prepares brief narratives, portrayals, product displays, graphs, etc. He finds out what is of value to his audiences and gathers expressions of worth from various individuals whose points of view differ. Of course, he checks the quality of his records, he gets program personnel to react to the accuracy of his portrayals; and audience members to the relevance of his findings. He does most of this informally—iterating and keeping a record of action and reaction. He chooses media accessible to his audiences to increase the likelihood and fidelity of communication. He might prepare a final written report, he might not—depending on what he and his clients have agreed on (p. 14.)

What organizes an evaluation utilizing the responsive approach? As Stake has alluded, it is the issues and concerns of those persons the evaluator has had conversations with that will receive the attention. He has referred to other evaluation approaches as *preordinate*. The following are suggested steps that Stake (1978) enumerated. They are to be used in progression, but also may interchange as the evaluation progresses.

1. The evaluator talks with program staff, clients, and anyone involved in the program to gain a sense of their posture with respect to the purposes of the evaluation.
2. The evaluator then places limits on the scope of the program. In addition, documents and official records will have been reviewed to help set these limits.
3. The evaluator personally observes the program in action.
4. As a result of Steps 1 through 3, the evaluator begins to discover, on the one hand, the stated and real purposes of the program, and

TABLE 7.2 Comparison of Preordinate & Responsive Evaluation Modes

Comparison Item	Type of Evaluation	
	Preordinate	**Responsive**
Orientation	Formal	Informal
Value perspective	Singular; consensual	Pluralistic; possibility of conflict
Basis for evaluation design (organizer)	Program intents, objectives, goals, hypotheses; evaluator preconceptions such as performance, mastery, ability, aptitude, measurable outcomes; the instrumental values of education	Audience concerns and issues; program activities; reactions, motivations, or problems of persons in and around the evaluand
Design completed when?	At beginning of evaluation	Never—continuously evolving
Evaluator role	Stimulator of subjects with a view to testing critical performance	Stimulated by subjects and activities
Methods	Objective; "taking readings," for example, testing	Subjective, for example, observations and interviews; negotiations and interactions
Communication	Formal; reports; typically one stage	Informal; portrayals; often two stage
Feedback	At discrete intervals; often only once at end	Informal; continuously evolving as needed by audiences
Form of feedback	Written report, identifying variables and depicting the relationships among them; symbolic interpretation	Narrative-type depiction, often oral (if that is what the audience prefers), modeling what the program is like, providing vicarious experience, "holistic communication"
Paradigm	Experimental psychology	Anthropology, journalism, poetry

Adapted from: Guba, E. & Lincoln, Y. (1981) *Effective Evaluation,* San Francisco; Jossey-Bass.

on the other hand, the concerns that various audiences may have with it and/or the evaluation.
5. The evaluator begins to conceptualize the issues and problems that the evaluation should address.
6. Once issues and problems have been identified, the design takes some form. (This occurs very late, as is not true of other evaluation approaches, and is called an *emergent design*.)
7. The evaluator selects methods for gathering data. Stake considers the instrument as humans, in that they will be observers.
8. The data collection procedures are accomplished.
9. Once the data have been collected and processed, the evaluator goes to an information-reporting mode. The information is organized into themes, and the evaluator prepares portrayals designed to communicate naturally, and provide as much direct personal experience as possible. Portrayals, in this sense, include case studies, plays, artifacts, and videotapes.
10. The evaluator matches issues and concerns to audiences in deciding what form the report will take.
11. The format of the report must be decided when reporting to each audience. The reports may be in the form of written statements, discussions, newspaper articles, and films.
12. The final step is completed when the evaluator assembles any formal reports (pp. 5–8).

It is obvious that this type of evaluation is continuous and interactive, in that at any point the evaluator could begin again because of the results found so far in the process. There may be new issues and concerns that have been discovered through the evaluation process. Table 7.2 summarizes the preordinate evaluation approaches in comparison to responsive evaluation.

Methodological Approaches in Evaluation Research

Although we have discussed the various methodologies utilized in other types of research, it is important that methodological approaches be explained, with specific respect to those utilized in evaluation research. The methods that will be discussed include: experimental and quasiexperimental, correlation, surveys, personnel assessment, expert judgment, and case study.

Experimental and Quasiexperimental Designs

True experimental designs will enable evaluators to assess absolute answers to questions they have conceived. If, for example, a curriculum were being evaluated for teaching students the cognitive skills in anatomy, then a true experimental design should be utilized. Randomization, an issue discussed at great length elsewhere in this text, also should be employed. The evaluator should decide to use the classroom, client, program, or school as the unit of randomization, because this provides a much stronger design than a nonrandomized study.

Quasiexperiments are usually used when randomization is not feasible. As an alternative to randomizing subjects, matching them or using a statistical technique (analysis of covariance) may suffice. Evaluators may want to generalize their results to other, similar groups, such as the success (or failure) of a preschool program. Therefore, in this instance, generalizability is very important and should be carefully considered when setting up the study design. Quasiexperimental designs include time-series and the pretest-posttest nonequivalent control group design. The regression-discontinuity design (Anderson, et al., 1975) is frequently utilized in evaluation research. Here comparison groups are chosen that differ from the treatment group in one significant and continuous dimension. An example of this would be a control group that differed significantly in family income.

Correlation

Correlational methods are utilized frequently by evaluators, and sometimes without justification for the reported results. Correlations do not imply cause and effect, and researchers must take precautions not to make such inferences. Regression analyses, however, have proven to be helpful in determining the formative evaluation aspects of a study in which the positive and negative aspects of the program can be compared.

Correlations can be utilized in the typical experimental control group design, when measures are compared to the pretest scores. In addition, correlations between costs and program-effectiveness indices across several programs, or even parts of a program, could be utilized to determine the continuation or modification of a program (Anderson and Ball, 1978).

Surveys

Surveys, which are a major type of evaluation research, are the primary instruments utilized to collect the necessary data in a needs assessment. Surveys can include interviewing (telephone, individual, group), observations, questionnaires, and analysis of program records. There are some general facets to interviewing, questionnaire design, and observations that should be regarded by evaluation researchers; these are discussed in greater detail in Chapter 5.

1. Provide the appropriate reading level in the questionnaire.
2. Avoid sensitive or ambiguous questions.
3. Match the interviewer with the interviewee.
4. Ensure that the questions are relevant and remain on task as to the purpose of the survey.

Personnel Assessment

Personnel assessment is especially useful for determining the context of the program being evaluated. The administrative structure and procedures of the program can be ascertained by surveying (as above) the personnel involved in the practice of administration. Data about staff roles, relationships, responsibilities, in-service training, hiring and firing procedures, policies for internal evaluation for remuneration, and the like can be gathered using personnel assessment.

The actual collection of this type of data varies from program to program and within the context of that program. There are many cognitive, affective, behavioral, psychological, and physiological instruments available for use. However, even though these tests may be standardized, we recommend them with caution, and ascribe to the tenet that most instruments for program evaluation should be tailored for each program.

Expert Judgment

Expert judgment can come in three or more forms: (1) the evaluators as experts, (2) the program staff as experts, and (3) outside panels of experts. The evaluation researcher and the evaluation team can and should be considered experts. They will have to make important decisions concerning design, data collection, interpretation, etc. With their experience and education, they should, and usually are, accountable and responsible for the decisions they render.

The program staff that is being evaluated can serve as experts as well. They can give firsthand observations, thoughts, and beliefs about the program. Although they at times may appear too close to the program to be objective, recurrent themes can be deduced from the many data sources. These themes will provide invaluable information to the evaluation team.

External experts can be very helpful to the evaluation process.

They can be especially useful when the goal is to estimate cost-effectiveness of programs. In these instances, economists or other social scientists familiar with cost-effectiveness determinations can be called upon for their expert advice and judgment. In addition, if documented support for the program is necessary, outside experts, political and professional, may be called upon to provide documention of the merits and the worth of the program.

Case Study

The case study approach has been discussed in detail elsewhere (Chapter 6). In evaluation research, as in other types of research, the case study is very valuable in determining the effectiveness, merit, and worth of programs or organizations. Usually, the evaluator or the team will determine how the case study should be conducted, when it should occur, and which elements are necessary for inclusion in this methodological approach.

A case study can help determine if a program should be initiated, continued, or expanded. It can also help diagnose weaknesses and strengths of a program so that modifications can be instituted. And finally, this methodology can enable the evaluator to establish the process of how and why the program operates.

The methodological approaches discussed in the preceding chapter were illuminated in light of evaluation research. While these approaches are useful and important in other types of research, their uniqueness is apparent to evaluation research. It should be noted here that several methods may be used in any one evaluation project, as they each contribute to the total process.

New Methodological Approaches

Evaluation researchers have recently begun to use several methodologies in their studies. These include simulation modeling, cost analysis, and contextual evaluation. While these methodologies may have been utilized in other types of research, evaluation researchers have seen the advantages of these methods.

Simulation Modeling. A simulation model enables one to understand how and why an intervention works or should work. Several characteristics make simulation modeling a valuable tool for evaluation research (Cooper and Huss, 1981). The first is that simulation modeling requires the investigator to make explicit assumptions regarding the system to be studied. Simulation modeling assists this effort by simulating alternatives or variations to raise assumptions.

The second characteristic is that the model can create conditions that would otherwise be difficult, hazardous, or unlikely to occur. These types of models are frequently used in nuclear reactor coding systems. A third use of simulation modeling is that events not under the control of social scientists can be studied. The barriers may be costs or ethics that are beyond the control of the investigator. And finally, the simulation model can be utilized to forecast future conditions, guide future allocations of funding, select optional populations for the program, or evaluate additional program alternatives before implementation. Simulation modeling usually begins from theory, builds up the causal links, and then produces results that can be compared with other data to test the reasonableness of the modeled theory.

An example of simulation models that have been utilized in the health science is the health risk appraisal. The health risk appraisal is a tool that can describe an individual's chance of becoming ill or dying from some cause over a period of time. Most health risk appraisals are statements of probability of a disease, rather than detection or diagnosis. These kinds of appraisals have been in existence since the eighteenth century, when health professionals began associating specific illnesses with certain occupations. These appraisals did not have a scientific base as they were made by observing patients. Since that time, the creators of the health risk appraisals have improved the scientific base of the tools in demonstrating the relationship between certain risk factors and specific causes of death or disability. A health risk appraisal is

1. A method or tool that describes an individual's chance of becoming ill or dying from a select cause over a specific period of time, as compared to either (a) the population as a whole or (b) some similar subset of the population such as those people of the same age, race and sex.
2. A technique that is in a relatively early stage of development and most useful for white middle-class people;
3. Is most often intended to
   a. Raise an individual's and/or group's level of awareness and knowledge of personal risk factors and potential health outcomes,
   b. Serve as a vehicle for health education and counseling in order to promote voluntary health-related behavior change,
   c. Serve as a group needs assessment instrument for planning health education/health promotion programs.

There are two major types of health risk appraisals: self-scored and computer-analyzed. The computerized health risk appraisal gives an estimate of risk based upon physiological (e.g., blood pressure), bio-chemical (e.g., cholesterol), and health habit (e.g., smoking) data. It can provide an estimate of the risk of dying and/or having a serious adverse health effect from a certain cause within a specified time pe-riod. The appraisal also compares risk with the "average" risk for the same age and sex and provides an appraised age as well as an achiev-able age. In addition, it also can provide group analysis based on par-ticipants in the appraisal process (Department of Health and Human Services, 1984).

Cooper and Huss (1981) recommend that an evaluator develop a simulation model with the help of a systems analyst if the evaluator is not familiar with computer capabilities. The steps in the construc-tion and utilization of a simulation model for evaluation purposes in-clude

1. Determine that a simulation model is an appropriate device. Where the system is simple and all interactions are clear, other techniques may be more cost/benefit effective. With a large number of observa-tions and few variables, standard causal analyses are a possible pre-liminary or alternative approach.
2. Define the boundaries of the simulation. The scope must draw the line between events to be simulated in the model and those assumed to be externalities or inputs to the model.
3. Specify the key interactive components. These may be the individual program participants, the service units, or any decision maker. If the reaction of a group as a group is a key event, then that group is a necessary component.
4. Define the actions (outputs) of each component as a list of possible "events." These become the effect of previous system events and the cause of other system events.
5. Specify which components will be affected immediately and directly by an event. An example from our model is that the event of gasoline purchase fills the automobile tank, lowers the tank level for the sta-tion, and occupies the station's availability to pump gasoline.
6. Define the effect, on a component, of the events that component "re-ceives." This frequently requires an assumption or working hypoth-esis. If a number of outcomes is possible, then assign a probability to each and have the program select at random to match the probabil-ities.
7. Begin simulating to see how the model operates. This involves mak-ing systematic changes in variables and any constants to see how the model responds. This process is sometimes referred to as a sen-sitivity analysis. (pp. 28–29)

Cost Analysis. Statistical significance of program benefits have long sufficed for determining the effectiveness of a program. Evaluation researchers began to realize that the public and the funding sources were not satisfied with numbers of statistical importance. Instead, what was wanted was a demonstration of the practical benefits of the program. To accomplish this, researchers showed that the benefits exceeded all adverse program effects, including budgetary costs; hence the term *benefit-cost analysis*. Thompson, et al. (1981) found that there was a problem using benefit-cost analysis in the realm of evaluation research. This problem concerned the evaluation of main program effects. For example, evaluators in hypertension control programs cannot value, monetarily, statistical decreases to control rates. In a situation such as this, researchers rely on the principle of cost-effectiveness even if we do not know the value of achieving an objective, we do know that we wish to achieve the objective in a way that minimizes costs.

Cost-effectiveness analysts determine the ratio of monetary to non-monetary program effects, e.g. the amount in dollars required per hypertensive patient who achieves control. These ratios do not determine if the programs should be implemented, but are used comparatively by decision makers who would choose the least expensive program that produces the same result.

The cost-effectiveness ratio for social programs is expressed as follows (Thompson, et. al. 1981):

$$\frac{ML - MG}{B - R}$$

ML = monetary losses—program costs plus some induced costs
MG = monetary gains—monetary costs that are averted
B = benefits
R = risks—adverse side effects of the program

For example, in a mammography screening program the costs (ML) could be $200,000; the monetary gains (MG) could be $20,000 in savings of hospitalizations for patients; 15 could be the breast cancer deaths prevented (B); and 2 could be the mortality number for those dying from the chemotherapy and radiation treatements (R). The ratio then is

$$\frac{\$200,000 - \$20,000}{15 - 2} = \$13,846 \text{ per lives saved due to the}$$
mammography screening program

In cost analysis the numerator of the ratio is the focus of attention. Determining the *costs* of a program is extremely important and can have important implications for program evaluation. In determining the costs of a program, the following must be considered: *direct costs,* which include budgetary and nonbudgetary direct costs; *indirect costs;* and *opportunity costs.* For a complete discussion of these main categories of costs see Thompson, et al. (1981).

Contextual Evaluation. Ethnography was discussed at length in Chapter 6. However, we have chosen to discuss it here within the context of program evaluation. To reiterate the difference between experimental and contextual evaluations: *experimental evaluations* validate simplified causes and effects through controlled comparisons, and *contextual evaluations* attempt to understand the complexity of a program.

Contextual evaluations assume that social interventions have several facets and relationships that relate to multiple outcomes (Britan, 1981). These evaluations seek to determine how programs work, how they fit into settings, how they achieve results, and how they can be improved. Contextual evaluations are inductive and describe program implementation; how treatments occur, and how program activities relate to formal rules, informal goals, participant understandings, and environmental pressures. The major methodology for a contextual evaluation is ethnography.

Ethnography encompasses the use of observations and interviews and relies very heavily on participant observation. The hallmark of ethnography is the observation, recording, and analysis of behavior in context. It includes systematic descriptions of social systems that look for interrelationships among particular behaviors, customs, rituals, beliefs, and values in terms of broader patterns of cultural understanding, social structure, and environment (Britan, 1981). The usual format for an ethnographer is a case study in which an analysis is conducted of program implementation and impact.

There are certain advantages to using experimental evaluations: when program goals are clearly stated, treatments are straightforward, and theoretical constructs are unambiguous. On the other hand, contextual evaluations are more useful when there are broadly stated goals, treatments are complex, and theoretical constructs are vague. Therefore, the choice of an evaluation methodology may depend upon the type and setting of the program.

Summary

This chapter has attempted to provide a condensed version of the field of evaluation research. This area of research generates much discussion and experimentation in the social sciences, with specific emphasis in educational evaluation. The case study depicted such a project where a program for gifted health science students was to be evaluated. A broad, general definition of evaluation research was established as the process of determining the effectiveness of a program.

The purposes of evaluation vary, depending upon the vantage point: administrator, consumer, evaluator, or organization. Almost anything can be evaluated, especially if there is support from one of the aforementioned groups.

There are many evaluation models, including behavioral objectives, systems analysis, decision-making, goal-free connoisseurship, case study, and the accreditation model. A discussion of the advantages and disadvantages of each model led us to the conclusion that perhaps a combination of models might be necessary for many program evaluations. The following steps were enumerated to aid the evaluator in conducting an evaluation: determine the client, the purposes of the evaluation, the methodology to be utilized, the nature of the contact, how the evaluation should be conducted, and who will use the results of the evaluation.

The major types of evaluation research used in the health sciences include need assessment, formative, summative, and responsive. Each type has its inherent strengths, weaknesses, and best area of suitability. It is generally up to the contractor to determine the type of evaluation, and this is accomplished by the nature of the evaluation research contract and the question that needs to be answered by the investigator.

Methodological approaches utilized in evaluation research are experimental, quasiexperimental, correlation, surveys, personnel assessment, expert judgment, and case study. Though these approaches are used in other research paradigms, they are discussed with specific reference to evaluation research. New and innovative research methodologies were discussed, including simulation, cost analysis, and contextual evaluation.

Evaluation research is a valuable tool for the health sciences. Programs have been asked to be accountable, and through a well designed evaluation, that accountability is enabled to be assessed.

Suggested Activities

1. Refer to the list on page 155, and add to the evaluation possibilities.
2. From the list in Activity 1, choose one topic and briefly describe the steps you would take in the evaluation process.

3. Compare and contrast two evaluation models. Use specific examples.
4. Interview a program administrator to assess that program's evaluation status (i.e., when was it last evaluated, by whom, why, and so on).

References

Anderson, S. and Ball, S. (1978) *The Profession and Practice of Program Evaluation,* San Francisco: Jossey-Bass.

Anderson, S., Ball, S., Murphy, R., and Associates (1975) *Encyclopedia of Education Evaluation,* San Francisco: Jossey-Bass.

Baker, E. (1974) Formative evaluation of instruction. In Popham, W. (ed.), *Evaluation in Education,* Berkeley: McCutchan.

Bloom, B. (1956) *Taxonomy of Educational Objectives,* New York: McKay.

Britan, G. (1981) Contextual evaluation: an ethnographic approach to program assessment. In Conner, R. (ed.), *Methodological Advances in Evaluation Research,* Beverly Hills: Sage.

Caro, F. (1977) *Readings in Evaluation Research,* New York: Russell Sage.

Chelimsky, E. (1978) Differing Perspectives of Evaluation. In Rentz, C. and Rentz, R. (eds.), *Evaluating Federally Sponsored Programs: New Directions for Program Evaluation,* 2 (Summer), San Francisco: Jossey-Bass.

Cook, T. and Campbell, D. (1976) The design and conduct of quasi-experiments in field settings. In Dunnette, M. (ed.) *Organizational Psychology,* Chicago: Rand McNally.

Cooper, R. and Huss, W. (1981) Simulation as an evaluation tool in Conner, R. (ed.), *Methodological Advances in Evaluation Research,* Beverly Hills: Sage.

Department of Human Services, State of Maine (1984) *Guidelines for Choosing Worksite Health Promotion Programs,* Maine: Health Promotion Department, Blue Cross & Blue Shield of Maine.

Eisner, E. (1979) *The Educational Imagination,* New York: Macmillan.

Guba, E. and Lincoln, Y. (1981) *Effective Evaluation,* San Francisco: Jossey-Bass.

Harless, J. (1973) An analysis of trend analysis, *Improving Human Performance: A Research Quarterly* 3:229–244.

House, E. (1980) *Evaluating with Validity,* Beverly Hills: Sage.

Mayer, R. (1962) *Preparing Objectives for Programmed Instruction,* San Francisco: Fearon.

Patton, M. (1978) *Utilization-Focused Evaluation,* Beverly Hills: Sage.

Popham, W. (1975) *Educational Evaluation,* Englewood Cliffs, New Jersey: Prentice-Hall.

Rossi, P. and Freeman, H. (1982) *Evaluation,* Beverly Hills: Sage.

Rossi, P., Freeman, H., and Wright, S. (1979) *Evaluation: A Systematic Approach,* Beverly Hills: Sage.

Rutman, L. (ed.) (1984) *Evaluation Research Methods,* Beverly Hills: Sage.

Scriven, M. (1967) The methodology of evaluation, *AERA Monograph Series on Curriculum Evaluation,* No. 1, Chicago: Rand McNally.

Scriven, M. (1973) Goal-free evaluation in E. House (ed.), *School Evaluation: The Politics and Process,* Berkeley: McCutchan.

Shortell, S. and Richardson, W. (1978) *Health Program Evaluation,* St. Louis: Mosby.

Stake, R. (1978) The case study method in social inquiry, *Educational Researcher* 7: 5–8.

Struening, E. (1983) Social area analysis as a method of evaluation. In Struening, E. and Brewer, M., (eds.), *Handbook of Evaluation Research,* Beverly Hills: Sage.

Stufflebeam, D. (1971) *Educational Evaluation & Decision Making,* Itasca, Ill.: Peacock.

Suchman, E. (1967) *Evaluative Research,* New York: Russell Sage Foundation.

Thompson, E., Rothrock, J., Strain, R., and Palmer, R. (1981) Cost analysis for program evaluation. In Conner, R. (ed.), *Methodological Advances in Evaluation Research,* Beverly Hills: Sage.

Tyler, R. (1949) *Basic Principles of Curriculum Instruction,* Chicago: University of Chicago Press.

CHAPTER **8**

Carrying Out Historical Research

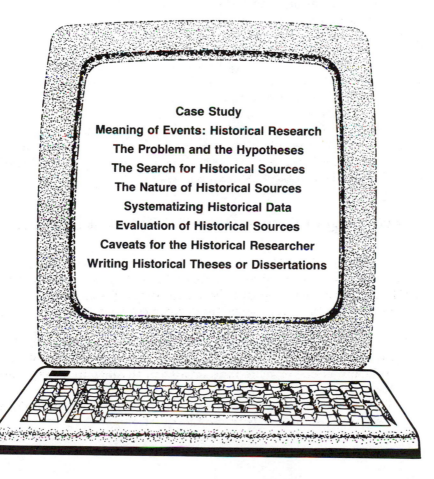

Case Study

Meaning of Events: Historical Research

The Problem and the Hypotheses

The Search for Historical Sources

The Nature of Historical Sources

Systematizing Historical Data

Evaluation of Historical Sources

Caveats for the Historical Researcher

Writing Historical Theses or Dissertations

Case Study_____

In thinking about potential topics for a thesis, Jan considered "wellness." He knew that everything seemed to be moving in that direction—especially jobs. There were many hospitals and clinics seeking wellness directors as well as several teaching openings for someone who could teach in the area of wellness, not to mention the wellness-health promotion activities being adopted by major industries. The more Jan thought about it, the more questions that came to mind, such as: Is wellness a fad? Will jobs be available in this area when I graduate? Is wellness really a part of the health sciences? Did someone in the health sciences start the wellness trend? Is wellness a better approach to health than any of several others? After much time and deliberation, Jan focused on the question, how did "wellness" get to where it is today? He felt that if he could answer this question, it may give him leads to several other answers and perhaps an idea for the future of wellness.

As he became more and more interested in this topic, Jan began to worry about whether or not something called historical research would qualify for a master's thesis. Because he was just in the process of taking courses in research and statistics, he wondered, if there was such a thing as historical research, and if so how it was done.

His major tasks were obvious—to find out whether historical research is in fact bona fide research, how it would be accomplished, and if he could trace the historical pathway of the topic, wellness.

The Meaning of Events: Historical Research_____

The question of whether or not there is such a thing as historical research has been debated for quite sometime. As pointed out by Best (1981), those who are skeptical about the merits of historical research (as compared to the scientific method) comment that

1. Since history is a result of natural, unplanned events, the historian is unable to generalize findings. The lack of controls and influence of one or more individuals fail to allow for predictability.
2. The historical researcher must rely on information from documents and witnesses; both may be questionable.
3. Data collection may be incomplete requiring tremendous inferences to fill the gaps.

On the other hand, the rebuttals made by those who believe the historian's activities are similar to those of scientific research are

1. The historical research has a problem statement, delimits the problem, develops hypotheses or at least raises rigorous questions, collects and analyzes primary data including hypothesis testing, and formulates conclusions or generalizations. Although it is true that variables are not controlled, this also characterizes much of the research in the health sciences, especially if it involves nonlaboratory investigation in school, public, or patient health settings.
2. The historian analyzes the reports of many witnesses and documents from several different vantage points so that the account of one person or document does not unduly bias the research effort.
3. To a nonhistorical researcher, it may appear that leaps are taken to arrive at conclusions; however, this is not the case. Only after the evidence has been critically analyzed for authenticity, accuracy, and veracity and after the principles of probability have been followed will conclusions or generalizations be developed.
4. Finally, even though quantitative measures are not employed, the scientific method is applied to bring about qualitative results.

Overall, historical research in the health sciences is important for several reasons. The findings of historical research enable health scientists to learn from past discoveries and errors. Also, historical research can offer roots to the entire field of health science, from medicine to health education—community, patient, and school. Further, this kind of research can provide information about barriers to professional growth and identify the needs for reform. Lastly, knowledge of events in the past may help in predicting future trends in the health sciences.

As a methodology, historical research has some advantages over other techniques. The most obvious one is that inaccessible subjects may be studied. For example, Jan can inquire about people who have contributed to the growth of wellness even if they are deceased. Researching documents allows him to be almost timeless. Concomitantly, historical research is suited to study the health sciences over a long period of time. This, of course, applies to Jan's situation very well because he wishes to follow the pathway of wellness over time to determine how it got where it is today. Another inherent advantage of historical research is that sample size can be much greater than it can be in experimental research. In studying documents over a long period of time, it would be a simple matter to have a sample as large as 2,000. Also, unlike experimental research, there is little likelihood that the data collection technique would change the data being collected. The researcher can observe and study spontaneous feelings and actions that have been recorded orally, in writing, or both. Frequently, the document expresses points of view untold to anyone when the person was alive. A distinct advantage to many researchers is that the monetary cost of historical research is relatively low, especially when compared to a large survey study. This does not imply poor quality, however; historical research can use documents of very high quality, often written by highly skilled writers in the health science field.

Nonetheless, like other research techniques, historical research does have drawbacks. Witnesses to as well as documents about particular events may exhibit a bias. Furthermore, many commonplace documents—diaries, letters, and so on—may not be available if they were not written by famous people. Consequently, Jan may have access only to the writings of those who have been seen as major contributors to the growth of wellness and not to the behind-the-scenes workers. If the documents are incomplete or assume prior knowledge about a preceding event, the historical researcher may have great difficulty filling in the missing parts. This is assuming that documents about the subject in question are even available—many events in the health sciences were not recorded. Jan would also have to be careful as to the nature of documents collected, as well as the people interviewed, to be sure sample bias did not occur. In other words, he would not be wise to seek only documents and people that were favorable to the wellness movement. Another disadvantage to historical research is that documents lack a standard format, which makes comparison difficult. In a related concern, data must be adjusted for comparability over time—writings about wellness, or any health topic, in the early days were much different than those of today. Because many impinging factors have taken place over the years, comparison of the documents may become impossible.

Historical research can be excellent if it is done in the correct way. It must go beyond the amassing of facts and descriptions to include hypotheses that may explain the occurrence of events and a relentless effort to collect, scrutinize, and interpret data. The general task of the historical researcher in the health sciences is to discover data contained in all types of documents, whereas most other research techniques allow for the creation of data from observations and tests.

Defining a Problem and Developing Hypotheses_____

In planning an historical investigation, it is necessary to define the problem as would be done for any other type of research endeavor. Consulting with historical researchers and reviewing the literature in the health sciences are important steps. As the problem takes shape, the researcher may recognize it as fitting into one of the five categories of historical research outlined by Beach (1969).

Current issues in health—wellness, health promotion, DRG's, role delineation, etc.—are often the impetus for historical research. A second category for historical research is the history of specific individuals or institutions (Thomas D. Wood, M.D., or ASHA, APHA, SOPHE). If the entire history of such a subject were not explored, a new portion could be.

A third category is to examine historically events or concepts that before appeared to be unrelated. For example, the concept of wellness and discontent with the medical model or research in health education and the changing emphases in health education journals could be investigated. The fourth category involves the synthesis of old data or the merging of new data with old.

Beach's fifth category is the reinterpretation of events that have been studied by other research historians. In this category, called revisionist history, the health science researcher works to revise existing histories within new frameworks.

Although the difficulty of defining and delimiting a problem exists for all research efforts, it is particularly so for historical research. The beginning health science researcher must understand that "The weapon of [historical] research is the rifle, not the shotgun" (Best, 1981). In other words, the effort should be a penetrating analysis of limited scope.

Once the problem is defined, the next step is to develop hypotheses that may be tested by gathering evidence and determining if the evidence supports each hypothesis. If the evidence is compatible with the hypothesis, then the hypothesis is confirmed. The hypothesis is rejected if the evidence is incompatible.

In Jan's situation, he may pose the problem, Why is the wellness movement so popular in the health science field today? Next, he may hypothesize that it is so popular because of

1. The rising cost of medical care over the years.
2. The desire of the general public for self-responsibility in health matters.

3. The disenchantment with the emphasis on physical health only, inherent in the medical model.
4. The coincident health education philosophy of prevention.

If Jan believed that these hypotheses were researchable, he would commence searching for historical sources.

The Search for Historical Sources

Before the search is begun, a plan of attack should be outlined. Brooks (1969) suggests that

> Resourcefulness and imagination are essential in the preliminary exploration as well as in the later actual study. One can suppose that certain kinds of sources would exist if he thinks carefully about his subject, the persons involved, the government or institutions concerned, and the kinds of records that would naturally grow out of the events that he will be studying. He should ask himself who would have produced the useful documents in the transaction he is concerned with. What would be the expected flow of events? What kinds of records would have been created? What would be the life history of the documents, from their creation through current use, filing, temporary storage, and eventual retention in a repository where he can consult them? What kinds of materials would one expect to be kept rather than discarded?

Chapter 3, Review of Related Literature, offers steps for a literature search by hand and by computer as well as sources of information with which to begin. Once the preliminary search begins, the historical researcher should be prepared to revise plans or alter directions as sources are revealed.

The Nature of Historical Sources

Historical data are usually categorized into two broad classifications, primary and secondary. *Primary sources* are reported by either a participant of the event or an observer of the event. In other words, these are eyewitness accounts. *Secondary sources* are not eyewitness accounts but rather reports by someone who may have talked with a participant or an observer or read a document produced by an actual observer or participant.

Primary Sources

Several types of primary sources are available to the health science researcher. Documents of a primary nature are the written records of actual participants or witnesses. These materials take many forms, such as constitutions, charters, official minutes or records, court testimony, periodicals, business records, contracts, wills, affidavits, notebooks, diaries, newspaper and magazine accounts, films, pictures, institutional files, computer diskettes, and the like. Documents can be further classified as handwritten or printed, published or unpublished, for public or private use. Also, a document may be distinguished by its preparation; whether it was prepared intentionally as a historical record or whether it was unpremeditated. The distinction between unpremeditated and intentional may be of great importance when the document is evaluated for authenticity.

Another important primary source is oral testimony. This is obtained in a personal interview, which may be recorded or transcribed as the witness relates the events. Jan could interview such people as John Travis and Don Ardell. This branch of investigation is called oral history and is so prominent that an organization, The Oral History Association, exists for all those interested in this technique. Ballads, tales, sagas and other forms of oral expression may convey information also. They may be primary or secondary sources.

Relics serve as a source to the historical investigator, also. Generally they include buildings, furniture, food, tools, weapons, paintings, coins, architectural plans and similar remains that were not deliberately intended to transmit historical information. A health science researcher investigating school health environment would observe school buildings, the physical plant, furniture, and the like as part of the research effort.

Secondary Sources

Secondary sources are documents or oral testimony by a person who was not present at the event but obtained the information from someone else, who may or may not have been an eyewitness. Consequently, secondary sources are usually of limited worth. Depending upon the research goals, an item may be a secondary source in one study, yet a primary source in another.

Systematizing Historical Data

As one would expect, a historical study can generate a great amount of data. The historical researcher must be well organized so that the hours of research in libraries, document rooms, offices, and archives will not be wasted.

As noted in Chapter 3, bibliography cards should be completed with foresight and in detail. Since several cards may be required for one document, it is suggested that each card be numbered in the corner, for example, *Card #2, One of 3 Cards.* Because many avenues lead to the same event, the historical researcher may wish to make multiple cards. This would allow the study of one event from several different angles. For example, in 1961 Dr. H.L. Dunn wrote the book, *High Level Wellness,* which has had a tremendous impact on people in the wellness movement and on later writings. Jan may wish to have four notecards about the book with separate headings—the information on the cards themselves would be identical except for some researcher remarks. He would simply make three copies of the same information by using paper cut to 3 × 5 or 4 × 6 and same size of carbon paper. Once the information is written, then the headings would be placed on each sheet. In Jan's case, the headings may look like these:

1961: "High Level Wellness" - written, H.L. Dunn
Physical Health only: "High Level Wellness'
Self-Responsibility: "High Level Wellness"
Medical Costs: "High Level Wellness"

This technique affords four different perspectives on one item of information. If this approach is used throughout the study, the researcher will have separate, but parallel files of the same data. To assist in file separation, the researcher may color-code the cards for different information. This method provides an efficient and rapid means of relating data from one category to another, thereby facilitating interpretation.

Meta-analysis may be used to synthesize research findings where the results of multiple studies are compared. This approach, presented in Chapter 9, may be of tremendous value to the historical researcher, depending upon the nature of the study.

A related approach in data gathering is one outlined by Cooper (1982). His concern is with conducting integrative research reviews.

In these reviews the health scientist is primarily interested in "inferring generalizations about substantive issues from a set of studies directly bearing on those issues" (Jackson, 1980). In other words, if Jan were to review several studies regarding wellness and attempt to draw conclusions from all of them, he would be conducting an integrative research review. Cooper contends that the health scientist "must recognize that the integration of separate research projects involves scientific inferences as central to the validity of knowledge as the inferences made in primary data interpretation" (Cooper, 1982).

To assist in this data collection technique, Cooper advocates that integrative research review be evaluated against scientific criteria. Consequently, the integrative research review is conceptualized as a process containing five stages: problem formulation, data collection, evaluation of data points, data analysis and interpretation, and presentation of results.

Stage one, problem formulation, examines what evidence should be included in the review, the constructing of definitions to distinguish relevant from irrelevant studies, and sources of potential invalidity such as narrow concepts and superficial operational detail. The second stage, data collection, involves procedures that should be employed to find relevant evidence, the sources of potentially relevant studies, the differences in the research contained in the sources, and the people used in each study as compared to the research target population.

Data evaluation, the third stage, is concerned with what retrieved evidence should be included in the present study, the separation of valid from invalid studies, and the examination of factors that might contribute to improper weighting of study results and omission of other results that might make conclusions unreliable. The fourth stage, analysis and interpretation, reviews what procedures should be used to make inferences about the literature as a whole, the synthesis of valid retrieved studies, differences in rules of inference, rules for distinguishing patterns, and review-based evidence to infer causality. The last stage, public presentation, comprises information to be included in the report, the application of editorial criteria, differences in guidelines for editorial judgment, the inclusion of review procedures and findings. Through this approach, reviews may be completed in a more scientific fashion and achieve greater objectivity.

Though systematization is important for all researchers, the historical health researcher should be particularly aware of techniques, such as meta analysis and Cooper's approach, to help in organization and in drawing unbiased conclusions. Sources of information are listed in the suggested readings at the end of the chapter.

Evaluation of Historical Sources

Historical data are subject to two types of evaluation. First, it must be ascertained whether or not the data are authentic. Second, if the data are authentic or genuine, they must still be evaluated for accuracy and worth. These approaches to data evaluation are called *external criticism* and *internal criticism,* respectively. Through evaluation, the historical researcher accumulates a body of validated, trustworthy facts and information that is known as *historical evidence.*

External Criticism

In establishing the authenticity or genuineness of data, the historical researcher raises several questions such as: Is it the original copy? Is it genuine? Who is the true author? When and where was it written? Under what conditions was it written? Is it a hoax?

Several methods may be employed in external criticism of data. Physical and chemical tests of parchment, paper, cloth, ink, paint, cloth, wood, or metal may be completed to determine the age and authorship of a data source. Also, tests of signature, handwriting, spelling, type, and script may be used. Finally, there must be consistency in language use, in knowledge and technology of the time, and in documentation, as well as among works done by the same person.

Internal Criticism

Though the data may prove to be authentic, the problems of accuracy and worth remain. Internal criticism explores statements within a document, the competence of the author(s), the accuracy of one account as compared to others, and author bias.

For example, Jan may discover a document about holistic health written over 50 years ago. He may determine the authenticity of the data, but question the worth of the statements in relation to wellness. Further, the accuracy of the medical statistics given by the author may be suspect. In addition, Jan would need to know about the competency of the writer. Was he involved in the medical field? Did he witness events personally? Was he an expert in holism? Did he write the document under unusual conditions?

In exploring some data, especially documents, Jan may find that there are several accounts of the same event—all of them slightly different. This is to be expected; even the classroom experience shows that a teacher speaks the same words to all students in the class, but not all students exit with the same message. This does not mean that Jan must believe one account or witness and ignore the others but rather that he must search for objective reality by scrutinizing all data carefully.

This scrutiny or internal criticism should be alert to bias or prejudice. A proponent of wellness may bias statistics or accounts of events to present the "wellness" side of an argument, whereas the skeptic may produce evidence prejudicial to the wellness movement. To some degree, this is to be expected. While it may not be intentional, the historical researcher must discern the truth.

Caveats for the Historical Researcher

In conducting historical research, the health scientist must be particularly careful in regard to the use of concepts, interpretation, causal inference, and generalization.

Concepts are very important for organizing information, people, and events. The concept of wellness employed by Jan does all of these things. However, one needs to be aware that a concept also places limits on the researcher's interpretation of the past. For example, if Jan believes that a defining attribute of wellness is that "self-responsibility is the major difference between wellness and the medical model," then he would omit much in his research effort. The other dimensions of wellness may be negated or at least reduced in importance, thereby limiting his search into the past for the foundations of the wellness movement.

Health science researchers frequently adopt concepts from other disciplines—psychology (e.g., motive, attitude), sociology (e.g., role) and anthropology (e.g., culture). This borrowing of concepts can be very beneficial, but the historical researcher in health must be cognizant of how the concepts are defined in the discipline from which they are borrowed and be certain that they are appropriate to the health science study.

The historical researcher continually **interprets** the data collected. In addition to using internal criticism to search for bias, the investigator must be aware of his or her own biases, personal interests, and values. We are all aware of selective perception, and the health researcher moving through years of data must not see only the things he or she wishes to be seen. Concomitantly, when reviewing historical data the researcher should be careful not to interpret past events with perspectives and concepts from the present, or at least very recent times. This is referred to as *presentism*. Jan may find some very early sources from physicians that to him reflect a concern for self-responsibility in wellness. However, this may not have been the intent of the physicians at that time—it could have had a very different meaning. Such findings must be interpreted in accordance with the time and conditions present when the source was written.

Causal inference means that the historical researcher views one set of events as bringing about, directly or indirectly, a subsequent set of events. For example, Jan may review the cultural, middle-class change in emphasis from people-orientation in the 1960s to me-orientation in the 1970s as causing an increase in interest in self-responsibility for health care. This may or may not be a correct interpretation. The idea must be fully explored with the underlying question, was it *the* cause? The longer the investigation continues, the more likely that additional antecedents will be discovered, each of which will face the same underlying question. In this case, it would be found that the rise in medical care costs may have served as an impetus for people to look after themselves. More often than not, the health scientist would note that an event was a contributing cause rather than *the* cause. The strength of the contribution can be denoted in the written report (e.g., a major influence).

Generalizing from historical evidence is fraught with several problems. First, the data collected are usually highly specific and limited and may not be representative. Second, even when one person is investigated, it must be realized that opinions stated in one major document may not be consistent with the same author's opinion at a later date. To overcome some of these problems, the researcher must increase the sample size of data collected. Otherwise, generalizations must be limited.

Writing the Historical Thesis or Dissertation

The writing of an historical thesis or dissertation presents a few more problems than the typical health science research effort; however, it also has a few more liberties. The organization of the historical report does not usually follow the general guidelines for theses and dissertations. Although this organization allows the researcher to depart from what might be seen as a presentation of bare facts in a monotonous, plain, unattractive style, it also challenges the writer, calling for creativity in organization.

The most obvious organizational format is chronological order. While this may be functional in a few instances, generally it is not. Therefore, the researcher may wish to consider presenting the data in a thematic format. For example, Jan may present his data according to each hypothesis developed.

When neither of these formats is workable, they might be combined. Herein, Jan could organize his thesis into chronological periods and within each period address the respective themes. This would allow the reader to grasp both the time periods and the continuity of themes as they progress from one era to another.

The methodology of the research effort may be presented in one chapter, especially if problems in external and internal criticism were found. Another chapter may contain the opinions of other historical researchers because their interpretation of events may be different from that of the current author. Another possible difference from the usual format is a chapter presenting the researcher's reaction to the interpretive process.

Though all theses and dissertations require careful writing, this is particularly the case for historical reports. Because interpretation is the key to historical research, every effort must be made to use words that accurately describe events, causal inference, and the like. If Jan notes that Halbert L. Dunn played a "major" role in promoting the wellness movement within the health sciences, he must ask why this adjective was employed. Is this his interpretation solely (perhaps he is in awe of Halbert L. Dunn), or does it reflect the opinion of experts in the field? While the use of adjectives in historical research adds life and color to the thesis, the ultimate goal is to report the truth in a style that is dignified and objective.

Summary

Historical research was seen not only to be bonafide, but also of great importance to the health sciences. Findings of historical research enable the health scientist to learn from the past, to provide roots to the field, to reveal barriers to future growth, and to assist in predicting the course of events. If done correctly, historical research has several advantages over other research methodologies. This requires the development of a problem statement, hypotheses, and a relentless effort to collect, scrutinize and interpret data.

Five categories for defining the problem were addressed: current issues in health, the history of specific individuals or institutions, exploration of unrelated concepts, the synthesis of old data or the merging of new data with the old, and finally the reinterpretation of events studied by other historians. The most important step was the definition of a problem in narrow terms. This was followed by the development of appropriate hypotheses to be tested by gathering evidence and determining whether the evidence supports the hypotheses.

Historical sources are primary or secondary in nature. Primary sources, reported by either a participant or observer of the event, include documents, oral testimony, and relics. Secondary sources are secondhand accounts of events, usually in written or oral form. Suggestions were given to systematize these data for ease in use.

Two approaches were discussed for evaluation of historical data: First, external criticism to determine authenticity; and second, internal criticism to evaluate accuracy and worth.

Four caveats were presented for the historical researcher: The use of concepts was discussed as being important but to be employed in an appropriate framework. Interpretation by the researcher must avoid personal bias, interest, or values. Further, every effort must be made to interpret events according to the times in which they occurred rather than from present or recent perspectives (presentism). Causal inference requires the collection of a large amount of data to confirm causation. Lastly, generalization from historical evidence was seen to be fraught with several problems.

Writing the historical thesis or dissertation was seen to be different from the usual health science investigation. Although more freedom was allowed the historical researcher, along with freedom came increased responsibility for organization. Chronological, thematic, and combined formats were discussed as well as suggestions for additional chapters. All in all, the historical researcher must be very careful in the selection of words and phrases so as not to distort the truth.

Suggested Activities

1. Select a voluntary health agency in your local setting and write a proposal for an historical study to include an appropriate title, problem statement, hypothesis, examples of primary and secondary sources, and methods of external and internal criticism.
2. List five reasons why historical research is needed in health education and indicate four specific topics that should be investigated.
3. Select an appropriate health science organization, such as Eta Sigma Gamma national health science honorary, and (1) name five people from whom you would want oral testimony (pick the best), (2) list four documents you would investigate, and (3) choose two relics you might pursue.
4. You are a new member of a health care team in the Ozarks country of Missouri and Arkansas. Over the past few months you have found that much of the health behavior of the rural residents is steeped in tradition

and folklore. This has presented a problem to the health care team because they have difficulty in both understanding and assimilating the behaviors.

You feel that knowledge of the origin and subsequent pathway of the health beliefs and behaviors of these people is necessary in order to facilitate better health care. You decide to find out.

What would be your first step? Write out a problem statement. Develop at least two hypotheses. Outline your plan of attack.

5. As a health scientist, you are acutely aware that your discipline has been subject to political influence. Because your interest lies in medicine, you would like to study the role of federal government in medicine in the United States. Your particular interest is the nature of that role (supportive or inhibitive) and the quality of health care. What would be your problem statement? List at least two hypotheses and ten sources of information for your historical research, and develop a time frame for conducting the study.

References

Best, J.W. (1981) *Research in Education,* 4th ed., Englewood Cliffs, NJ: Prentice-Hall, Incorporated.

Beach, M. (1969) History of education, *Review of Educational Research* 39:561–76.

Brooks, P.C. (1969) *Research in Archives: The Use of Unpublished Primary Sources,* Chicago: University of Chicago Press.

Cooper, H.M. (1982) Scientific guidelines for conducting integrative research reviews, *Review of Educational Research* 52:291–302.

Dunn, H.L. (1961) *High Level Wellness,* Arlington, VA: R.W. Beatty.

Jackson, G. (1980) Methods for integrative reviews, *Review of Educational Research* 50:438–460.

Suggested Readings

Barzun, J. and Graff, H. F. (1977) *The Modern Researcher,* 3rd ed., New York: Harcourt, Brace, Jovanovich.

Cutler W. W. (1971) Oral history: its nature and uses for educational history, *History of Education Quarterly,* 189–94.

Fischer, D. H. (1970) *Historians' Fallacies: Toward a Logic of Historical Thought,* New York: Harper and Row.

Glass, G. V. (1978) Integrating findings: the meta analysis of research. In Shulman (ed.), *R. Educ. Res.,* Vol. 5, Itasca, IL: Peacock.

Glass, G. V., McGraw, B., and Smith, M. (1981) *Meta Analysis in Social Research,* Beverly Hills: Sage.

Gottschalk, L. (1969) *Understanding History: A Primer of Historical Method,* New York: Alfred A. Knopf.

Hahn, D. B. (1982) The Malden studies: the first experimental research project in school health education, *Health Education* 14(4):8–9.

Iverson, B. K., and Levy, S. R. (1982) Using meta analysis in health education research, *Journal of School Health* 52:234–239.

Johns, E. B. (1977) Graduate health education: past, present, and future. Paper presented before Eta Sigma Gamma (National Health Science Honorary) Annual Meeting, Atlanta, October 14.

Lussier, R. (1984) History of health education. In Rubinson, L. and Alles, W. (eds.), *Health Education: Foundations for the Future,* St. Louis: Times Mirror/Mosby College Publishing

Means, R. K. (1963) The historical development of health education in the United States. In Veenker (ed.), *Synthesis of Research in Selected Areas of Health Instruction,* Washington, D.C.: School Health Education Study.

Weber, N. B. (1982) Historical research as it applies to groups and institutions, *Health Education* 13:10–11.

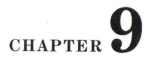

CHAPTER **9**

Analyzing and Interpreting Data

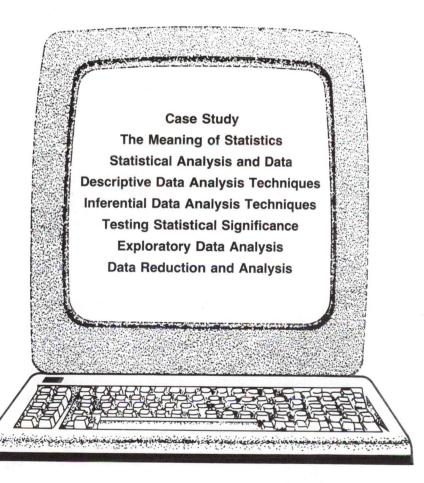

Case Study
The Meaning of Statistics
Statistical Analysis and Data
Descriptive Data Analysis Techniques
Inferential Data Analysis Techniques
Testing Statistical Significance
Exploratory Data Analysis
Data Reduction and Analysis

Case Study

According to the reports reviewed by Jon, chief health educator for the city, the incidence of autoimmune deficiency syndrome (AIDS) was increasing at an alarming rate. Several health care professionals were requesting information about the population that was contracting the disease. They wanted to know how many there were, the ages involved, the average age, their sexual orientation, the average number of sexual contacts, the range of sexual contacts, the relationship of weight loss to AIDS, the relationship of persistent unexplained diarrhea, and a host of other questions.

Jon was aware that medical records would contain the raw information, but it would need to be analyzed and interpreted. He would need to take all the data from the medical records and compile, analyze, and interpret it in a fashion comprehensible to the health care professionals. In short, Jon had to decide what statistics should be used to describe the data and had to answer all the inquiries he received.

The Meaning of Statistics

Statistics is a language that can be employed to express concepts and relationships that cannot be communicated in any other way. To the neophyte health researcher, it is a language to be in awe of or to fear; in contrast, the seasoned health scientist who understands the logic of statistics and appreciates its expressive power views it as a language to organize, analyze, and interpret numerical data.

Another approach to looking at statistics is in terms of its functional aspects. On the one hand, it can function to describe data. That is, to explain how the data look, the center point of the data, how spread out the data may be, and how one aspect of the data may be related to one or more other aspects. For example, Jon wants to describe the total number of victims, the average age of the victims, the age range, and how AIDS relates to unexplained weight loss and diarrhea. His primary concern is to describe the group of people who have contracted AIDS in his jurisdiction. Subsequently, this branch of statistical analysis is called descriptive statistics. No conclusions can be extended beyond this immediate group and any similarity to those outside the group cannot be assumed.

A different function of statistics is to infer. Inferential statistical analysis involves observation of a sample taken from a given population. Conclusions about the population are inferred from the information obtained about the sample. Suppose you were to observe the health habits of a random sample of poor inhabitants of the Appalachian region. You could then make inferences about the health habits of the total population of poor persons in the Appalachians. Unlike descriptive data analysis, generalizations can be made from the sample to the respective population. Note that Jon is unable to do this in his study since he is not dealing with a sample and is using descriptive data analysis.

Also, inferential data analysis can be used for estimation and prediction. For example, scores obtained on the Graduate Record Examination may predict how well an incoming candidate may perform in a graduate health science program. Extrapolation is a component of inferential statistics but not of descriptive statistics.

Statistical Analysis and Data: Parametric and Nonparametric

Two types of data are recognized in the application of statistics, parametric and nonparametric. Parametric data are either interval data (no true zero, measured equal intervals) or ratio data (true zero, measured equal intervals, ratio relationship). Further, parametrical statistical tests assume that the data are normally or near normally distributed. In comparison, data that are either counted (nominal scale) or ranked (ordinal scale) are called nonparametric data. Nonparametric statistical tests, often referred to as distribution-free tests, do not require the more restrictive assumption of a normally distributed population.

Frequently, parametric tests are considered the more powerful of the two. However, this is only the case when all the assumptions and restrictions of parametric data have been met. If there is lack of homogeneity of variances, unequal n's, and oppositely skewed distributions, the t-test is not as powerful as converting the data to ordinal scale and applying nonparametric tests. Generally, nonparametric statistical tests have wider applications and are less difficult to compute.

Descriptive Data Analysis Techniques

There are several statistical techniques available to the health science researcher who wishes to describe the observed research group.

- Measures of central tendency
    Mean
    Median
    Mode
- Measures of spread or variation
    Range
    Variance
    Standard deviation
- Measures of relationship
    Coefficient of correlation

It is the responsibility of the health science researcher to select the technique that best fits the data and will explain the data in a manner comprehensible to the intended audience.

Measures of Central Tendency

Jon, in the AIDS example, was asked to describe the group using averages—average age, average number of sexual contacts, and so. This is a typical request because most people wish to find a value about which the observations tend to cluster. The three most common measures used to describe the centering point of a set of data are the mean, median, and mode. Collectively, they are called measures of central tendency.

The Mean. The mean of a set of data is commonly referred to as the arithmetic average. It is computed by summing all the observations in the group and dividing by the number of observations. The formula is

$$M = \frac{\Sigma X}{N}$$

where:

$$M = \text{mean}$$
$$\Sigma = \text{sum of}$$
$$X = \text{scores in a distribution}$$
$$N = \text{number of scores}$$

For example, if Jon recorded the ages of sixteen AIDS victims and were to compute the average age, it might be as shown below:

$$\overline{X}$$
24
34
21
56
28
44
42
34
51
29
38
18
25
34
27
36

$\Sigma X = \overline{541}$

$$N = 16$$

$$M = \frac{541}{16} = 33.81$$

The arithmetic mean, which may be considered the fulrum or balance point of a distribution, is one of the most useful statistical measures because it provides much information, is affected by all scores, and serves as a basis for the computation of other important measures, such as variability.

The Median. The median is a measure of position in that it is the point above and below which one-half of the scores fall. In other words, it is the middle-most position. If Jon examined the number of sexual contacts for an odd number AIDS victims to determine the median point, he would find that it is the midscore. For example:

```
7
6            2 scores above
4 – median
3            2 scores below
1
```

If Jon had an even number of subjects, the median would be the middlepoint between the two middle scores.

$$\begin{array}{c} 10 \\ 8 \\ 7 \\ 3 \end{array} - \text{median 7.50}$$

10   2 scores above

8

7   — median 7.50

3   2 scores below

The median is not influenced by extreme scores as the mean is. Therefore, in some instances it may be a more realistic measure of central tendency than the mean. However, the median is usually reserved for a quick measure of central tendency or when distributions are markedly skewed.

The Mode. The mode is simply the most frequently occurring score. By examining the ages of the sixteen AIDS victims in Table 9.1, it can be seen that the most frequently occurring score or age is 34. Subsequently, the modal age for that particular group is 34. The mode is the quickest estimate of central value and shows the most typical case.

Measures of Spread or Variation

The measures of central tendency are useful, but sometimes not enough so. This is particularly true in a comparison of two groups whose means are identical. In such situations, it is important to know whether the scores or observations for each group tend to be quite similar (homogeneous) or spread apart (heterogeneous). Measures of variation, to include range, variance, and standard deviation, may be employed to show the degree of spread or variation among scores.

As an example, Jon reviewed the data for two groups of AIDS victims. The first group comprised victims without a committed relationship and the second group were committed to a relationship. Their

TABLE 9.1 Commitment and Casual Sexual Contact

Group 1 Committed	Number of Contacts	Group 2 Uncommitted	Number of Contacts
Jack	75	Bill	52
Ken	60	Fred	48
Ron	45	Chuck	47
Bob	40	Clark	53
Tom	30	Mike	50
$\Sigma X =$	250	$\Sigma X =$	250
Mean =	50	Mean =	50

number of casual sexual contacts within the last 6 months were compared and they were identical.

The Range. The range is the simplest measure of variation. It is
the difference between the highest and lowest scores. For example, in
Group 1 the range is 45 (75 − 30), and Group 2 has a range of 6 (53
− 47). The range may be used justifiably as a hasty measure of variability, but because it takes into account only the extremes and not
the bulk of observations, it is not generally employed.

Variance and Standard Deviation. The most useful measures of
variation are standard deviation and variance. In a study dealing
with a sample, the variance is the sum of the squared deviations from
the mean, divided by N − 1. The formula is

$$s^2 = \frac{\Sigma(X - M)^2}{N - 1} \quad \text{or} \quad \frac{\Sigma x^2}{N - 1} \text{ where } x = (X - M)$$

From Table 9.1, Group 1, the following calculations would result in
obtaining the variance, with the mean being 50. The calculations are
shown in Table 9.2.

$$M = \frac{250}{5} = 50$$

$$s^2 = \frac{\Sigma x^2}{N - 1} = \frac{1250}{4} = 312.50$$

The standard deviation is computed by obtaining the square root of
the variance. By formula, it is:

$$s = \sqrt{\frac{\Sigma x^2}{N - 1}}$$

TABLE 9.2   Variance of Group 1: Committed

X	x or (X − M)	x^2
75	+ 25	625
60	+ 10	100
45	− 5	25
40	− 10	100
30	− 20	400
ΣX = 250	Σx = 0	Σx^2 = 1250

Therefore, the standard deviation from Group 1 would be:

$$s = \sqrt{\frac{\Sigma x^2}{N - 1}} = \sqrt{\frac{1250}{4}} = \sqrt{312.50} = 17.68$$

The variance and standard deviation measure variation within a set of data. The larger they are, the greater the variation or heterogeneity. Through similar computation, the variance and standard deviation of Group II, Uncommitted, are 6.50 and 2.55 respectively. Subsequently, Group I has much greater variance than Group II. Standard deviation units are identical to the units of the raw data (centimeters, sexual contacts, etc). This point, combined with accuracy and ease of computation, make standard deviation the preferred measure of variation.

When the health science researcher is working with data from an entire population, there is a slight change in the formula along with different symbols. The population mean, μ (mu), is the sum of all values divided by N (the total number in the entire population). By comparison, the sample mean, $\overline{X}$, is an estimation of the population mean. Similarly, the sample variance is an estimate of the population variance which is determined by the formula

$$\sigma^2 = \frac{\Sigma x^2}{N}$$

The standard deviation of the population is ascertained by

$$\sigma = \sqrt{\frac{\Sigma x^2}{N}}$$

The difference between formulas for populations and samples is the use of N − 1 for division in the sample formula rather than N. The reason for employing N − 1 in the sample formula is to provide an equation that gives an unbiased sample variance. In other words, N − 1 allows for a more accurate estimate of the population variance and standard deviation.

Measures of Relationship

Some of the most interesting questions posed in health science research revolve around the relationship of one variable to another, such as smoking and lung cancer. The method used most frequently to describe the relationship between two or more variables or between two or more sets of data is linear correlation. The degree of relationship is expressed by the coefficient of correlation, symbolized by r.

Some of the unique characteristics of the correlation coefficient are that it is a pure number, it is nondimensional, and it may take on values between −1.00 and +1.00. A correlation coefficient of zero indicates no relationship between the variables in question. The closer the r is to 1.00 (negative or positive), the stronger the relationship. A perfect positive correlation of +1.00 specifies that for every unit increase in one variable there is a proportional unit increase in the other variable. Concomitantly, a perfect negative correlation of −1.00 means that for every unit increase in one variable there is a unit decrease in the other variable. Perfect correlations are highly unlikely in dealing with human health concerns.

The scattergram is a means of displaying the relationship between variables and is developed by graphically plotting each pair of variables that correspond to the X and Y axis respectively. The line drawn through or near the coordinate points is referred to as the line of best fit or regression line. Fig. 9–1 demonstrates several correlations and their regression line.

The beginning health science researcher must be careful not to fall into the trap of attributing a cause-and-effect relationship to variables that might be related. For instance, Kuzma (1984) reports a strong relationship between a child's foot size and handwriting ability. As explained, however, it is likely because both increase with age rather than being a direct cause-and-effect relationship. Spurious relationships must be viewed with caution and interpreted judiciously.

Spearman Rank Order Correlation. The Spearman Rank Order Correlation is used to determine the relationship between two ranked variables (rather than interval or ratio variables). That is, the Spearman Rank Order Correlation, signified by r_s, is designed for nonparametric data. Frequently, a health science investigator may employ it to compare judgments by a group of judges of two objects or the scores of a group of subjects on two measures (for further information on this usage, consult Siegel, 1956). A less frequent, but valuable usage is to compare judgments by two judges of a group of objects or items. Hays (1973) discusses the Spearman Rank Order Correlation for assessing inter-judge equivalence. In cases of multiple judges and multiple objects the Friedman two-way analysis of variance or Kendall Coefficient of Concordance would be used.

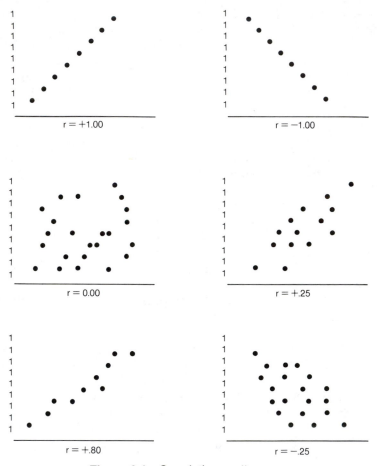

Figure 9.1 Correlation scattergrams.

The equation for the Spearman Rank Order Correlation coefficient is:

$$r_s = 1 - \frac{6\Sigma d^2}{n(n^2 - 1)}$$

where:

    n = number of pairs
    d = difference between paired ranks
    Σd^2 = sum of the squared differences between ranks

If Jon, in the example case, were to have ten AIDS victims ranked according to the severity of the disease by two independent physi-

TABLE 9.3   Ranking Severity of AIDS by Two Independent Physicians

Victim Number	Physician #1 Rank Order (X)	Physician #2 Rank Order (Y)	d (x − y)	d² (x − y)²
1	1	2	1	1.00
2	4	1	3	9.00
3	7.5	9.5	−2.5	6.25
4	2	3	−1	1.00
5	7.5	8	−0.5	0.25
6	3	4	−1	1.00
7	5	9.5	−4.5	20.25
8	9	5	4	16.00
9	6	6	0	0.00
10	10	7	3	9.00
				$\Sigma d^2 = 63.75$

cians, he would use the Spearman technique. Table 9.3 shows the data. Note that ties in rank are handled by averaging the ranks. Using the formula, Jon would obtain:

$$r_s = 1 - \frac{6(63.75)}{10(99)} = .62$$

The Spearman Rank Order Correlation procedure is an acceptable method for parametric data when there are fewer than 30 but greater than 9 paired variables. The ease of computation allows it to be used by health science teachers for a single classroom of students.

Pearson Product-Moment Correlation. The Pearson Product-Moment Correlation, the most often used and most precise coefficient of correlation, is used with parametric data. The basic formula for the Pearson Product-Moment Correlation coefficient, symbolized by r, is:

$$r = \frac{N \,\Sigma XY - (\Sigma X)(\Sigma Y)}{\sqrt{N \,\Sigma X^2 - (\Sigma X)^2 \; N \,\Sigma Y^2 - (\Sigma Y)^2}}$$

This is the raw score equation that is convenient for both calculator and computer use. Statistics books can be explored to obtain equations written in a different format (Kuzma, 1984).

Jon wished to investigate the relationship between the victims' age and number of sexual contacts since their diagnosis of AIDS. Table 9.4 displays the data and necessary calculations for sixteen victims. The process involves five columns.

TABLE 9.4   Victim Age and Number of Sexual Contacts Since Diagnosis

Variable X Age	Variable Y Contacts	X^2	Y^2	XY
18	30	324	900	540
21	18	441	324	378
24	24	576	576	576
25	17	625	289	425
27	22	729	484	594
28	12	784	144	336
29	15	841	225	435
34	10	1156	100	340
34	11	1156	121	374
34	10	1156	100	340
36	6	1296	36	216
38	4	1444	16	152
42	1	1764	1	42
44	3	1936	9	132
51	1	2601	1	51
56	0	3136	0	0
$\Sigma X = 541$	$\Sigma Y = 184$	$\Sigma X^2 = 19965$	$\Sigma Y^2 = 3326$	$\Sigma XY = 4931$

$$r = \frac{16(4931) - (541)(184)}{\sqrt{16(19965) - (541)^2}\sqrt{16(3326) - (184)^2}}$$

$$r = \frac{78896 - 99544}{\sqrt{319440 - 292681}\sqrt{53216 - 33856}}$$

$$r = \frac{-20648}{\sqrt{26859}\sqrt{19360}}$$

$$r = \frac{-20648}{(163.58)(139.14)}$$

$$r = \frac{-20648}{22760.52} = -.90$$

$$r = -.90$$

Inferential Data Analysis Techniques_____

Inferential statistics have two principal functions: (1) to predict or estimate a population parameter from a sample statistic, and (2) to test statistically based hypotheses. By comparison, the previous section discussed statistical techniques to describe a given sample or population.

Meta-Analysis

Meta-analysis is a method developed by Glass (1977) that synthesizes quantitative data from many primary sources. The data focus on the same question and use similar variables. The purpose of using meta-analysis is to statistically integrate the findings from a broad population of individually conducted projects. The statistic used to integrate the findings of these studies is the magnitude of the effect of the treatment. The *effect size* (Δ) is computed by subtracting the mean score of the control group on the dependent variable from the experimental group mean and dividing by the control group standard deviation:

$$\Delta = \frac{Xe - Xc}{SDC}$$

Δ = effect size
E = experimental group
C = control group
SD = standard deviation

The mean of the effect sizes for all studies included in the research review is then calculated to estimate the typical effect of the problem being studied. For example, a meta-analysis of pretext sensitization effects in experimental design was conducted by Wilson and Putnam (1982). The authors wished to investigate if subjects' posttest scores were affected by a pretest. They gathered results from 32 studies and computed those outcomes as standardized differences between pretested and nonpretested groups. The average effect size was +.22 indicating a general positive (elevated) effect of pretest on post-test. Cognitive results were elevated .43, attitude results .29, and personality .48. Of all effects 64 per cent were positive, and 81 per cent of the cognitive effects were positive. The investigators concluded that researchers should use the pretest as a design variable (if present) and should estimate its effect.

There are several limitations of meta-analysis, including (1) inclusion of poorly conducted studies in the equation, (2) cost of conducting the study, (3) criteria being used for including primary sources are difficult to agree upon, and (4) incomplete data are sometimes used because they are the only data available. However, meta-analysis has been and will continue to be a valuable aid in helping scholars keep up with the relevant research. Although it will not replace the literature review, it does provide a method for reviewing the studies mentioned in the literature review.

Regression Analysis and Prediction

An important use of the Pearson Product-Moment Correlation coefficient is for prediction. The regression line (line of best fit) can be used to predict the value of a dependent variable (Y) from a known independent variable (X) value. To illustrate, when Jon asked, "How strong is the association between victim age and the number of sexual contacts since diagnosis of AIDS?" the technique of choice was the correlation coefficient. However, if he asked, "What would be a victim's predicted number of sexual contacts since diagnosis of AIDS based on the victim's age?" linear regression analysis would be the method of choice.

The formula for predicting Y from X is:

$$\tilde{Y} = r \left(\frac{s_y}{s_x} \right) (X - M_x) + (M_y)$$

where:

r = correlation coefficient between X and Y
s_y = standard deviation of Y distribution
s_x = standard deviation of X distribution
M_x = mean of X distribution
M_y = mean of Y distribution
X = independent variable
$\tilde{Y}$ = dependent variable to be predicted

As an example, suppose Jon had the following information and desired to predict the number of sexual contacts since diagnosis.

Victim age (X) = 43 r = −.90
Victim age (X) = 20
          s_x = 10.55 s_y = 8.98
          M_x = 33.81 M_y = 11.50

The prediction for the victim aged 43 would be

$$\hat{Y} = -.90\left(\frac{8.98}{10.55}\right)(43 - 33.81) + (11.50)$$

$$\hat{Y} = -.77(9.19) + (11.50)$$

$$\hat{Y} = -7.08 + 11.50$$

$$\hat{Y} = 4.42$$

The prediction for the victim aged 20 would be

$$\hat{Y} = -.90\left(\frac{8.98}{10.55}\right)(20 - 33.81) + (11.50)$$

$$\hat{Y} = -.77(-13.81) + (11.50)$$

$$\hat{Y} = 10.63 + 11.50$$

$$\hat{Y} = 22.13$$

For the older victim, the predicted number of sexual contacts since diagnosis is well below the mean though for the younger victim it is well above the mean. These results are consistent with the coefficient of correlation obtained in Table 9.4.

When the coefficient of correlation, r, is less than perfect ($+1.00$ or -1.00) an error in prediction will exist. On the other hand, there is no error in prediction when a perfect correlation occurs, so that for every increase in X there is a proportional increase in Y (perfect positive r) or for every decrease in X there is a proportional decrease in Y (perfect negative r). Recalling the scatter diagrams in Fig. 9.1, the regression line failed to pass through all the coordinate values in relationships that were not perfect. Subsequently, there was not a direct proportional increase or decrease in the variable Y based on the variable X.

The health science researcher can estimate just how precisely the regression line describes the relationship between the two variables. The measure for estimating the prediction error is called the standard error of estimate and is determined by

$$s_{est}y = s_y\sqrt{1 - r^2}$$

Note that in using the formula, when $r = 0$ the standard error of estimate is s_y based on:

$$s_{est}y = s_y\sqrt{1 - 0^2} = s_y(1) = s_y$$

Subsequently, in this situation the standard deviation of Y is considered the standard error of estimate.

In the example predictions used by Jon the standard error of estimate would be:

$$\begin{aligned}
s_{est}y &= s_y\sqrt{1 - r^2} \\
&= s_y\sqrt{1 - .90^2} \\
&= s_y\sqrt{1 - .81} \\
&= s_y\sqrt{.19} \\
&= .44\ s_y
\end{aligned}$$

The standard error of the estimate is interpreted similar to the standard deviation. When $r = \pm.90$, an actual performance score of Y would likely fall within a band of $\pm .44\ s_y$ from the predicted Y 68 per cent of the time.

Testing Statistical Significance_____

The beginning health science researcher should keep in mind that scientific conclusions are statements that have a high probability of being correct rather than statements of absolute truth. Subsequently, the researcher must ascertain how high the probability has to be before he or she can declare that a relationship exists between two variables or denote that the difference between the two is greater than chance. To accomplish this, appropriate statistical tests must be used. Before the examination of several such tests, it is necessary to discuss some basic concepts and terminology surrounding testing for statistical significance.

The Null Hypothesis

The null hypothesis (H_0) is a claim that there is no significant difference or relationship between two or more variables. In other words, any difference or relationship that appears to exist is caused only by chance.

Alternative Hypothesis

The alternative hypothesis (H_1) is a statement that disagrees with the null hypothesis such that if the null hypothesis is rejected, the health scientist must accept the alternative of a significant relationship or significant difference between the two variables.

Critical Region

The critical region is the far end of the distribution (Fig. 9.2) as seen in the normal curve. In a one-tailed test, in which only one end of the distribution is used, whereas in a two-tailed test both ends of the distribution are used. For example, if Jon were to hypothesize that knowledge about AIDS is the same for AIDS victims as for the general public (null, no difference), a two-tailed test would be employed. On the other hand, Jon could hypothesize either of the following:

1. AIDS victims have greater AIDS knowledge than the general public, *or*

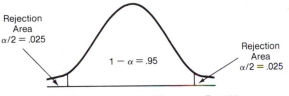

Z=−1.96   Two-tailed test: No difference   Z=1.96

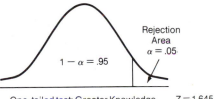

One-tailed test: Greater Knowledge   Z=1.645

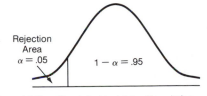

Z=−1.645   One-tailed test: Less Knowledge

Figure 9.2 Two-tailed and one-tailed regions.

2. AIDS victims have less AIDS knowledge than the general public.

Both hypotheses indicate direction of difference and would therefore require a one-tailed test.

Level of Significance

The acceptance or rejection of a hypothesis is based upon a level of significance (alpha level, α) which corresponds to the area in the critical region (Fig. 9.2). Many research efforts in health science establish the level of significance at the 5 per cent (.05) alpha level, although it may be set at the .025, .01, or .001 levels. Rejecting the null hypothesis at the .05 alpha level suggests a 95 per cent probability that the differences between the two variables is real, that is, not the result of chance. In other words, there is a less than 5 per cent probability that the differences are caused by error or chance.

In a two-tailed test of significance, the 5 per cent area of rejection is split between the upper and lower tails of the curve (Fig. 9.2) since the null hypothesis is nondirectional. By comparison, in the directional one-tailed test, the 5 per cent area of rejection is either at the upper end or the lower end of the curve (Fig. 9.2). As a general rule of thumb, the following probabilities and interpretations are widely accepted by health science researchers (Kuzma, 1984):

Probability Value	Interpretation
>.05	Result not significant
<.05	Result is significant
<.01	Result is highly significant

Type I and Type II Errors

Type I error is the rejection of a null hypothesis when it in fact is true. The alpha level of significance determines the probability of a Type I error. If the health science researcher rejects a null hypothesis at the .01 level there is a 1 per cent risk of rejecting it when it is actually true. Similarly, using the .05 alpha level of significance the researcher is taking a 5 per cent risk of rejecting the null hypothesis even when it is true.

However, if the null hypothesis is accepted when in fact it is false, a Type II error occurs. Therefore, if the health science researcher establishes the alpha level of significance as high as .01 the possibility of a Type I error is reduced, but the chance of a Type II error increases.

As an example, suppose that Jon compared two educational techniques to be used with the AIDS victims—Technique A and Technique B. If he rejected the null hypothesis and claimed that Technique B was the preferred method for teaching, new equipment may be purchased and additional personnel budgeted. Later, in subsequent experimentation or in actual programs, it may be found that Technique B failed to bring about the expected results. Although the ultimate truth about the falsity of the null hypothesis would still be unknown, evidence supporting the null hypothesis would be abundant, leaving Jon humiliated and with a depleted budget. He probably committed a Type I error.

On the other hand, if he accepts the null hypothesis and it is later found that there is a difference between Techniques A and B in that one brings about better results, he again may be embarrassed. Typically, Type I errors lead to unwarranted changes whereas Type II errors maintain the status quo when a change should occur.

The t-Test for Two Independent Sample Means

Health science research workers frequently draw two samples from a population and assign them to a control group or to an experimental group. After the experimental group has been exposed to the treatment, the researchers may wish to compare the experimental to the control group. Because the mean is likely the most satisfactory measure for characterizing a group, health scientists find it important to determine if there is a difference between the mean of the experimental group and the mean of the control group. To accomplish this, a t-test is used to determine the probability that the difference between the means is a real difference rather than a chance difference.

In such a situation, the null hypothesis is expressed as:

$$H_0: M_1 = M_2 \text{ or } H_0: M_1 - M_2 = 0 \tag{1}$$

The alternative hypothesis is:

$$H_1: M_1 = M_2. \tag{2}$$

The formula for the t-test is as follows:

$$t = \frac{M_1 - M_2}{\sqrt{\dfrac{s_1^{\,2}}{N_1} + \dfrac{s_2^{\,2}}{N_2}}} \tag{3}$$

where:

M_1 = mean of experimental group
M_2 = mean of control group
N_1 = number in the experimental group
N_2 = number in the control group
s_1^2 = variance of experimental group
s_2^2 = variance of control group

When the samples are greater than 30 subjects, the t critical values are expressed as z scores. Therefore, the obtained t-value from the formula is compared with the z distribution for acceptance or rejection of the null hypothesis. If the obtained t-value exceeds the z score of 1.96 (two-tailed test), the researcher may conclude that a significant difference exists between the two means at the .05 level (Illustration 9.3)B. Concomitantly, an obtained t-value greater than a 2.58 z score (two-tailed test) allows the researcher to reject the null hypothesis at the .01 level of significance.

One of the concerns that Jon may have about an educational program for AIDS victims is a reduction in the fear and panic displayed by many such victims. If he had two randomly selected groups with one being experimental and the other being control, he could compare the mean of the two groups on a measure designed to reflect fear. The necessary data to test the null hypothesis that there is no difference between the experimental and control groups at the .01 level would be:

Experimental Group	Control Group
$N_1 = 34$	$N_1 = 32$
$M_1 = 75.25$	$M_2 = 70.25$
$s_1^2 = 21$	$s_1^2 = 22$

$$t = \frac{M_1 - M_2}{\sqrt{\dfrac{s_1^2}{N_1} + \dfrac{s_2^2}{N_2}}} = \frac{75.25 - 70.25}{\sqrt{\dfrac{21}{34} + \dfrac{22}{32}}}$$

$$t = \frac{5}{\sqrt{.62 + .69}} = \frac{5}{\sqrt{1.31}} = \frac{5}{1.14}$$

$$t = 4.39$$

Because the obtained t-value from the formula exceeds the z score of 2.58, Jon may reject the null hypothesis at the .01 level of signifi-

**TABLE 9.5   Critical Values for
Large Samples**

	.05 Level	.01 Level
Two-tailed test	1.96	2.58
One-tailed test	1.64	2.33

cance. Table 9.5 shows the t-critical values for the rejection of the null hypothesis in samples with an N greater than 30.

When the samples are fewer than 30 in number (small samples), a t-table is used rather than the normal probability table. The reason for this is that the distribution curves of small samples are different from the normal curve.

The formula for testing the significance of the difference between two small sample means is:

$$t = \frac{M_1 - M_2}{\sqrt{\dfrac{(N-1)s_1^2 + (N-1)s_2^2}{N_1 + N_2 - 2}\left(\dfrac{1}{N_1} + \dfrac{1}{N_2}\right)}}$$

The t-value, which is obtained from the formula, is then compared with the t-value from a t-table with $N_1 + N_2 - 2$ degrees of freedom. If the t-value obtained through the formula exceeds the Table t-value at a specific probability level, then the null hypothesis is rejected at that level.

The t-Test for Two Nonindependent Sample Means

Often the health science researcher is involved with samples in which the composition of one group has bearing on the composition of the other group. For example, the subjects may be matched on one or more characteristics or the same subjects may be in a pretest-posttest experiment. In such cases, the two groups are no longer independent, so a special t-test for nonindependent or correlated means is required. The measure to be analyzed is the difference between the paired scores.

The formula used is

$$t = \frac{M_D}{\sqrt{\dfrac{\Sigma D^2 - \dfrac{(\Sigma D^2)}{N}}{N(N-1)}}}$$

where:

$$D = \text{the difference between the paired scores}$$
$$M_D = \text{the mean of the differences}$$
$$ED^2 = \text{the sum of the squared difference scores}$$
$$N = \text{the number of pairs}$$

The t-value obtained is compared to those in the t-table with $N - 1$ degrees of freedom at the appropriate level of significance.

Analysis of Variance

When comparing the mean of two groups the health science researcher employs the t-test. However, if two or more groups are involved, one of the most powerful methods for comparing means is analysis of variance (ANOVA). For example, a health science investigator may want to determine whether there is a significant difference in blood pressure among three groups of students—those under conditions of high stress, moderate stress and no stress (assuming there are students with no stress!). It is possible to compute a t-test between the means of each pair, but the problems with this approach are (1) ascertaining a level of significance to compensate for "overtesting," (2) the necessity of computing several tests, and (3) the possibility of errors in calculating so many tests. This is particularly so if several groups are involved—five different groups would require ten separate t-tests. ANOVA is able to avoid these problems.

In analysis of variance, as in the t-test, a ratio of observed differences/error is used to test hypotheses. The ratio, called the F-ratio, uses the variance of group means as a measure of observed differences among groups. The within-groups variance (V_w), simply the sum of the variances of each of the groups, is the denominator in the F-ratio. The between-groups variance (V_b), which measures the variation among the means of the groups, is the numerator in the F-ratio.

$$F = \frac{V_b}{V_w} = \frac{\text{between groups variance}}{\text{within groups variance}}$$

The total groups variance (V_{vt}) equals the scores for all groups combined into one composite group.

The rationale of the F-ratio is as follows. The between-groups variance shows the influence of the experimental variable or treatment, while the within-groups variance represents the sampling error in the distributions. If the between groups variance fails to be much greater than the within groups variance, the health scientist would conclude that the difference between the means is likely caused by sampling error. On the other hand, if the F-ratio is substantially greater than 1, it would appear that the difference is likely the result of the treatment.

To determine whether the F-ratio is great enough to reject the null hypothesis at the predetermined level of significance, the researcher must consult an F-table. Like the t-table, it contains the critical values necessary for testing. In entering an F-table, the appropriate degrees of freedom must be used. The between groups variance (V_b) has k − 1 degrees of freedom (where k is the number of groups) and the within groups variance (V_w) has k(N − 1) degrees of freedom (where N is the number of observations in each group).

The analysis of variance is the first step in the analysis of such designs. If a significant F-ratio is obtained, it is only known that somewhere in the data something other than chance is operating. The researcher must employ a special form of the t-test to isolate the presence, nature, and extent of the influencing variable. Examples of such special t-tests are Duncan's multiple range test and tests by Newman-Keuls, Tukey, and Scheffe.

Because ANOVA is a complex tool with several applications, variations, and limitations, it is suggested that the health science investigator consult statistical texts that outline it in detail. The only additional comment to make here is a delineation of the assumptions made when using ANOVA.

1. Observations must be independent.
2. The observations in each group must be normally distributed.
3. The variances of the groups are homogeneous, that is, the variance of each group must be equal to that of any other group.

These can usually be accomplished with well-planned random sampling.

Analysis of Covariance

On occasion intact rather than random groups must be used by the researcher. For example, in an educational setting the health science investigator must employ intact classes for research rather than selecting students randomly and assigning them to control and experimental groups. In such situations, without several pretests, it is difficult to know the initial differences between the groups. To work around this, the analysis of covariance (ANCOVA) can be used to equate the pre-experimental status of the groups. That is, ANCOVA statistically removes the differences in initial status of the groups so that they are equal with respect to one or more control variables. Therefore, if a difference is found between the groups after experimentation, the control variables(s) cannot be used to explain the effect.

Analysis of covariance is useful to the health science researcher when comparison groups can only be matched on the principal variable and not on others. It is a post hoc technique of matching on such variables as prior education, age, and socioeconomic status. Because it requires complex mathematical computations and the demands of several assumptions, the inexperienced health scientist is advised to consult a statistician and complete additional reading such as the volume by Hopkins and Glass (1970).

Test of Significance for Correlation Coefficient

Previously in this chapter the correlation coefficient was discussed as showing the degree of relationship between two variables. The Spearman nonparametric technique and the parametric Pearson Product-Moment technique can be followed by a precedure to determine the statistical significance of the correlation coefficient derived.

In such cases, the null hypothesis states that there is no relationship between the two variables, i.e., correlation is zero. The test of significance of r is through the formula:

$$t_1 = \frac{r - 0}{\sqrt{(1 - r^2)/(N - 2)}}$$

with $N - 2$ degrees of freedom, where N is the number of paired observations. The correlation coefficient is considered significant if the obtained t-value is equal to or greater than the t-value in the t-distribution table.

For example in the Spearman rank order correlation obtained in Table 9.3 the following would apply.

$$t_r = \frac{.62}{\sqrt{[1 - (.62)^2]/(10 - 2)}}$$

$$= \frac{.62}{\sqrt{(1 - .38)/8}} = \frac{.62}{.28} = 2.21$$

$$t_r = 2.21$$

On a two-tailed test at the .05 level of significance with 8 degrees of freedom, the null hypothesis is accepted since the obtained t-value fails to equal or exceed the t-critical value of 2.306.

Nonparametric Tests of Significance

When the health science researcher is working with nonparametric data, nonparametric or distribution-free statistical techniques must be used.

The advantages of nonparametric tests are (1) that they do not have the many restrictions required for parametric tests, (2) they are very suitable for health surveys and experiments in which outcomes are difficult to quantify, and (3) the ease of computation. On the other hand, they (1) are less efficient, (2) are less specific, and (3) fail to deal with all the special characteristics of a distribution.

Some of the most frequently used nonparametric tests are presented in this section.

The Chi-Square Test. The chi-square test (X^2) is generally employed in causal comparative studies and in comparison of observed and theoretical frequencies. As a test of independence, it is not a measure of the degree of relationship but rather used to estimate the likelihood that some factor other than chance accounts for the apparent relationship.

The Mann-Whitney Test (U-test). The Mann-Whitney test is the nonparametric counterpart of the parametric t-test. Simply, it is designed to test the significance of the difference between two randomly drawn samples from the same population. Usually each sample has less than 20 subjects, because more than that allows the sampling distribution of U to approach a normal distribution wherein the t-test may be used.

The Sign Test. The sign test is a procedure for determining the significance of the differences between two correlated or nonindependent samples. For example, experimental and control groups may be matched on several variables or the subjects may be matched with themselves in a pretest-posttest situation wherein they act as a control group in one instance and an experimental group in another. The sign test is particularly useful when the treatment effect cannot be measured but only judged to result in inferior or superior performance.

The Median Test. The median test, a nonparametric test, determines the significance of the difference between the medians of two independent groups, whereas the sign test operates with two correlated groups. It is an application of the X^2 test with a 2×2 table and one degree of freedom.

Wilcoxen Matched-Pairs Signed Rank Test. The Wilcoxen Matched-Pairs Signed Rank Test is employed by the health researcher to ascertain whether two samples differ from each other to a significant degree when there is a relationship between the samples. Although similar to the sign test, it is more powerful because it tests not only direction but also magnitude of difference between matched groups.

The Kruskal-Wallis Test. Developed along the same lines as the Mann-Whitney U-test, the Kruskal-Wallis test is the nonparametric correspondent to the parametric one-way analysis of variance procedure. This would be used when the researcher wished to determine the significance of differences among three or more groups.

The Kendall Coefficient of Concordance. This Kendall coefficent of concordance, frequently referred to as Kendall's concordance coefficient W or the concordance coefficient W, is used in research efforts involving rankings made by independent judges. The Kendall coefficient shows the degree to which such judges agree in their assignment of ranks.

Exploratory Data Analysis

Often the health science researcher retrieves the data and immediately analyzes it through one or several of the techniques previously discussed. According to Borg and Gall (1983), such data are "untouched by human hands" in that they are punched onto computer cards and placed into the computer, and the computer program delivers the requested descriptive or inferential statistics. The failing of this sequence of events is that important patterns and phenomena revealed by the individual scores are overlooked.

Tukey, in his 1977 text *Exploratory Data Analysis,* proposed a practical approach to data analysis that minimizes prior assumptions, allowing the data to guide the choice of appropriate methodology. The statistical techniques, collectively called exploratory data analysis, assist the researcher to gain new insights about the nature of the data and about unexpected or unforeseen patterns.

The four major ingredients of exploratory data analysis are

- *Displays:* reveal the behavior of the data as well as the structure of analyses.
- *Residuals:* bring attention to the data that remain after some analysis.

- *Re-expressions:* simplify behavior and clarify analyses by means of simple mathematical functions such as square root and the logarithm
- *Resistance:* ensures that a few extraordinary data values do not overly affect the results of analysis.

As a means of introduction into this complex form of data analysis, a stem and leaf display is presented using scores from a group of learning-disabled students who participated in an experimental reading curriculum (Leinhardt-Leinhardt, 1980). Table 9.6 shows the data as provided by a computer program. Review of data in this fashion makes it difficult to depict patterns or departures from patterns.

The first column in Table 9.6 is the identification number for each student. The second number is the code for the curricular approach received by each student, and the third column displays the school identification code. The fourth column, titled words, is the number of words read by each student over a three-day period. The fifth column is a measure of silent reading time, and the sixth column is a teacher prediction measure.

In a stem and leaf display, the data values are sorted into numerical order and brought together graphically to reveal patterns and deviations therefrom. For example, the raw data from column 5 of Table 9.6 is summarized in a stem and leaf display in Table 9.7. The basic concept is to let the digits of the data values do the work of sorting into numerical order and graphic display. Generally, a certain number of digits at the beginning of each data value serve as the basis for sorting (herein, the first digit) and the next digit (herein, the second digit) appears in the display to the right of the vertical line. For example, the first score in column 5 of Table 9.6, 0.33, is displayed in the fourth line of Table 6.7, stem and leaf display. Each "leaf" in the display can be converted to a regular score by placing the stem label to the left of it and then multiplying by the unit, .01.

The researcher can view the stem and leaf display of Table 9.7 to find that the scores fail to form a normal distribution. Most of the scores cluster around .30 at the lower end of the scale. Consequently, the researcher is alerted to the need for statistics that do not require a normal distribution.

Another advantage is that the researcher can raise questions and form hypotheses as to why the majority of students scored at the lower end of the scale. Appropriate tests can be made to test the hypotheses developed from viewing the stem and leaf display. Such hypotheses and tests may not be conducted by the researcher who does not use exploratory data analysis.

Further, as in this case of an experimental curriculum, outliers are readily detected. An outlier is simply a research subject whose score

TABLE 9.6   Raw Data Experimental Reading Curriculum

Sequential Location	CUR	School	Words	Silent	Overlap
1	0.00	1.00	2489.00	0.33	48.65
2	0.00	1.00	3755.00	0.80	94.59
3	0.00	1.00	3346.00	0.58	95.95
4	0.00	1.00	3057.00	1.27	44.59
5	0.00	1.00	7002.00	0.84	93.24
6	0.00	1.00	748.00	1.04	97.30
7	0.00	1.00	1462.00	0.36	54.05
8	0.00	1.00	9562.00	1.63	90.54
9	0.00	1.00	4434.00	0.44	91.89
10	0.00	1.00	4295.00	1.15	94.59
11	0.00	2.00	4426.00	0.82	86.49
12	0.00	2.00	1632.00	0.02	6.76
13	0.00	2.00	1626.00	0.92	54.05
14	0.00	2.00	2886.00	0.83	44.59
15	0.00	2.00	484.00	0.35	52.38
16	0.00	2.00	483.00	0.35	53.57
17	0.00	2.00	1867.00	0.25	83.43
18	0.00	2.00	1437.00	0.10	4.05
19	0.00	2.00	1162.00	0.35	6.76
20	0.00	2.00	1676.00	0.38	2.70
21	0.00	2.00	1218.00	0.44	6.76
22	0.00	3.00	0.00	0.52	87.84
23	0.00	3.00	0.00	0.32	81.08
24	0.00	3.00	4713.00	0.27	94.59
25	0.00	3.00	2823.00	0.23	89.19
26	0.00	3.00	1093.00	0.16	25.68
27	0.00	3.00	2560.00	0.17	22.97
28	0.00	3.00	3036.00	0.38	94.59
29	0.00	3.00	4423.00	0.75	98.65
30	0.00	3.00	5811.00	1.13	94.59
31	0.00	3.00	2948.00	0.19	71.62
32	1.00	4.00	198.00	0.48	100.00
33	1.00	4.00	198.00	0.66	97.30
34	1.00	4.00	293.00	0.42	82.43
35	1.00	4.00	293.00	0.25	87.84
36	1.00	4.00	198.00	0.77	85.14
37	1.00	4.00	253.00	0.69	100.00
38	1.00	4.00	253.00	0.64	100.00
39	1.00	4.00	32.00	0.13	64.86
40	1.00	5.00	20.00	0.35	39.19
41	1.00	5.00	999.00	0.62	58.11
42	1.00	5.00	20.00	0.11	52.38
43	1.00	5.00	67.00	0.16	18.82
44	1.00	5.00	20.00	0.35	5.41
45	1.00	5.00	0.00	0.06	39.29
46	1.00	5.00	0.00	0.09	42.86
47	1.00	5.00	67.00	0.48	32.43
48	1.00	5.00	419.00	0.17	24.32
49	1.00	6.00	88.00	0.27	20.27
50	1.00	6.00	212.00	0.44	52.70
51	1.00	6.00	88.00	0.32	10.81
52	1.00	6.00	212.00	0.69	44.59
53	1.00	6.00	212.00	0.49	39.19

TABLE 9.7 Stem and Leaf Display of Experimental Curriculum Scores
Unit = .01 for scale of display

	0	6 9 ←————————————————Stem
	1	0 3 6 6 6 7 7 9
	2	0 3 5 6 7 7
	3	2 2 3 5 5 5 5 5 6 8 8
	4	2 4 4 4 8 8 9
	5	2 8
————→	6	2 4 6 9 9 ←—————————Leaf
Stem label or	7	5 7
starting part	8	0 2 3 4
(leading digits	9	2
used in sorting)	10	4
	11	3 5
	12	7
	13	
	14	←—————————————Separation bar
	15	for starting parts
	16	3 and leaves
N = 53		

differs markedly from those of the other subjects, for example, the student who scored 1.63 (eighth student of column five in Table 9.6). The stem and leaf display in Table 9.7 reveals the outlier very quickly. If an error in calculation was not made, the researcher should seek a plausible explanation as to why this score was obtained. In this instance, Leinhardt and Leinhardt (1980) found that this student was not under the control of the teacher and was therefore not exposed to the same treatment as other members of the class. The decision to remove an outlier from the research study is a problematic one; however, there are statistical techniques that yield quantitative decision rules for identifying outliers. The investigator should report the number of outliers and the technique for handling them in analysis.

Exploratory analysis is relatively new to the health science field, with the result few computer programs are available for use. In order to assist the neophyte, Velleman and Hoaglin (1981) have written a text containing both BASIC and FORTRAN programs for microcomputers or mainframes. If the health science researcher does not have access to software or such a text, the very least that could be done would be to either generate stem and leaf displays by hand or inspect the individual scores for pattens (normal distribution) and outliers. Needless to say, computer programs make the task less demanding and less prone to error.

The Computer for Data Reduction and Analysis_____

Today and even more so in the future, the health science researcher must have computer literacy. It is particularly important for data reduction and subsequent data analysis. Data reduction refers to the process of reducing the data to some form suitable for analysis, whereas data analysis means conducting statistical tests on the data, frequently by computer.

Suppose that Jon, the chief health educator for the city, administered a questionnaire to all the AIDS victims to ascertain their knowledge about AIDS and to determine their usage of health care facilities in the city. He would need to perform data reduction in order to subject the data to computer analysis. To begin, Jon must understand that the answers on the questionnaire must be transferred to computer punch cards and that all the data must be coded in some fashion so that it can be entered onto the cards. Then, via the cards, the data must be analyzed using a computer program that will perform the desired analysis.

The 80-Column Computer Card

More often than not, as in Jon's case, data are transferred from the original documents or from computer recording forms to 80-column computer punch cards. These cards are recognized by almost everyone because they are commonly used for paying bills, registering for classes, or even purchasing concert tickets. Fig. 9.3 shows a standard 80-column punch card. Note that the card has 80 vertical columns

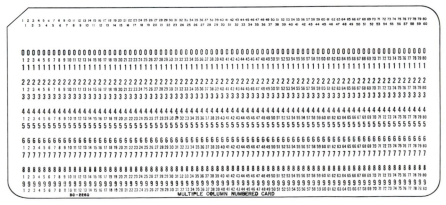

Figure 9.3 Standard 80 Column Punch Card

(identified by numbers at the bottom of the card and between the 1 and 0 punches) and 12 horizontal rows in which 0 through 9 are printed on the card and 11 and 12 are blank. Rows 1 through 9 are called "digit" punches, while rows 0, 11, and 12 are known as "zone" punches. Generally, numerical data are punched into rows 1 through 9.

The first step in working with the computer punch card is to develop a card format. This format is like a road map in that it explains to the computer and researcher where things are located. For example, Jon would need to assign identification numbers to each questionnaire, which would then be punched onto the computer card. This should be done even if the questionnaires were anonymous so that if a keypunching error occurred, the researcher could easily go back and compare the punched card to the actual questionnaire. Because computer cards are addressed from left to right, Jon would designate the first three columns for an identification number. Assuming he had 115 respondents, the first ID number would be 001, the second 002, and so on until 115 was reached. If he had less than one hundred respondents, then only two columns would be necessary.

The next bit of information from the questionnaire may be the gender of the respondent. The potential number of responses is less than ten, consequently only one column needs to be set aside for this information, column four. Columns five and six may denote the ward in which they reside within the city (assuming there are more than 10 but less than 100 wards).

This process continues until all the information on the questionnaire is transferred to the computer punch card. If more than one card is required for each person, the separate set of cards is called a deck. In Jon's case, deck 1 would consist of 115 cards containing the first 80 columns of information from the questionnaire. Deck 2 would be 115 cards containing the second 80 columns of information. Each card should have a deck identification number as well as a respondent ID number.

Because errors can be made in keypunching, it is suggested that all the cards be put through the keypunch machine a second time to verify their accuracy. The keypunch operator simply performs all the same operations and the keypunch machine jams when there is a discrepancy between the number previously punched on the card and the one being punched during the verification process. The operator then checks to determine if the data were entered incorrectly the first time or during the verification process. A related suggestion is to have a duplicate deck of cards produced in case the original is lost or damaged.

Another option open to the researcher is to place the data on computer tape. The data can be transferred from cards to tape very quickly and easily. This is highly recommended if there is a great amount of data. Also, the computer tape can be left at the computer center so that the researcher does not have to carry the cards around all the time. However, professional assistance should be employed if this route is chosen.

Coding for Data Reduction

The principal task of data reduction is coding, wherein a code number is assigned to each answer category so that the answers may be entered onto computer punch cards. This step was briefly mentioned in Chapter 5 in the section on Survey Flow Plan. It is preferable to precode a questionnaire rather than postcode it. The latter may be applicable to open-ended questions.

Returning to the example of Jon, the first three columns of the 80 column punch card are the ID numbers of the respondents. This is an obvious numeric code. However, column four was reserved for gender and the possible codes herein are 1 = male, 2 = female, 9 = no answer. The questionnaire would read as follows:

Gender: (circle one) Male   1   4/

Female 2

The numbers used most often for nonresponse are 9 or 0. If two columns are involved the number is simply repeated e.g. 99, or 999. Note that to the right of the question is a "4/" which tells the keypunch operator which card column is applicable to this answer.

For some questions, the actual numbers may be keypunched onto the cards. For example:

Age at last birthday _____   31–32/

Because two numbers are likely, two columns on the computer card are assigned to the age field.

Another example from Jon's questionnaire could read:

Which of the following health care facilities, if any, do you often use concerning AIDS? (Circle all that apply)

Student health center	1	45/
University hospital	2	46/
St. Mary's hospital	3	47/
General hospital	4	48/
City clinic	5	49/
HMO clinic	6	50/
Other	7	51/

In this example, the respondent is asked to circle all that apply, therefore more than one column is needed. If the respondent was requested to circle only the one most used, only one response would occur and only one card column would be needed. However, because the respondent could circle as many as he or she wished, a separate column for each response is allotted. Herein, if the respondent circled University hospital (2) and HMO clinic (6) the keypuncher would punch a 2 in column 46 and a 6 in column 50. The researcher should be aware that questions such as this take up valuable computer card space and may necessitate the use of more than one card per person. Further, assurances must be made that the blank columns are not treated as nonresponses. In such instances, 0 = inapplicable could be used.

Precoding is very important and has the advantages of eliminating a code book and the need for the researcher to read all questionnaires and mark a code for each answer.

Computer Programs for Data Analysis

Data obtained by the researcher may be analyzed by hand, by calculator, or by computer—desktop or mainframe. If the number of subjects is small and the necessary calculations simple, the researcher may choose to do the work by hand or with a calculator. For example, a calculator was used to determine the Pearson Product-Moment correlation between victim age and number of sexual contacts since diagnosis for Jon's subjects in Table 9.4. This took about 20 minutes. Needless to say, a computer would be able to accomplish several such correlations within one minute; however, the time of preparation and cost in dollars did not make it feasible. The neophyte researcher should understand that the cost of programming for a few subjects is about the same as for studies involving a great many subjects. However, if Jon wished to perform several analyses on his data of 115 respondents, he should make appropriate use of computer programs.

The computer programs most commonly used are in SPSS (Statistical Package for the Social Sciences), SAS (Statistical Analysis System) and SAS/Graph. SPSS is a collection of statistical procedures for data analysis and data management. SAS and SAS/Graph are an integrated system of programs for data analysis and presentation of the results in numeric and graphic form. If an established computer program such as these is to be used, the researcher should learn the demands of the program before keypunching the cards, because different programs may require a specialized format. Further, programs have established limits on both the number of subjects and the number of variables to be analyzed. If these are ignored, the program will not run and the data will not be analyzed.

Once a computer program or statistical package has been selected, it is simply a matter of adding the control cards to the data deck and submitting it as "input" to the computer center for processing. The control cards are standard 80-column computer cards that contain such information as number of respondents, number of variables, and appropriate fields in the card format. For established programs, such as in SPSS or SAS, a handbook or manual will describe the construction of control cards. The beginner should seek out a consultant for assistance—usually one or more are available at university computer centers.

The output from the computer can be received within minutes or days depending upon the nature of the analyses, the backlog at the computer center, and of course computer malfunction. As any computer user can tell you, it is very frustrating to wait for your output and then discover that it did not run because of an error in the control cards or the data cards. To avoid this problem, be certain to check the deck of cards carefully before submitting it. The output or computer printout is usually interpreted easily. If difficulty does arise, either the handbook or a consultant should be sought out for advice. It is recommended that the researcher not write on the computer printout because it may later be photoreduced for use in a research report, master's thesis, or doctoral dissertation. This saves money for retyping and eliminates the possibility of error in transferring the data to a typed page.

The increase in the number of personal computers (PC's) may make it more convenient to complete analyses as opposed to a large mainframe computer. On occasion, the purchase of a computer includes software that can be used for statistical analysis. If not, there are several excellent software packages ranging from very inexpensive to very expensive that can be purchased or even leased. Another option is that the health science researcher may have a modem on the personal computer that will allow connection to a university mainframe. This may allow either the seasoned researcher or the research student to sit in the office or at home to conduct complex analyses. Small hand-held computers are currently available; however they are much more limited in data analysis applications than desktop PC's.

Checking for Accuracy in Data Analysis

As noted in the section on exploratory data analysis, the researcher often fails to know the data. That is, he or she lacks a "feel" for what the data are about. The same holds true for data analysis. The researcher should be able to understand how the data are handled and manipulated to bring forth the results. When using a calculator, the researcher may repeat the calculations or check the printed tape output for error. However, when a computer is used this is not possible. Therefore, it is mandatory that the research student have adequate knowledge of what the results should look like. As an obvious example, Jon should know that his Pearson Product-Moment correlation should not read -1.25. After obtaining the computer printout, Jon may wish to check one of the calculations by redoing it with a calculator. If everything works out, then he may be more assured that the computer program is correct.

Summary

Chapter 9 began with a discussion of statistics—a language to organize, analyze, and interpret numerical data—including descriptive and inferential statistics. Descriptive statistics function to describe data, whereas inferential statistical analysis involves observation of a sample taken from a given population. Conclusions about the population are then inferred from the sample. Statistical techniques were found to vary with the nature of the data, either parametric or nonparametric.

Specific descriptive data analysis techniques were presented as measures of central tendency, measures of spread or variation, and measures of relationship. The mean, median, and mode were the three measures of central tendency. The measures of spread were the range, variance, and the standard deviation. Both the Pearson Product-Moment correlation and the Spearman Rank Order correlation were discussed for parametric and nonparametric data. The correlation coefficient was presented as a pure, nondimensional number that may take on values between -1.00 and $+1.00$.

Inferential data analysis techniques included regression analysis and prediction, tests of statistical significance (t-tests), analysis of variance, analysis of covariance, and tests of significance for a correlation coefficient. In regard to tests of significance, the null and alternative hypotheses were discussed as were the critical region, levels of significance, and Type I and II errors. Nonparametric tests of significance reviewed were the chi square, the Mann-Whitney Test U-test, the sign test, the median test, the Wilcoxen matched-pairs signed rank test, the Kruskal-Wallis test, and the Kendall coefficient of concordance.

Exploratory data analysis was seen to be important in helping a health science researcher to gain new insights about the nature of the data and about unexpected or unforeseen patterns. Stem and leaf displays were discussed and an example presented. It was recommended that health science researchers perform some type of exploratory data analysis before subjecting the data to complete analysis.

Data reduction was discussed as a preparatory step for computer data analysis. The 80-column computer punch card was presented in regard to formatting and data entry. Coding was viewed as an essential component in data reduction, and precoding was recommended over postcoding.

Data analysis began with the notation of two major computer programs: SPSS and SAS. The steps for arranging input data were discussed as well as potential problems with output. Microcomputers may serve as a tool for data analysis depending upon the software available and the possible use of a modem to connect to a mainframe. Checking for accuracy was seen as an important procedure no matter what data analysis technique was used.

Suggested Activities

1. You have administered a health knowledge test to two different groups (N = 20) with the scores listed below. Calculate the mean, median, range, and standard deviation for each group. Compare the means of the two groups using a t-test. The highest possible score is 100.

Group A		Group B	
95	45	91	86
87	67	97	81
91	81	88	79
75	63	81	96
56	77	77	72
59	49	83	88
61	72	87	93
45	76	79	79
58	80	84	89
78	82	90	78

2. Visit the university computer center and become familiar with all the steps necessary to submit a data deck.
3. Consult with a faculty member, personal computer club, or PC magazine to determine what software is available for PCs for data analysis. Make a brief list of such software, including the type of operating system necessary. Be able to explain the difficulties in ascertaining such information and the factors that may play a role in selecting particular software.

4. Review the handbooks for SPSS and SAS to learn what types of programs are available to you for data analysis and what limitations or restrictions they have for keypunching and analysis.

5. You have been asked to serve as a consultant to the school superintendent for a project involving students who have taken health education and those who have not. The students were randomly selected and assigned to control and experimental groups, with the experimental group receiving health education. The data have been collected by means of a health knowledge test, an attitude scale toward healthful living, and a behavior inventory. Both the attitude scale and the behavior inventory can be compiled to have one score per student. The superintendent wants your advice on

   a. what can be done to determine if there is a significant difference between the two groups in regard to (1) knowledge, (2) attitude, and (3) behavior.

   b. writing out the respective null and alternative hypotheses appropriate to this research project.

   c. what tests of significance you would recommend to the superintendent and why.

   d. what level of significance you would recommend and why.

6. As patient education and wellness coordinator at the hospital, you administered two different health risk appraisals (HRAs) to a group of 45 people taking part in your weight loss classes. The data of most interest to you are appraised age, achieveable age, and the recommended weight in pounds. You wish to determine if there is a significant difference between the two HRAs on all three variables. How would you proceed? What would be the appropriate null hypotheses? What level of significance would you set? What tests of significance would you use?

   As a further point of data analysis, you would like to ascertain the relationship between achievable age and the number of pounds of weight to be lost by the participant. How would you go about this? Which correlation technique would you employ? Why?

References

Borg, W. R. and Gall, M. D. (1983) *Educational Research,* New York: Longman.

Glass, G. (1977) Integrating findings: the meta-analysis of research. In Schulman, L. (ed.), *Review of Research in Education,* Vol. 5, Itasca, Il: F. E. Peacock.

Hays, W. L. (1973) *Statistics for the Social Sciences,* 2nd ed., New York: Holt, Rinehart and Winston.

Hopkins, K. D. and Glass, G. V. (1970) *Basic Statistics for the Behavioral Sciences,* Englewood Cliffs, NJ: Prentice-Hall.

Kuzma, J. (1984) *Basic Statistics for the Health Sciences,* Palo Alto, CA: Mayfield Publishing Company.

Leinhardt, G. and Leinhardt, S. (1980) Exploratory data analysis: new tools for the analysis of emperical data. In Berlinger, D. C. (ed.), *Review of Research in Education,* Washington, D.C.: American Educational Research Association.

Siegel, W. (1956) *Nonparametric Statistics,* New York: McGraw-Hill.

Tukey, J. W. (1977) *Exploratory Data Analysis,* Reading, MA: Addison-Wesley.

Velleman, P. F. and Hoaglin, D. C. (1981) *Applications, Basics, and Computing of Exploratory Data Analysis,* Boston: Duxbury Press.

Wilson, V. and Putnam, R. (1982) A meta-analysis of pretest sensitization effects in experimental design, *American Journal of Research* 19 (2): 249–258.

CHAPTER 10

Presenting the Data

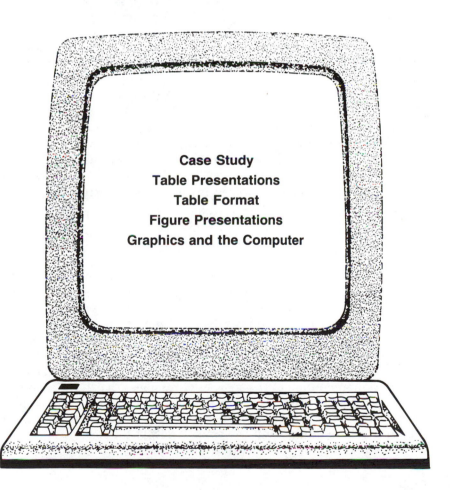

Case Study
Table Presentations
Table Format
Figure Presentations
Graphics and the Computer

Case Study_____

Jonathon, a senior at Newtown University, is enrolled in a health sciences research course. The major semester assignment is to conduct a research study using the components learned in the course. In other words, Jonathon was to state the problem, derive hypotheses, conduct a literature search, conceive the methodology, actually carry out the experiment, present and analyze the data, and summarize the project including conclusions and recommendations. If he has read the text to this point, Jonathon will be equipped with the necessary knowledge to complete the assignment. This chapter will enable Jonathon to present the data he collects for his study. Usually the form of data presentation includes tables, figures, and graphics.

Table Presentations_____

The first part of this chapter will discuss the presentation of tables in manuscripts for publication, reports, books, term papers, master's theses, and doctoral dissertations. The purpose for including tables and several types of tables will be described. In addition, we will discuss the relationship between the table and the text, which is a very important consideration. Finally, the format of tables will be detailed so that you can construct a proper table. The section concludes with guidelines for including tables.

Purpose of Tables

Tables usually represent quantitative material (numbers) and sometimes words that present qualitative comparisons or descriptive information. As an example of a word table, Jonathon could use a table to depict some of the questions and their responses in the questionnaire he used. Word tables should not repeat what has been discussed in the text, but rather illuminate that discussion. Using tables to depict collected data enables the reader to have a clear understanding and comprehension of the masses of numbers that have been collected during the project. The analysis of original data should be presented in these tables so that readers are not burdened with long lines of numbers that disrupt the smooth flow of the text. Data should be presented so that their significance is easily recognized by the reader.

Tables are used to present information in the form of totals and subtotals, rank-order relationships, and results of statistical analyses (Campbell, Ballou, and Slade, 1982). Once you have decided what data belongs in the table, there are a few additional considerations (American Psychological Association, 1983):

1. Rounded-off values may display patterns more clearly than precise numbers.
2. A reader will be able to compare numbers down a column more easily than across a row.
3. Row and column averages can provide a visual focus that allows the reader to inspect the data easily.
4. Ample spacing between rows and columns can improve a table because the white space creates a perceptual order to the data. (p. 84)

It should be noted here that some institutions of higher education suggest or mandate use of a particular style or publication manual. You should consult with the appropriate personnel to determine which, if any, style manual is utilized. Many health science departments utilize the *Publication Manual of the American Psychological Association* (APA), because it is preferred for most journals to which potential social sciences authors might submit their projects for publication.

Relating the Tables to the Text

A good table should supplement the text of the paper. However, you should refer to all tables and their data in the text. A discussion of the highlights of the table is all that is necessary in the paper, and each table should have a brief introduction that explains the manner in which the data are presented and suggests their general meaning. Two rules apply to the inclusion of tables:

1. Each table should be understandable without reference to the text.
2. The text should be complete so that the reader may follow it without referring to the tables.

In the text, tables are referred to by their numbers. They are numbered consecutively, using arabic numerals; for example:

Table 4 shows . . .
. . . behavioral scores with no pretest (see Table 4)

TABLE 10.1 Mean Knowledge Scores of Pretested and Unpretested Students

This summarizes the mean knowledge scores of the students who took the health science test. The students were asked their health knowledge in regard to smoking, nutrition, and exercise. In both the pretested and unpretested groups, girls achieved slightly higher scores on the test. However, scores of both groups were very similar and showed no difference between the pretested and unpretested groups.

Group	n	Health Science Test
Girls		
Pretested	120	18
Unpretested	110	20
Boys		
Pretested	118	17
Unpretested	108	19

Note: Maximum score was 30.

The actual placement of the table is sometimes a difficult decision. Should it go after the analysis? Before? Here are some rules that may be helpful:

1. Each table should be placed entirely on one page.
2. Text material may be placed on the same page with a table about one-half page or less.
3. A table should be separated from the text by three spaces above and below (Table 10.1).
4. A table containing both a table and text should begin with the text material.
5. If all the preceeding conditions cannot be met, a table should be placed between paragraphs (Pelegrino, 1979).

Single-Variable Tables

Single variables are usually used in a descriptive or explanatory study. Measurements such as the range, mean, mode, or median may be depicted in such a table. In addition, frequency distributions and grouped data may be presented. Table 10.1 is an example of a single-variable table in that one score was reported. Table 10.2 depicts the frequency distribution for the scores on the health science knowledge test.

TABLE 10.2 Frequency Distribution of Scores on Health Science Knowledge Test

Score	Frequency	Score	Frequency	Score	Frequency
1	0	11	18	21	38
2	0	12	20	22	20
3	0	13	22	23	17
4	0	14	20	24	14
5	0	15	25	25	13
6	0	16	35	26	7
7	6	17	36	27	4
8	7	18	40	28	0
9	15	19	41	29	0
10	14	20	44	30	0

Percentage Tables

Percentages can provide an efficient way to summarize information. These data can be reported in single or multiple variable form. The listing of percentages as presented in Table 10.3 should be summed. An indication of sample size is also important so that the percentages will not be misleading. There is an important question you might be asking here: What happens to the nonrespondents? Should they be included in the computation for the percentages? There are two methods that you could choose to answer this dilemma. The first is to subtract the number of nonresponses from the total sample size and use this new figure as the base for the percentages. In our example, Jonathon may have a sample size of 456, but only 411 students reported their gender. In this case the 45 nonrespondents would be omitted and 411 rather than 456 would be the base for computing the respective percentages. A second method of dealing with nonrespondents is to use the total sample size (456) as the base and include the nonrespondents as a percentage. In our case study of 456, assume that 205 were males, 206 were females, and 45 were nonrespondents. If we used the first method (using 411 as a base) we

TABLE 10.3 Sex Distribution for Students Taking Health Science Knowledge Test

Sex	Percentage
Males	45
Females	55
	100.0
	(456)

would be able to write that 50 per cent were males and 50 per cent females. By the second method (456 as base) we would have 45 per cent males, 45 per cent females, and 10 per cent nonrespondents (Bailey, 1982). If we continue to use nonrespondents as part of the analysis, the base number remains constant and adds stability to all the analyses.

Contingency (Bivariate) Tables

Health science studies, as well as other social science investigations, sometimes focus upon the relationship between two variables. Tables are used to display the way the values of the variables are associated. Interrelationships are examined and are thus called cross-tabulations or contingency tables. In these kinds of tables, all combinations of categories of all the variables are presented. However, the most usual form is the two-variable table, each variable being dichotomous. Therefore, two dichotomous variables present a table with four cells, sometimes labeled a fourfold table.

Through evolution, one variable has been termed the *column variable* and is labeled across the top so its categories form vertical columns down the page and usually represent the independent variable. The other variable, the *row variable,* is labeled on the left margin, forming categories of rows across the page and thus the dependent variable. The intersections of the categories of these two variables form the interior of the table. An easy way to construct this contingency table is to list the total frequencies in each category for each variable. The simplest dichotomous variables and most frequently used are gender and race. If we had 100 respondents to a survey concerning health risk factors we would have 100 as a total for gender and race (each person has a gender and race). Table 10.4 shows that we have 50 males, 60 blacks, and 40 whites.

The numbers outside the square are referred to as *marginals.* The row marginals are 60 and 40, and the column marginals are 50 and

TABLE 10.4   Race by Gender

Race	Male		Female		
Black	30	a	30	b	60
					a+b
White	20	c	20	d	40
					c+d
	50		50		
	a+c		b+d		
			100 = a+b+c+d		

50. The row and column marginals provide no information about each other, but are found in the interior of of the cells. You should, once again, be sure to note the N (100) in the lower right-hand corner, which is attained by adding either the row or column marginals.

Absolute numbers should be used in the cells when a statistical analysis will be conducted. This analysis is always placed at the bottom of the table. If, however, no statistical analysis will be used, then percentages should be used in the cells. Usually, the independent variable is presented in percentages, thus the columns become percentaged.

Multivariable Tables

Multivariable tables contain three or more variables, and are similar to those presented in the previous sections. Jonathon would use such a table in his paper if he wanted to report on a number of variables and their association or correlation. The format is typically a correlation matrix, which presents the correlations between all the pairs of variables in the analysis. If we had five variables we would want to show the relationship between each pair of variables. The matrix as in Table 10.5 would list all the variables along the left-hand margin of the table, except for the last one. At the top of the table, the variables are listed beginning with the second variable. The obtained correlations are presented once for each pair of variables.

You might wonder why there is a blank space in the lower left-hand corner of Table 10.5. If these correlation coefficents were in-age of those already included in the table. The same is true for the omission of the last variable from the row listing and the first variable from the column listing (Abrahamson, 1983). The dependent variable should be placed in the last column, column E in Table 10-5. Now you can easily determine the relationship between the dependent variable and each of the independent variables.

Another type of multivariable table that is frequently used is the

TABLE 10.5 Correlation Matrix-Multivariable Table

Variable	B	C	D	E
A	.10	.30	.40	.35
B		.72	.50	.62
C			.21	.41
D			.48	.48
E				.22

TABLE 10.6   Analysis of Variance Table

Source of Variance	SS	df	MS	F	Level of Significance
Between groups	261.1	2	100.1	21.0	.01*
Within groups	687.8	144	477.7		
Total	888.9	146	577.8		

*<p.01.

analysis of variance table (ANOVA). Table 10.6 is an example of how to set up the ANOVA table.

Table Format

As we have mentioned previously, each institution will have a set of guidelines for students and professors to use when submitting reports, articles, and the like. The following discussion should enable you to ascertain the many different terms associated with constructing a table. Table 10.7 has been devised to depict these many terms.

TABLE 10.7—*table number*
Mean Scores of Students with Pretesting and without Pretesting—*table title*

stub head— **Group**	n^a	**Grade**—*column spanner*		
		7	**8**	**9**—*column heads*
Knowledge Tests—*table spanner*				
Boys *row stubs*				
Pretested	118	17	18	20
Unpretested	108	19	22	21
Girls				
Pretested	120	18	19	20
Unpretested	110	20	21	20
Body *Attitude Tests* —*table spanner*				
Boys				
Pretested	118	18	20^b	22
Unpretested	108	20	22	23
Girls				
Pretested	120	19	20	21
Unpretested	110	22	24	23

stub column   *columns*

Note. Maximum score on each test was 30.—*note to table*
[a]Numbers of students out of 125 in each group who completed both tests.
[b]Two boys had identical answers.

Table Numbers

All tables should be numbered consecutively with arabic numerals. In a book chapter, use sequential numbers preceded by the chapter number and a decimal point. We have used this method throughout this book. In the text of your report, paper, or thesis, refer to the tables by number, not by the title. If your manuscript includes an appendix with tables, identify the tables of the appendix with capital letters and arabic numerals: Table B.1 would be the first table of Appendix B.

Table Titles

The title of a table should be clear and brief and should explain the table. *Avoid* using information contained in the headings of the table; for example:

> Relation Between Attitude and Knowledge Tests

This would be unclear and not tell what data is contained in the table. Another bad example is:

> Mean Health Science Knowledge and Attitude Scores of Girls and Boys
> in Grades 7, 8, & 9 Who Were Pretested and Not Pretested

This is too detailed and duplicates the information in the table headings. A better example is:

> Mean Scores of Students With Pretesting & Without Pretesting

This is a *good* table title in that it explains clearly what the data will tell the reader.

Table Body

The body of a table contains the data. Mullins (1977) suggests the following guidelines when constructing the body of a table:

1. Use as few entries as possible without eliminating vital information.
2. Within each table, use the same rules for retaining decimals and for rounding.
3. Arrange entries so that the most important comparisons are between adjacent numbers.
4. To prevent confusion of percentages and numbers, place a percent sign (%) after the first number in a column of percentages

that add up to 100 per cent. Also use "percentage" in the column heading.
5. If a column head does not apply to an item in a row stub (this is called a *cell*), leave the cell blank.
6. If rounding prevents the sum of percentages in an additive column from being 100 per cent, use a footnote to explain.
7. Do not use intersecting lines to connect items in different columns.

Stub

Stub is the name for the rows in the far left-hand column of the table. The names of these columns should be short, clear, and grammatically consistent. The stubs usually present the independent variables. If you use abbreviations, use them consistently in all tables and use a note to explain the abbreviations in your first table.

Stub Column

The stub column is the column of row stubs and their subcategories. In Table 10.7 these rows are denoted by *Boys, Girls, Pretested, and Unpretested*. The subcategories should be indented at least one space from the margin to distinguish them from the row stubs.

Stubhead

The stubhead is the title of the stub column. In Table 10.7 *Group* is the stubhead.

Column Head

The column head names the column and should be grammatically consistent. These heads usually name the dependent variables, dependent upon the discipline and guidelines followed. In Table 10.7, for example, *7, 8,* and *9* are the column heads.

Column Spanner

The column spanner identifies two or more columns, each of which has its own column head. In Table 10.7 *Grade* is the column spanner.

Table Spanner

Table spanners cover the entire width of the body of the table, allowing for further divisions within the table. *Knowledge Tests* and

Attitude Tests in Table 10.7 denote table spanners. Table spanners can also be utilized to combine two tables into one as they are in Table 10.7.

Notes

Tables have three types of notes: general notes, specific notes, and probability notes. These are always placed below the table. *General note.* General notes explain, qualify, or provide information relating to the entire table. This may include an explanation of abbreviations, symbols, and so on. These notes are designated by the word <u>Note.</u> (underlined, followed by a period). In Table 10.7, it reads:

<u>Note.</u> Maximum score on each test was 30.

In addition, general notes indicate that a table is reprinted from another source. To do this, you must obtain permission to reproduce or adapt all or part of a table from a copyrighted source. Give credit to the original author and to the copyright holder.

Example of Note from Book

<u>Note.</u> From *Health Education: Foundations for the Future* (p. 120) by L. Rubinson and W. Alles, 1984, St. Louis: Mosby Times/Mirror. Copyright 1984 by Mosby Times/Mirror. Reprinted by permission.

Example of Note from Article

<u>Note.</u> From "Hypertension Compliance" by T. Chval, 1980, *Journal of Compliance,* 1, p. 1. Copyright 1980 by *Journal of Compliance.* Reprinted by permission.

Specific Note. A specific note refers to a particular column or to an individual entry. Specific notes are indicated by superscript lowercase letters (superscript a in Table 10.7, for example). Within the headings and body of the table, the superscripts are ordered horizontally from left to right across the table by rows, beginning at the top left. Each table is independent of any others; therefore notes always begin on each table, with superscript a.

Probability Level Note. A probability level note indicates the results of significance tests. Asterisks indicate the probability levels of tests of significance. When more than one level appears in a table, use one asterisk for lowest level, two for the next, and so on. These levels and the number of asterisks do not have to be consistent from table to table. Table 10.8 is an example of utilizing the probability level note.

Note Format. The ordering of the notes in a table is general first, specific second, and probability level third.

Example of Order of Notes

> *Note.* Maximum score on each test was 30.
> [a]Numbers of students out of 125 in each group who completed both tests.
> *p<.05.   **p<.01.

Each type of note begins at the margin on a new line, beginning with the general note. The first specific note begins flush left on a new line and all subsequent specific notes follow one after the other on the same line. The first probability level notes follow one another.

These parts of a table have been presented so that you can easily construct a good, coherent, and useful table. The following are some guidelines you might use when constructing your tables (American Psychological Association, 1983):

1. Is the table necessary?
2. Is the entire table, including the title and headings, doublespaced?
3. Are all similar tables in the manuscript consistent in presentation?
4. Is the table brief, but explanatory?
5. Does every column have a column heading?
6. Are all probability level values correctly identified, and are asterisks attached?
7. Are the notes in the proper order: general, specific, probability level?
8. If all or part of a copyrighted table is reproduced, do the table notes state this?
9. Is the table referred to in the text? (p. 94)

TABLE 10.8 Example of Probability Level Note

E
1.70*
3.86**

*p.<.05
**p<.01

Figure Presentations

This section describes how figures should be utilized in a manuscript. The various types of figures will be discussed, as well as how to cite figures in the text. A general discussion of instructions for preparing figures with an accompanying list of guidelines completes the section. We have determined, for use in this text, that figures encompass any type of illustration other than a table. These may be in the form of charts, graphs, photographs, maps, or drawings. The author provides these materials for the publisher to photograph.

Purpose of Figures

Figure, as mentioned, refers to charts, graphs, drawings, maps, and photographs. They are used to present data very clearly and concisely. The inclusion of a figure should be carefully considered, because figures are expensive to produce, both for the author and publisher. Therefore, figures should be used only when they actually contribute something to a paper. Some points to consider when including a figure are

1. Is the figure important and necessary?
2. Does it efficiently present information?
3. What idea do you need to convey?
4. What type of figure is best for your paper? (American Psychological Association, 1983, p. 95)

Sometimes it becomes confusing to decide if you should use a table or a figure. A good rule of thumb might be, if the data shows trends, it could be better augmented by a figure rather than a table. Remember that a good figure should not duplicate what is contained in the text, should be easy to read and understand, and should be carefully prepared. You can employ a professional artist to do the work, or you can attempt the project yourself. Check the guidelines from your college or university, or from the journal (if you are submitting a manuscript for publication).

Types of Figures

There are many types of figures. Those we will discuss here include graphs, charts, dot maps, drawings, and photographs.

Graphs. Graphs usually show how things are compared or distributed. These come in the form of percentages or absolute values.

There are several types of graphs: line graphs, bar graphs, scatter graphs, and circle graphs.

Line graphs. Line graphs are used to show trends or results of a line series experiment. The independent variable is plotted on the x axis (horizontal) and the dependent variable is plotted on the y axis (vertical). See Fig. 10.1 for an example. The length of the y axis should be approximately two thirds the length of the x axis. The grid marks (dashes) on the axes denote the units of measurement. If changes on the axes are disproportionate, the differences will be distorted. Thus, the curve or slant of the line must accurately depict the data. Notice the double slash on the axes in Fig. 10.1. This indicates that the origin of the coordinates is not zero.

Bar graphs. Bar graphs are easy to read and construct (see Fig. 10.2). Solid vertical or horizontal bars present one kind of data. There are also subdivided bar graphs (each bar shows two or more kinds of data); multiple bar graphs (whole bars represent different variables in one data set); and sliding bar graphs (bars are split by a vertical line that serves as the reference for each bar).

Circle graphs. Circle or pie graphs show percentages and proportions (see Figure 10.3). A general rule to follow, for clarity, is to depict only five or fewer items. The segments should be ordered from large to small, with the largest segment beginning at the 12:00 position and moving clockwise to the smallest. The differences in segments should be highlighed from light to dark, with the smallest por-

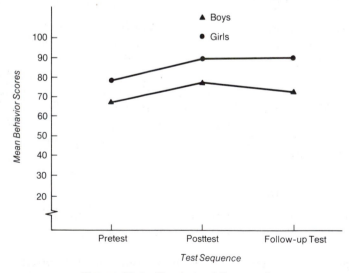

Figure 10.1   Example of line graph.

Mean Scores of Sixth, Seventh, & Eighth Grade Students
on the Comprehensive Health Science Test, 1986-87.

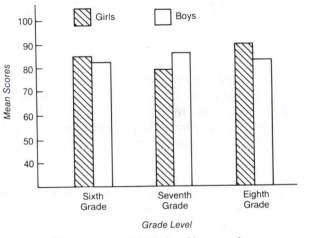

Figure 10.2   Example of bar graph.

Time Alloted for Health Science Classes:
Newbury High School, 1978-1987.

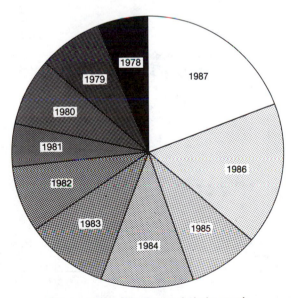

Figure 10.3   Example of circle graph.

tion being the darkest. Using different patterns of lines and dots shows the shaded patterns.

Scatter graphs. Scatter graphs consist of single dots that are plotted as on a line graph, but the dots are not joined together (see Fig. 10.4). The dots represent where the variables intersect, and a cluster of dots along a diagonal indicates a correlation.

Charts. Charts can describe relationships between group segments on the sequence of operations in a process. These are usually depicted by boxes that are connected by lines. Examples include charts of organizations (see Fig. 10.5), flow charts showing a step-by-step process, and schematics that show components in a system (e.g., a television circuit board).

Drawings. Drawings are usually prepared by a professional artist because they are difficult to accomplish. The drawing should be as simple as possible so that the author's idea can be easily conveyed. A drawing enables the author to augment the manuscript by providing ideas and images from different viewpoints: two-dimensional and side views.

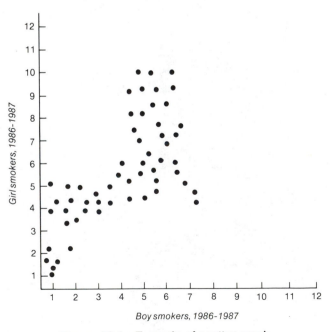

Figure 10.4 Example of scatter graph.

DEPARTMENT OF HEALTH AND SAFETY STUDIES
Organizational Chart

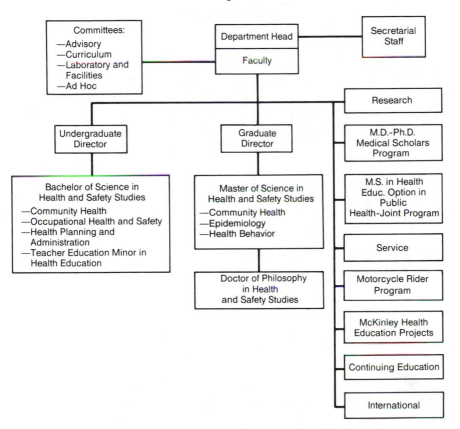

Figure 10.5 Example of organizational chart.

Photographs. Professional photography is important when photographs are used in a manuscript. They can provide focus and interest points and add something of value to the words in a manuscript. Inform the photographer that there should be a strong contrast between the subject and the background. The use of black-and-white film is mandatory, because color prints are difficult to reproduce accurately. When photographing people, attempt to get a signed consent form from those people. When using a photograph from another source (book, journal, or other), obtain the original picture (because photographs of photographs do not reproduce adequately). You must also obtain written permission to reprint from the coypright holder and must acknowledge the holder in the figure caption (American Psychological Association, 1983).

Citing of Figures

When using a figure, it should be placed as close as possible to the first reference made to it in the manuscript. The figures should be consecutively numbered with arabic numerals in the order as they are mentioned, e.g. *Figure 1, Figure 2, Figure 3*. The number should be written lightly in pencil on the back of the figure, near to the edge. In addition, note the top of the figure and write the figure's title (again, lightly). In the manuscript refer to figures by numbers, for example,

Figure 1 shows, . . .

The data are related (see Figure 1).

Avoid writing "see the figure above or below" on a specific page. This is because the placement of figures cannot be determined until the manuscript is typeset. The printer should be apprised of the approximate placement of the figure by a break in the text and a note:

Insert Figure 1 about here

The same procedure is used for noting the placement of tables.

Captions and Legends

The *caption* is the explanation of the figure and is placed below it. The caption describes the contents of the figure in a sentence or a phrase.

Example of Figure Caption

Figure 1. Time and set point between attitude and behavior surveys.

Information that is needed to clarify the limits of measurement should be placed in the caption in parentheses after the caption. It is important that all terminology used in the text and the figures agree.

The *legend* is a key to the symbols in the figure. There are some standard legend symbols: ■, ●, and ▲. Fig. 10.6 is an example of a figure with a legend. The legend is put into the figure and should have the same kind and size of lettering that is utilized in the figure.

All figure captions should be typed (double-spaced) on a separate page. The notation *Figure Captions* should appear in the top center of the page, and each caption should be flush to the left margin. Under-

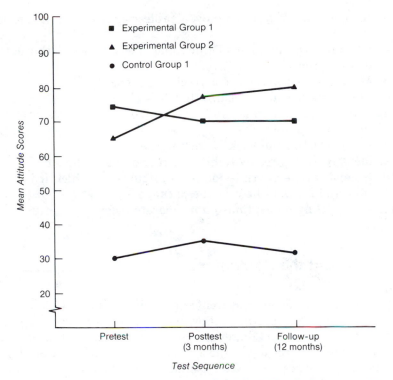

Figure 10.6 Mean attitude scores of eighth grade students over 12 months.

line *figure,* and capitalize only the first word and proper names. Double-space if there is more than one line.

Example of Figure Page

Figure 1 The relationship of skills and attitudes to health science knowledge.

Instructions for Preparing Figures

The following list provides some general instructions for preparing figures for manuscripts, reports, term papers, theses, dissertations, and so on.

1. Place each figure on a separate page measuring 8½″ × 11″. Sometimes you will have to use larger paper. In these cases, check with your local format procedures.
2. Check to make sure that the figure is necessary.

3. Do not type letters; employ a professional or use a lettering stencil.
4. Minimize the number of lines and check to see if the data is plotted properly.
5. Make sure all words are correctly spelled.
6. Check the legend to ensure that it is clear.
7. Use arabic numerals, and be sure that all figures are mentioned in the text.
8. Write *TOP* on the back of each figure.
9. Identify all figures by lightly writing on back of each.
10. Receive written permission for all figures for which it is necessary and include them in the package.
11. Write all figure captions on a separate page.

Graphics and the Computer

Computers have given researchers a distinct advantage: speed and accuracy. Computer programs allow us to use word processors to prepare reports, theses, and dissertations. We can also use the computer to help prepare figures and tables. This section will give a brief overview of computer graphics. We recommend that you consult computer experts on your campus and microcomputer software programs for a specific review of graphics for your own computer. Much of the following information has been taken from Demel and Miller's *Introduction to Computer Graphics*.

The Impact of Computer Graphics

Pictures, charts, and graphs have always added to the written word by enhancing or explaining sometimes complex thoughts and ideas. With the advent of computer graphics, we have more efficient ways of producing these enhancements.

Applications of Computer Graphics

Many fields such as engineering, business, art, education, and the chemical and biological sciences have utilized computer graphics. Engineers have used the computer to provide graphics in five areas: design, analysis, drawing, manufacturing/construction/processing, and quality control. Chemical scientists who study the structure of chemical substances use x-rays to determine the location of atoms in molecular structures. Using computer graphics allows chemical scientists to complete more complicated structure determinations and provides a faster way to determine the structures.

In the business world, computer graphics have enabled companies to send reports to management that aid in making decisions concerning selling, buying, or expansion. Graphics can be presented in color or black and white and even integrated with the text, which saves time when producing a report. Computers have also provided businesses with *modeling,* which is a type of program that simulates the action of the marketplace.

In the field of art, computer graphics are utilized for illustration, for creating images and repetitive patterns, for animation, and for dynamic displays. When the many and repetitive drawings animators have to make to merely change the movement of a leg are considered, the computer certainly has offered an opportunity for the artist to be more efficient and productive in her or his work.

Education has benefited from computer graphics in that the learner can interact with the computer, and dynamic motion enables complicated concepts to be more easily presented. Objects appear more real and three-dimensional, which enhances the learning of students. New graphics systems can provide pictures of real objects for the user to point to or select. These are called *icons,* for example, a picture of a trash can to indicate the action of throwing something away. The icon allows the user to think in real terms about the electronic information and its actions.

The benefits of computer graphics are wide and varied. They enhance productivity, allow for greater creativity, and speed up the process. While some graphics programs may still be expensive, their use is becoming commonplace, and supposedly their cost will decrease.

Programming Languages

There are several computer languages used for computer graphics. These include BASIC, FORTRAN, and PASCAL. BASIC is the language that is used by many microcomputers, with FORTRAN being utilized in the mainframe computers. Dependent upon the computer software you use, the language may be any of the three mentioned. The use of a well-written program can give the developer (you) a relatively easy way to create graphics.

Computers Using Graphics

Several types of computers have the capacity for using graphics. These include mainframes, minicomputers, and microcomputers. *Mainframe* computers are large and can accommodate several users at once. These types of computers are usually found in large universities, financial institutions, large companies, and other multiuser places of employment. The *minicomputer* is smaller than a mainframe and usually slower. It is lower priced and more simple to operate and can be assembled in different ways for various applications. These attributes enabled the minicomputer to lead the way in computer graphics. *Microcomputers* are even smaller and lower priced than the minicomputer. However, again, they are slower and do not allow as many users as other computers. The microcomputer has been a big boon for computer graphics because many software programs are available for these computers.

Summary

This chapter gave an overview of how to present tables and figures in a term paper, research report, thesis, or dissertation. Each student should check with his or her college's or university's required format before embarking upon writing. The use of a guide makes writing and working with tables and figures much easier.

Tables are usually representative of quantitative material. However, words may be used in a table to present qualitative comparisons or descriptive information. When deciding to utilize a table, make sure that the table enhances the manuscript and gives the reader a clearer understanding and comprehension of the numbers mentioned in the manuscript. A good table *supplements* the text and must be mentioned or referred to in the body of the paper.

There are several types of tables that you may need to use in a paper; single variable, percentage, contingency (bivariable), and multivariable. Regardless of the type, the format is the same for any kind of table. Formatting is dependent upon the particular style you or your institution adheres to and should be carefully followed. Several guidelines in constructing a table were mentioned.

Figures are more difficult to construct because they require professional lettering and spacing. Figures include charts, graphs, drawings, maps, and photographs. A cautionary note: make sure that the figure is necessary and that it augments the text. When submitting figures along with a manuscript, include a separate page listing the figures because this ensures correct captions. Each figure should be titled in light pen or pencil on its reverse, along with a notation as to which end is the top. Legends denote the symbols used in the figure. Symbols are used to differentiate between groups, sexes, and so on. It is important that these symbols remain consistent within and between the figures in the manuscript.

The final part of Chapter 10 deals with computer graphics. There have been many applications for graphics especially in the fields of engineering, chemical sciences, arts, education, and business. Computer graphics are available for a large variety of computers: mainframes, minicomputers, and microcomputers. Graphics enhance the text, allow for faster productivity, and can include a variety of interactive activities.

Suggested Activities

1. Prepare the following types of tables, using data from any journal article: single variable, percentage, contingency, and multivariable.
2. Using a different article than the one you used in Activity 1, prepare a figure to illustrate an apparent trend.
3. List and explain the advantages of using a computer for your graphics.

References

Abrahamson, M. (1983) *Social Research Methods,* Englewood Cliffs, New Jersey: Prentice-Hall.

American Psychological Association (1983) *Publication Manual of the American Psychological Association,* 3rd ed., Washington, D.C.: Author.

Bailey, K. (1982) *Form and Style,* Boston: Houghton Mifflin.

Demel, J. and Miller, M. (1984) *Introduction to Computer Graphics,* Belmont, California: Wadsworth.

Mullins, C. (1977) *A Guide to Writing & Publishing in the Social and Behavioral Sciences,* New York: Wiley

Pelegrino, D. (1979) *Research Methods for Recreation & Leisure,* Dubuque, Iowa: Wm. C. Brown.

CHAPTER 11

Scaling

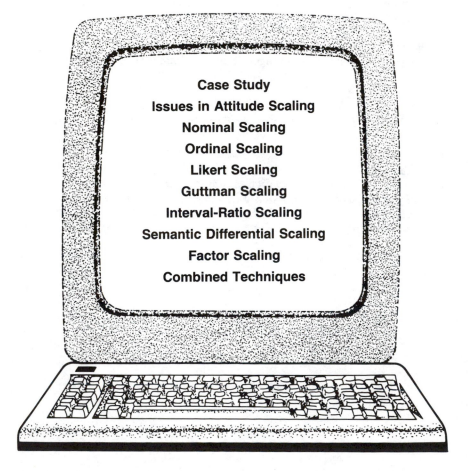

Case Study

Issues in Attitude Scaling

Nominal Scaling

Ordinal Scaling

Likert Scaling

Guttman Scaling

Interval-Ratio Scaling

Semantic Differential Scaling

Factor Scaling

Combined Techniques

Case Study

Michael, a patient education coordinator in a large metropolitan hospital, is developing a program for patients with spinal cord injury (SCI). One of the major concerns expressed by most SCI patients—about 80% are male—is sexual functioning. Experience has taught Michael that this issue can play havoc with the recovery of both the individual and the partner. A goal of the patient education program is not only to impart knowledge but to develop a positive attitude toward sexuality and sexual relations. The problem confronting him was how to develop an instrument to evaluate sexual attitudes in order to measure the effectiveness of his program.

Issues in Attitude Scaling

At the outset of Michael's project, it is important that he differentiate and comprehend several terms that are often used interchangeably. Generally, an *attitude* is viewed as possessing both an affective component and an action tendency. That is, it not only indicates how people feel but also how they may respond (Allport, 1935). Further, attitudes embody direction—a favorable or unfavorable component—as well as magnitude and intensity that imply a strength of feeling or degree of favorableness or unfavorableness. Needless to say, measurement is difficult at best. Researchers and practitioners must depend upon what people say are their feelings. In short, opinions—which are verbal manifestations of an attitude (Hovland, Janis, and Kelley, 1953)—are obtained, and from these opinions an inference is made about attitudes.

Though the process of inferring attitude from expressed opinion has some limitations, it should be realized that all methods of observation are inferential. Different methods vary only in the degree of objectivity they possess (Isaac and Michael, 1981). To complete the task, Michael must construct an attitude scale which, simply put, is a measuring device for the assignment of symbols or numbers to the concept or behavior being observed. If the concept is sexuality, sexuality must be assigned a range of possible values so that each patient who completes the scale will have a particular scale score or value.

Nominal Scaling_____

A nominal scale is the lowest level method of quantification. Basically, it is the creation of mutually exclusive and exhaustive groups that are as homogeneous as possible. For example, patients can be assigned categories according to gender, male or female. This would be a nominal scale of gender. While nominal scaling is appropriate in many instances (race, occupation, educational level, or religious affiliation), it is not suitable for the complexity of scale required by Michael. He will no doubt be more interested in higher-level methods of quantification that reveal the degree of feeling. Rather than finding out whether or not the SCI patient wishes to engage in sexual relations (yes/no) on the nominal level, it would be beneficial to discover the intensity of desire and feelings. (How much do you wish to engage in future sexual relations on a scale of 5?)

Ordinal Scaling_____

The ordinal scale is capable of signifying both differences (favorable/unfavorable) and the degree of difference (very favorable to very unfavorable). However, ordinal measures have no absolute values so the differences between adjacent ranks may not be equal. For example, Michael may construct an item on a scale of five that reads:

A man who cannot have sex is not a "real" man.   1 2 3 4 5
(Circle one number)

A ranking of 1 may be assigned the "very unfavorable" category, while the ranking of 5 would be "very favorable" in so far as having a positive attitude about sexuality. Subsequently, if a patient who had circled number 1 before attending the Sexual SCI Program may circle number 5 at the conclusion of the program. It is readily apparent in this case that a change in attitude has taken place because the later score is quite different from the original score. Nevertheless, it cannot be said that the patient's attitude is five times as favorable at the end of the program. Ordinal scales only permit ordering into *more than* or *less than* categories. Therefore, it could be reported that the patient had a more favorable attitude than at the commencement of the program.

Likert Scaling_____

Rensis Likert (1932) employed ordinal scaling and summated rating techniques to develop an attitude scale. *Summated rating* refers to the fact that several items are used in an attitude scale and, to ascertain an individual's score, the researcher adds (sums up) each item score circled. If the attitude scale comprises ten items and the person circles 1 for every item the summated rating score would be ten, whereas the summated rating score of 50 would be obtained by the person who circles 5 for each of the ten items.

One of the major problems of summated rating is that all the items may fail to measure the same concept. Perhaps some of the items in the ten-item scale just mentioned really do not measure what the others measure, in this case attitude toward sexuality. Likert created a technique to eliminate such items and thereby improve internal consistency. This will be discussed in more detail later.

In constructing a Likert-type scale, the first step is to assemble a large number of items considered relevant to the attitude under investigation. These items or statements should fall in approximately equal numbers with respect to their relative favorableness or unfavorableness toward the object of interest.

Next, each statement must be weighted from 1 to 5, with 3 as the neutral position. It makes no difference whether a rank of 1 is the favorable or unfavorable end of the continuum, as long as the weighting is consistent. For purposes of illustration, however, let us allow the higher score to indicate a stronger agreement with the attitude being scaled. Therefore, a positive statement would be scored by the following key:

Strongly Agree	Agree	Undecided	Disagree	Strongly Disagree
5	4	3	2	1

A negative statement would be scored as follows:

Strongly Agree	Agree	Undecided	Disagree	Strongly Disagree
1	2	3	4	5

The reason for reversing the negative items or statements is to provide a total score that reflects positiveness toward the object in question. In other words, in Michael's scale the SCI patients with a positive sexual attitude would agree with positive statements and disagree with negative ones, while patients with an unfavorable (negative) sexual attitude would disagree with positive items and agree with negative ones. To obtain a total score, the relative weightings of each response are summed. Subsequently, in this example the higher total score represents a more positive sexual attitude than a lower total score.

Now, all of these items should be administered to a sample of the population for whom the scale is intended. As a general rule, the sample size should be at least twice the number of statements desired in the final scale, and most Likert-type scales have 20 to 22 items.

Selection of statements for the final scale is based on an objective check for internal consistency and statement differentiation between the highest and lowest scores. If selection is being done by hand, the scores can be separated into quartiles so the the upper 25 per cent can be compared with the lower 25 per cent. The median score for each statement is calculated. If any statement has the same median score for both the high and low groups, it should be eliminated from the scale. For best differentiation, only those statements that have widely different median scores for the highest and lowest groups are retained. When a computer is available, it is suggested that internal consistency be checked by an item-total correlation. Herein, the responses for *each* statement are correlated with the *total* scores obtained by the subjects on the whole test. This technique reveals the amount of agreement between each individual item and the total test; that is, the degree to which each item measures what the total test measures. Those statements receiving a low correlation should be eliminated.

As a final note, retain items with a high correlation and be certain to have approximately an equal number of positive and negative statements covering a range of topics within the attitude being measured.

Some of the advantages of Likert scaling are (1) it is simple to construct; (2) each item is of equal value so that respondents are scored rather than the item (unlike Thurstone scaling, discussed under Interval-Ratio Scaling); (3) it permits the use of latent attitudes in that items can be employed that are not manifestly related to the attitude being measured; (4) it is likely to produce a highly reliable scale.

The disadvantages of include: (1) the lack of reproducibility [discussed in Guttman scaling], (2) the absence of unidimensionality or homogeneity present in the Guttman scale.

Guttman Scaling

Another major type of attitude scale is commonly called cumulative scales developed by Louis Guttman (1944). The name is derived from the cumulative relation between items and the total scores of the individuals. Items or statements can be ordered from low to high according to difficulty or value-loading so that to approve or correctly answer the last item implies approval or success of all prior ones. If a middle item is incorrect or disapproved, it implies that all following items are incorrect or disapproved. Therefore, in a cumulative scale, knowledge of a subject's total score allows the answering pattern to be predicted. The technique of analysis used to accomplish this is termed *scalogram analysis* (Edwards and Kilpatrick, 1948). The word that describes this capability is *reproducibility,* i.e., the ability to reproduce a person's responses to each item in the scale based solely upon the total score he or she earned.

For example, suppose that Michael was concerned about what sexual behavior the SCI patients would find acceptable now that they have severe limitations to their sexual abilities. He may incorporate several behaviors such as eye-to-eye contact, holding hands, hugging, kissing, petting, and intercourse. Because each behavior requires a greater depth of intimacy and inherent risk, he assigns values of 1, 2, 3, 4, 5, and 6, respectively. Therefore, a patient who receives a total score of 3 would have approved of eye-to-eye contact, holding hands, and hugging while rejecting the other three behaviors. In essence, a patient would obtain one point for each behavior he or she found acceptable, allowing the health science researcher to reproduce the pattern of response. This cannot be done with other attitude scaling techniques because they are not unidimensional (measuring one and only one attribute) to the degree obtained through scalogram analysis.

To begin construction, the researcher accumulates a list of items that have face validity for unidimensionality. That means a group of attitude statements that appear to be homogeneous in measuring one factor so that the scale is univocal. Unlike the Likert scale, which uses a scoring system of 1 to 5, a simple binary coding system of 1 or 0 is used to score responses. Therefore, each respondent either agrees or disagrees with the statement by viewing it as favorable or unfavorable.

The next step is to administer the attitude statements to a large number of respondents for whom the scale is intended. The large number, approximately 100, is necessary so as to avoid the possibility of forming an error-free scale by chance. A score is obtained for each respondent by summing the weights (1 or 0) according the the responses given (agree–disagree).

One of several procedures may be employed to evaluate the scalability of the set of statements. Guttman suggested the "Cornell technique," in which a table is constructed with one column for each response category for each statement and one row for each subject. As an example, suppose that Michael had the following four attitude statements:

Sexual Attitude Statements for SCI Patients

1. Absence of sensation does not mean absence of sexual feelings.
2. The inability to perform does not mean the absence of desire.
3. Sexual experimentation with a partner should be encouraged.
4. Sex only serves as another source of frustration.

Starting with the person who has the highest score, the responses of each patient to each statement are recorded by placing an "x" in the appropriate cell of the table. Table 11.1 illustrates how this would be done for twenty patients responding to Michael's four attitude statements.

To determine reproducibility Guttman developed the "coefficient of reproducibility," which is supposed to indicate the percent age of accuracy with which responses to the various statements can be reproduced from the total scores. This is accomplished by producing cutting points for the response categories (1 to 0) of each attitude statement. A *cutting point* marks that place in the rank order of subjects where the most common response shifts from one category to another. Rules for determining cutting points are: (1) locate so as to minimize error, and (2) no category should have more error than nonerror. Error refers to those responses that fall outside the column or category (1 to 0) in which they theoretically belong. The total number of errors are then calculated and introduced into the formula for the coefficient of reproducibility.

The formula expresses the total number of errors as a proportion of the total number of responses, subtracted from unity. It is as follows:

$$C = 1 - \frac{E}{R}$$

where:

E = the total number of errors
R = the total number of responses (# items × # respondents)

TABLE 11.1   Cornell Technique Scalogram Analysis: Sexual Attitudes

	Statements				
	1	2	3	4	
Subjects	1–0	1–0	1–0	1–0	Scores
1	x	x	x	x	4
2	x	x	x	x	4
3	x	x	x	x	4
4	x	x	x	x	4
5	x	x	x	x	4
6	x	x	x	x	4
7	x	x	x	x	4
8	x	x	x	x	4
9	x	x	x	x	3
10	x	_x_	x	_x_	3
11	x	x	x	x	2
12	x	x	_x_	x	2
13	x	x	x	x	1
14	x	x	x	x	1
15	x	x	x	x	1
16	x	x	x	x	1
17	x	x	x	x	1
18	x	x	x	x	1
19	x	x	x	x	1
20	_x_	x	x	x	1
Errors		1 1	0 1	0 0	
Total	0 1				
Errors = 4					

In Table 11.1 the four-statement scale devised by Michael shows the Cornell Technique for producing the coefficient of reproducibility. The horizontal lines in the body of the table are possible cutting points for the statements. The total number of errors is seen to be 4. The total number of responses is 80 (4 items multiplied by 20 respondents). Therefore, the coefficient of reproducibility would be:

$$C = 1 - \frac{4}{80} = .95$$

According to Guttman, any coefficient of reproducibility above .90 is adequate to indicate unidimensionality and scalability such that responses can be reproduced from knowledge of the total score. However, critics such as Edwards (1959) claim that a coefficient of .90 is insufficient as a sole criterion for scalability. He suggests that the researcher needs to know how low such a coefficient can go in order to determine whether or not the coefficient is in fact adequate. To accomplish this, a minimal marginal reproducibility (MMR) coefficient needs to be computed through the formula

$$\text{MMR} = \sum_{i=1}^{N} \frac{(\% \text{ responses in modal category})}{N}$$

where N = number of items.

With the data in Table 11.1, the MMR can be computed to ascertain the adequacy of the .95 coefficient of reproducibility. There are four categories or statements each with an alternative of 1 or 0, and it is necessary to tabulate the modal response in each. In reviewing each statement it can be observed that the modal response for the first statement is 1, because there are nineteen "x's" in column 1 and only one in column 0; it is 1 for the second statement, with ten "x's"; 1 for the third statement, with eleven; and 1 for the final statement with ten. To calculate the proportion of responses in the modal categories, a denominator of 20 is used because there are a total of twenty responses. Therefore, the formula would read

$$
\begin{aligned}
\text{MMR} &= \frac{(19/20 + 10/20 + 11/20 + 10/20)}{4} \\
&= \frac{(.95 + .50 + .55 + .50)}{4} \\
&= \frac{2.5}{4} \\
&= .63
\end{aligned}
$$

According to the MMR of .63, it can be seen that the .95 coefficient of reproducibility is not high solely because of the modal frequencies, and that it could be considerably lower and still be a scale with reproducibility.

Some of the advantages of Guttman scaling are (1) reproducibility so that the pattern of responses may be traced from the total score, and (2) it may be more unidimensional than Likert scaling. On the other hand, some of the problems include (1) it is quite difficult to construct, (2) unidimensionality may not really exist (Smith, 1951), (3) scalogram analysis may be too restrictive in that only a narrow universe of content can be used, (4) the Cornell technique and use of cutting points is questionable (Clark and Kriedt, 1948) (5) and the detailed analysis and scoring procedures may produce no better results than the summated-rating (Likert scaling) technique (Green, 1954).

Needless to say, there appear to be many more drawbacks than advantages to using Guttman scaling techniques. This does not mean that health science researchers should abandon the approach but rather determine its appropriateness according to the objectives of the research effort. One evaluation instrument in the health education field that uses the Guttman technique was developed by Olsen (1970) for appraising the health-related attitudes of college students. Overall, there are twenty-two different subscales each with a small number of items to be used in the college setting.

Interval-Ratio Scaling

Another method of quantification is the interval scale. Based on equal units of measurement, the interval scale demonstrates how much of a given characteristic is present. Further, the difference in amount of the characteristic present in persons with scores of 25 and 26 is assumed to be equivalent to the difference between persons with scores of 75 and 76. In other words, interval scales indicate the relative amount of a trait, which is something that neither nominal nor ordinal scales permit. However, because a true zero fails to exist in ordinal scales, it is inappropriate to claim that a score of 75 is three times a score of 25.

In contrast, a ratio scale possesses not only the equal interval properties of an interval scale, but also a true zero. For example, a zero on a pharmacy weight scale shows the complete absence of ounces or grams. Moreover, a ratio scale has the properties of real numbers, which can be added, subtracted, multiplied, divided, and expressed in ratio relationships. Therefore, a pharmacy scale that measures 10 grams has twice as much weight on it as one that measures 5 grams.

The most precise ratio scales are common in the physical health sciences, e.g., for measuring blood pressure. The behavioral health sciences, which measure characteristics such as attitudes are limited to interval scales or even less precise types, such as ordinal or nominal scales.

Thurstone and Chave (1929) developed the Thurstone technique of scaled values, frequently referred to as the method of equal-appearing intervals. Herein, a large number of attitude statements are collected and entered on separate cards. The statements, via the cards, are then submitted to a panel of judges who are required to rank the statements into eleven equidistant piles. The eleven piles represent a continuum from extremely favorable to extremely unfavorable, with the middle pile being neutral.

The scale value for any particular statement is the median of the frequency distribution by the judges. If more than one statement had the same scale value, then the statement with the smaller Q statistic or interquartile range was retained for the final scale. It is believed that the smaller interquartile range, the greater the degree of agreement among the judges with respect to that particular statement's position along the continuum.

The general goal is to obtain 20 to 22 statements to form the final scale. The 20 or 22 statements are then randomly arranged and administered to a group of respondents who can either agree or disagree with each item. To score, the mean or median value of those statements with which the respondent agreed is calculated. In other words, the respondent is asked to only check those items to which he or she agrees, and the mean or median value of the checked statements is the scale score for that respondent.

If Michael followed these steps to construct a Thurstone-type attitude scale for SCI patients, a portion of the scale may appear thus:

Sexual Attitude Statements for SCI Patients

1. The worst thing about SCI is inability to function sexually. (10.0)*
2. Hoping for a sexual relationship is senseless. (8.2)
3. Sex may or may not be important in a relationship. (5.0)
4. Partners should try new and different sexual approaches. (2.5)
5. Sex is the most essential part of a relationship. (1.0)

*This is the scaled value for the statement. The patient checks the statements with which he or she agrees and the scale values of the statements checked are used to ascertain a scale score by finding the average or the median score.

Some of the statements are unfavorable toward sexuality (statements 1 and 2) while others are favorable (statements 4 and 5) and still others neutral (statement 3).

One of the advantages of the Thurstone scale is that the statements are weighted or valued rather than the respondents. Also, it is easier to construct than the Guttman scale. Nevertheless, the Thurstone scale is disadvantageous in that it is much more cumbersome to construct than the Likert scale. Further, there is the question about the dependence of the scale values upon the opinions of the judges (Murphy and Likert, 1937). Moreover, it has been shown that this method is no more reliable than the Likert technique (Ferguson, 1941).

Some Thurstone-type scales have been produced for current use in the health science field. One such instrument is a scale to appraise the attitudes of college students toward euthanasia (Tordella & Neutens, 1979). Another scale measures attitudes toward smoking marijuana (Vincent, 1970). These and other such scales are of great value to the practitioner who lacks either the expertise or time for construction.

Semantic Differential Scaling

The semantic differential scale was developed by Osgood, Suci, and Tannenbaum (1957) to measure attitudes. The semantic differential (SD) has three elements: (1) the attitudinal concept to be measured; (2) a pair of opposite adjectives; and (3) a series of undefined scale positions, usually seven in number, between each of the polar adjective pairs. For example, for the concept of research the polar adjective pairs forming the opposite ends of the seven categories could be "good-bad," or "complex-simple". If this were the case, then the SD might look as follows:

Research

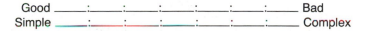

Good _____:_____:_____:_____:_____:_____ Bad
Simple _____:_____:_____:_____:_____:_____ Complex

The polar adjective pairs should be selected according to the objectives of the study. In addition to the polar adjective pairs developed by the originators of the SD, Jenkins, Russell, & Suci (1958) created an atlas of semantic profiles for 360 words. In both instances, Osgood and Jenkins, the pairs of polar adjectives can be used to measure three dimensions—evaluative (e.g., good-bad), potency (e.g., hard-soft), and activity (e.g., fast-slow).

Heise (1970) has researched question format to find that there is no difference whether one concept is presented followed by all adjective-pair scales, or one concept followed by one pair only, or all concepts rated on one polar adjective pair. Further, if one concept is followed by all adjective pair scales, the ordering of concepts makes no difference. However, it is recommended that evaluation, potency, and activity scales be mixed or combined to prevent response sets. Concomitantly, the polar adjective pairs should be randomly arranged so that left and right positions on the total scale do not encourage a response set.

Sorokin (1976) has developed a semantic differential to measure attitudes toward aspects of sexuality. Two of the concepts in his scale are shown for illustration.

Sexuality Scale
Concept 9: Getting Married

pleasing	___:___:___:___:___:___	annoying
constructive	___:___:___:___:___:___	destructive
desirable	___:___:___:___:___:___	undesirable

Concept 10: Having Sexual Relations with the One You Love

pleasing	___:___:___:___:___:___	annoying
constructive	___:___:___:___:___:___	destructive
desirable	___:___:___:___:___:___	undesirable

These concepts could be used in our case study by by Michael to develop his scale for SCI patients. If he wished, different polar adjective pairs could be selected, such as

Concept: Having Sexual Relations with the One You Love

important	___:___:___:___:___:___	unimportant
constrained	___:___:___:___:___:___	free
active	___:___:___:___:___:___	passive
approach	___:___:___:___:___:___	avoid

The three principal factors or dimensions are represented as well as a fourth, situational dimension. "important-unimportant" represents the evaluative factor and "constrained-free," and "active-passive" reflect the potency and activity dimensions, respectively. The situational component is rendered by the adjective pair, "approach-avoid."

In administering and scoring the SD, the patients or subjects should be instructed to put down their initial impression. The scale positions are converted to numerical values so that various statistical assessments can be completed.

important __7__:__6__:__5__:__4__:__3__:__2__:__1__ unimportant

The scores can be analyzed for differences between concepts, between scales, between subjects, or any such combination. Subsequently, a semantic differential generates a large amount of data. For information on analysis techniques, consult Kerlinger (1964), Nunnally (1962), Snider and Osgood (1969), and Osgood, Suci, Tannenbaum (1957).

Two advantages of the semantic differential are that it is simple to construct and easy for the respondent to complete. Further, it allows for several types of analyses to take place. However, that also serves as a disadvantage because some analyses can be very complex. If the researcher employs this method of attitude scale construction, it is important to outline the scoring technique in detail for the practitioner.

Factor Scaling

Factor analysis is a procedure used to determine the number and nature of variables underlying given measures. For example, if Michael had 45 statements planned for a scale to measure attitudes toward sexuality and SCI, it would be advantageous for him to know whether or not all the statements or items are measuring that particular concept or if underlying concepts exist. In other words, is the scale unidimensional? Through factor analysis, Michael might discover that a number of statements have some variance in common such that they correlate highly with some underlying dimension. If so, this dimension will appear as a "factor" or construct, which can be considered as a separate scale. In essence, factor analysis is a method for extracting common factor variances from sets of measures.

An instrument developed to measure attitudes about heterosexual relationships of educable mentally handicapped teenagers (Neutens, 1975) can be used as an example of factor analysis. Initially, 70 statements about dating and premarital and marital relations were obtained from a large population of educable mentally handicapped students. After they were edited these statements comprised a preliminary instrument, which was administered to 257 educable mentally handicapped teenagers. All 70 statements were intercorrelated, yielding an R matrix (statement 1 correlated to statements 1 through 70, statement 2 correlated to statements 1 through 70, and so on until all statements were correlated with one another to form a matrix). This matrix underwent factor analysis with the principal components solution and varimax orthogonal rotation to reveal three underlying concepts or dimensions within the 70 items. In other words, some of the 70 items correlated highly with one of the extracted factors or dimensions, others highly with a second factor and still others correlated highly with a third factor. Statements that failed to correlate at .300 were eliminated; this produced an instrument with 37 statements that measured three factors. Table 11.2 shows the three factors and the *factor loadings* (which can be considered the correlation between the statement and each of the three factors).

TABLE 11.2   Rotated Factor Loadings of Heterosexual Relations Statements

Factors and Statements	Factor Loadings		
	I	II	III
I			
1.	.529	.122	−.184
2.	.524	−.068	.002
3.	.511	.101	.073
4.	.473	−.012	.267
5.	.456	.014	.117
6.	.442	.098	.135
7.	.438	.229	.038
8.	.424	.055	−.026
9.	.419	.142	.248
10.	.417	.251	.086
11.	.394	−.028	−.190
12.	.390	.080	−.011
13.	.369	.253	−.060
II			
14.	.078	.582	.156
15.	.068	.479	−.103
16.	.023	.479	−.009
17.	.249	.475	.105
18.	.072	.458	.145
19.	.228	.455	.007
20.	.180	.432	.053
21.	−.031	.431	.196
22.	.191	.382	.089
23.	.286	.312	−.026
24.	.178	.301	−.105
25.	.130	.300	.194
III			
26.	.218	.059	.440
27.	−.123	.136	.436
28.	.030	.201	.434
29.	−.083	−.182	.415
30.	.064	−.043	.410
31.	−.344	.184	.389
32.	.151	−.121	.385
33.	.052	.246	.375
34.	.032	−.301	.373
35.	−.314	−.023	.351
36.	.297	.166	.331
37.	−.236	−.023	.312

The factor structure is almost perfect. All I statements are loaded significantly on Factor I, all II statements on Factor II, and all III statements on Factor III. The only questionable statements are 31,

34, and 35, which have rather substantial negative loadings. Overall, the factor loadings are evidence for construct validity of the scale.

Unlike the Likert, Guttman, or Thurstone scaling techniques, the scales are not named until after factor analysis rather than before construction. The factor scale name is usually derived from the content or theme of the statements contained within it.

In Neutens' heterosexual relations attitude scale, factor analysis was employed to validate attitude statements. If factor analysis is the only method employed in scale development and the scale is scored accordingly, the following rules apply. An individual's total score on a scale is calculated by taking the score on each statement in the scale (scored from 1 to 5 and corrected for negative items) and weighting it by the factor loading on that scale. For example, from Table 11.2, if a respondent scored, for Scale I, 2 on statement 1, 4 on statement 5, and 3 on statement 10, the total score for Scale I would be

$$2(.529) + 4(.456) + 3(.417) = 1.06 + 1.83 + 1.26 = 4.15$$

Some of the advantages of factor scaling are (1) unidimensionality of each scale, (2) weighting of statements and continuous scores such that each statement is not of equal value (i.e., one statement may be weighted more according to its factor loading on the factor or dimension). The continuous score occurs when the discrete score (5, 4, 3, 2, or 1) is multiplied by the factor loading. Also, with the availability of computer programs to do the computations, construction is now easy. The disadvantages are the difficulty in hand computation and the necessity to name scales after their construction. A scale so developed may have descriptive value, but very little theoretical value.

Combined Techniques

A health science researcher, such as Michael in our case study, could develop an attitude scale that employed a combination of scaling procedures. Michael would thus attempt to strengthen the instrument by circumventing some of the disadvantages of each scaling procedure. For example, he could originate statements concerning sexuality and SCI through an attitude object test rather than construct the statements himself. Herein, he would have SCI patients write out a sentence telling how they feel about particular attitude objects such as marriage, sexual intercourse, oral sex, sexual experimentation, and so on. These statements would be edited to formulate a preliminary instrument.

Next, the statements could be submitted to a group of judges in the areas of sexuality and SCI, as well as the area of attitude scale construction. Rather than the eleven categories as developed by Thurstone, the judges could rate across five categories from strongly favorable to strongly unfavorable.

The judged preliminary instrument would then be given to a representative sample of SCI patients for scoring and analysis. The scoring could be done with either the Likert or Thurstone techniques of a five-point or three-point scale. These responses could then be factor analyzed to discover underlying concepts or dimensions each. These dimensions could then be subjected to the point biserial item analysis to determine differentiation of statements as well as monotonic quality. The Cronbach alpha for internal consistency (1951) can be applied to determine the interpretability of each subscale. Further, Michael can perform an intercorrelation of the subscales to ascertain the independence of each. Finally, the completed attitude scale with inherent subscales can be checked for reliability through a test-retest procedure.

In other words, the researcher needs to examine the objectives for the study and determine which method or methods would be most appropriate to construct an attitude scale which will accurately measure the desired attitudes. The scoring technique of the final product should be relatively easy for the practitioner; otherwise the instrument will not be used.

Summary

It was seen that attitudes, which comprise affective and action components, are difficult to measure. However, direction, magnitude and intensity dimensions may be assessed, depending upon the approach employed by the health science researcher. The approaches presented were nominal scaling; ordinal scaling, including the Likert and Guttman techniques; interval-ratio scaling—the Thurstone technique; semantic differential scaling; and factor analytic scaling.

Each method of scaling possesses advantages and disadvantages. It was discovered that a combination of scaling techniques could be employed to construct the best scale possible. Overall, the nature of the study, the respondents, and the practitioners who are employing the scale should influence the direction taken by the researcher in developing an attitude scale.

Suggested Activities———————————————————

1. Match the items on the left with those on the right.
    a. nominal measurement   1. more patients, less patients
    b. ordinal measurement   2. two patients, three patients
    c. interval measurement 3. patients, patient educators

2. Ordinal measures are capable of signifying both _____ and _____.
3. Three advantages Likert scaling has over Thurstone scaling are:
    a. _____
    b. _____
    c. _____
4. To circumvent the problems of a single scaling technique, what would you "pull" from each of the techniques discussed in the chapter to combine into a unique technique?
5. Go to the library and prepare to discuss the Cronbach coefficient alpha as it pertains to attitude scale construction.
6. What are two reasons that a semantic differential scale would be good to use with children? What are two reasons that an SD would be inappropriate for this population?
7. Write out five studies for which a Guttman scale would be most applicable.
8. As a community health educator, you are requested to ascertain the attitudes of children and parents who are participants in a local latchkey program. The program has been in existence for 7 months and appears to be operating quite smoothly. Hopefully, the development of an attitude scale will afford periodic evaluation of attitudes over the next few years as the program continues to grow.
    What issues do you need to consider in constructing such a scale? Would you plan on devising one or two scales (one for children and a separate one for parents)? Why?
    Outline the necessary steps you would use to construct such a scale(s). Develop thirty attitude statements or attitude objects applicable for measuring attitudes toward a latchkey program.
9. An elementary school teacher has decided to teach about smoking and health in her two fifth-grade classes. However, she wishes to use the lecture-discussion method in one class and a facilitator–values clarification approach in the other. She asks you to construct an instrument to measure the attitudes of fifth graders toward smoking so that it can be employed in the experiment. Ultimately, she is wondering which approach is most likely to bring about a more positive change in attitudes toward smoking.
    As a consultant, you plan the steps required to develop an instrument that would be appropriate for her to use. She does not have access to a computer for scoring. Further, you outline a time frame for each stage of

development so that she can see how much time the task of developing such an instrument will require.

References_____

Allport, G. (1935) Attitudes. In Murchinson, C. (ed.), *Handbook of Social Psychology,* Worcester, Massachusetts: Clark University Press.

Clark, K.and Kreidt, P. (1948) An application of Guttman's new scaling techniques to an attitude questionnaire, *Educational and Psychological Measurement* 8:215–23.

Cronbach, L. (1951) Coefficient alpha and the internal structure of tests, *Psychometrika* 16:297–334.

Edwards, A. (1959) *Techniques of Attitude Scale Construction,* New York: Appleton-Century-Crofts.

Edwards, A. and Kilpatrick, F. (1948) A technique for the construction of attitude scales, *Journal of Applied Psychology* 38:375.

Ferguson, L. (1941) A study of the Likert technique of attitude scale construction, *Journal of Social Psychology* 13:51–7.

Green B. (1954) Attitude Measurement. In Lindzey, G. (ed.), *Handbook of Social Psychology, Volume One,* Cambridge, Massachusetts: Addison-Wesley.

Guttman, L. (1944) A basis for scaling qualitative data, *American Sociological Review* 9:139–50.

Heise, D. (1970) The semantic differential and attitude research. In Summers, G. F. (ed.), *Attitude Measurement,* Chicago: Rand McNally.

Hovland, C., Janis, I., and Kelley, H. (1953) *Communication and Persuasion,* New Haven, Connecticut: Yale University Press.

Isaac, S. and Michael, W. (1981) *Handbook in Research and Evaluation,* San Diego: Edits Publishers.

Jenkins, J., Russell, W., and Suci, G. (1958) An atlas of semantic profiles for 360 words, *The American Journal of Psychology* 71:618–99.

Kerlinger, F. (1964) *Foundations of Behavioral Research,* New York: Holt, Rinehart, & Winston.

Likert, R. (1932) A technique for the measurement of attitudes, *Archives of Psychology* 21:140.

Murphy, G. and Likert, R. (1937) *Public Opinion and the Individual,* New York: Harper.

Neutens, J. J. (1975) Measuring attitudes about heterosexual relationships of educable mentally handicapped adolescents. Paper presented at the National Council on Family Relations, Salt Lake City, Utah.

Nunnally, J. (1962) The analysis of profile data, *Psychological Bulletin* 59:311–19.

Olsen, L. (1970) An evaluation instrument for appraising the health related attitudes of college students. Unpublished Ph.D. dissertation, University of California, Los Angeles.

Osgood, C., Suci, G. and Tannenbaum, P. (1957) *The Measurement of Meaning,* Urbana: University of Illinois Press.

Smith, R. (1951) Randomness of error in reproducible scales, *Educational and Psychological Measurement* 11:587–96.

Snider, J. and Osgood, C., (eds.) (1969) *Semantic Differential Technique,* Chicago: Aldine.

Sorokin, W. (1976) *Personal Health Appraisal,* New York: John Wiley and Sons, Inc.

Tordella, M. and Neutens, J. (1979) An instrument to appraise attitudes of college students toward euthanasia, *Journal of School Health* 49(6):351–52.

Thurstone, L. and Chave, E. (1929) *The Measurement of Attitudes,* Chicago: University of Chicago Press.

Vincent, R. (1970) Attitude toward smoking marijuana, *Journal of School Health* 40(9):454–56.

CHAPTER **12**

Considering Ethics in Research

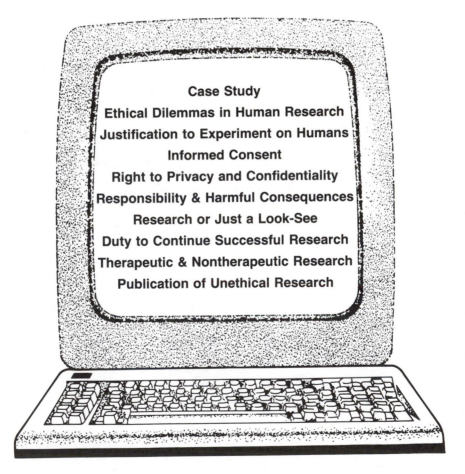

Case Study

Ethical Dilemmas in Human Research

Justification to Experiment on Humans

Informed Consent

Right to Privacy and Confidentiality

Responsibility & Harmful Consequences

Research or Just a Look-See

Duty to Continue Successful Research

Therapeutic & Nontherapeutic Research

Publication of Unethical Research

Case Study

Carol, a doctoral candidate in Health Sciences, has worked the past year and a half as an in-house health promoter for a medium-sized corporation. Her zeal for stress reduction in the workplace won her approval from the chief executive officer (CEO) to study the effect of stress reduction techniques on the physiologic, psychologic (work satisfaction), and productivity variables of middle-management executives. The productivity variable was the idea of the CEO, and the appropriate information would be obtained by him and forwarded to Carol.

She felt this would make an excellent doctoral dissertation and wrote her proposal accordingly. The proposed study would comprise an experimental group, which would take stress reduction classes and perform exercises, and a control group, which would continue their current pattern of stress management, if any. The study would be conducted over a nine-month period. The CEO would inform all potential middle-management executives that they could use their flex-time lunch hour to work with Carol for stress reduction purposes if they wished. Neither the CEO nor Carol would mention to the managers that their work output was to be monitored over the next 9 months; They also would not mention that a study was being conducted. Carol reasoned that the Hawthorne effect would be eliminated in this fashion. As far as the participants were concerned, it would simply be another program offered by Carol, because she has offered several since her arrival.

Carol's proposal contained all the required information as well as her plans to use the information at work to enhance stress reduction and work productivity. Further, Carol hoped to publish the results in a prestigious journal.

In reading the proposal, the doctoral committee members were alarmed by the breach of ethics in several instances of her proposal. What do you see as a potential breach of ethics in Carol's planned dissertation? What could she do to correct these problems?

General Ethical Dilemmas in Human Research

Research on human subjects has been conducted since the time of the ancient Greeks. However, not until the atrocities of Nazi research became known was an effort made to protect research subjects. (Hastings Center, 1976) The Nuremberg medical trials documented such charges as:

1. August, 1942 until May, 1943, some Dachau prisoners were severely chilled or frozen in either a tank of ice water for 3 hours or forced to stand outside, naked, at below freezing temperatures.
2. December, 1941 until February, 1945, prisoners at Buchenwald and Natzweiler were injected with spotted fever virus to keep it alive.
3. July, 1942 to September, 1943, prisoners were deliberately given wounds infected with *Streptococcus,* tetanus, and gas gangrene, which were then irritated by forcing wood shavings or ground glass into them. After the blood vessels to the wounds were tied off, the wounds were treated with sulfanilamide to check for its effectiveness.

Yet, even as the Nuremberg trials of 23 physicians were being conducted in postwar Germany, the United States Public Health Service supported a research project in the rural south with complete disregard for the rights of subjects.

The study, known as the Tuskegee syphilis study (Brandt, 1978) commenced in 1929 in Macon County, Alabama where Tuskegee is located. This county was found to have the highest syphilis rate in the United States, and it was believed that it merited special attention. The project was regarded as a study in nature rather than an experiment because the purpose was to follow the natural course of the disease. The researchers at the time felt that because so many blacks had syphilis anyway, it was simply a matter of taking advantage of a natural situation. No formal protocol was written, but letters between Dr. Taliaferro Clark, Chief of the U. S. Public Health Service (U.S. PHS) Venereal Disease Division, and his colleagues revealed that, in addition to observing the natural course of the disease, the researchers desired to show that antisyphilitic treatment was unnecessary. This was because many blacks experienced a spontaneous cure, and 70% of the remainder were not inconvenienced by the disease. It was admitted that 30% of the subjects were highly contagious and seriously affected. Nevertheless, the U.S. PHS chose not to treat the disease with arsenic and bismuth, which was recognized as a treatment at the time.

The male subjects, between the ages of 25 and 60, were not told about the nature of the study but believed they were being treated for the disease. The study continued indefinitely so subjects could be watched until they died, then an autopsy could be performed. Incentives were used throughout the 40-year period to keep everyone participating. Moreover, the USPHS gave the U.S. Army a list of 256 names of men who were in the study and subseqently drafted, requesting that they not be treated for syphilis. The Army complied.

Although articles about the Tuskegee syphilis study appeared in the medical press as early as 1936, news about the study did not reach the national public press until 1972—the study was still ongoing at the time. The Department of Health, Education, and Welfare (DHEW) (now called the Department of Health and Human Services) formed a committee to investigate criticisms. Three basic issues arose: (1) should the study have been conducted and should the men have been informed, (2) should the men have been treated when penicillin became available, and (3) should the study be terminated? Needless to say, many still believe that the incident was handled too casually and that a myriad of ethical issues were not addressed.

The beginning researcher should realize that the Tuskegee study was carried out by supposedly forthright Americans through a branch of the federal government. It was supported through tax dollars and generally accepted by portions of the medical community. Only with the hue and cry from the public did the study stop. As a health scientist, like Carol, the objectives, justification, and methodology of your study should be scrutinized with ethical eyes. Any researcher may mean well, but failure to consider ethical dilemmas is inexcusable.

Some of the major issues are (1) justification to experiment on humans, especially children, the handicapped, the elderly, or prisoners; (2) informed consent of the subject: (3) confidentiality through the right to privacy; (4) truthtelling and deception: (5) the degree of organization that qualifies a procedure as experimental; (6) the researcher's responsibility for harmful consequences; (7) the duty to continue a successful experiment or research effort; (8) the relationship of therapeutic to nontherapeutic research; (9) sponsored research; and (10) the publication of research. As to be expected, these ten issues hold inherent ethical problems that tend to compound the research endeavor. To simplify matters, this chapter addresses the major issues only.

Justification to Experiment on Humans

In any research effort, there must be substantial justification for the need to experiment with humans, including the implications for usage of results. The *Nuremberg Code* was devised as a result of the trials at Nuremberg to prevent future atrocities in human research (Fromer, 1981). It suggests ten principles to be addressed in justification and methodology. Simply, they are

1. Voluntary consent of the participant is absolutely essential. The subject must be capable of giving consent without coercion and full responsibility rests with the principal investigator.
2. The experiment must be designed to bring forth results that will benefit society and cannot be obtained in any other manner.
3. Human experimentation should be based on animal research results as well as knowledge of the natural course of events, disease, or problem.
4. All unnecessary mental or physical harm should be avoided.
5. When there is reason to believe that death or disabling injury may occur, no experiment should be conducted except perhaps when the experimenting physicians also serve as subjects.
6. The degree of risk should never exceed the humanitarian importance of the problem to be solved.
7. All precaution should be taken to protect subjects from even remote possibilities of injury or death.
8. Only qualified personnel should be allowed to conduct experiments.
9. The subject must be able to withdraw from the experiment at any time if a point is reached which may bring about physical or mental harm.
10. The principal investigator must be ready to terminate the experiment at any stage if it appears that injury, or death will result.

On the surface the Nuremberg Code appears to embrace all the necessary components. However, at least three flaws are evident. First, too much onus is given the principal investigator, especially in regard to informed consent. Concomitantly, the overall tone is that as long as the investigator possesses positive intentions, no harm will come to the subject. It may be asked, who knows what is good for society and who knows how much risk is worth that good? Finally, no one monitors the principal investigator to determine whether or not his or her actions and decisions are in fact ethical ones. Nevertheless, the Nuremberg Code provided a start in protecting the rights of the human subjects.

Frequently, argument about justification revolves around (1) the interests of health sciences, (2) the interests of the subjects or patients, and (3) the interests of the community (Beecher, 1970). While it may be noted in the first issue that acquisition of knowledge and full understanding of any truths are not morally objectionable, it must be realized that not every method is allowable simply because it potentially increases knowledge and understanding. Health science, like other sciences, must be placed in line with other life values. When this is done, it can be readily witnessed that the interests of health science are not the highest values to which all others must be subordinated.

Regarding the interests of the subject or patient as justification, the health science researcher must be cognizant of the myriad of questions raised through consent. For example, what limits should a competent adult be allowed to take? Should the subject or the researcher set the limits? These inquiries become more complex when a researcher deals with special target groups such as the children, the ill, the elderly, or prisoners.

The third issue, the interests of the community (i.e., human society, the common good) as justification, introduces more questions. Can public authority endow the researcher with the power to experiment on the individual in the interests of the community when such experimentation may transgress individual rights? Does the person exist for the community or does the community exist for the person? Keep in mind the experiments of World War II in Germany as well as those conducted in Tuskegee. Was there a well-meaning community in both instances?

In Carol's study of stress reduction in the work place, what would be an acceptable justification? Is the acquistion of knowledge about stress reduction and stress reduction techniques in the workplace adequate? Is benefit for the workers in the experimental group and potential benefit for others appropriate? Is authority from the CEO to augment work productivity enough to overrule the executives' individual rights?

Vulnerable Target Groups: Children

Justification of research on human beings is always demanding, but particularly so for those target groups who are especially vulnerable. Children are often selected for studies in the health sciences field because they are a captive audience in the school system as well as in pediatric wards across the country. Neither the 1947 Nuremberg Code nor the 1949 International Code of Medical Ethics mentions children or other "imcompetents" in nontherapeutic research. The 1964 Helsinki Declaration requires parental or guardian consent for nontherapeutic research on children. This was endorsed by the American Medical Association in 1966. Although it appears plausible on the surface, giving parents or guardians total freedom to submit children to experiments is somewhat frightening. Further, there may be direct or indirect coercion on the parents to "volunteer" their children.

The most famous example of experimentation on children is the Willowbrook experiment (Veatch, 1977) Willowbrook State Hospital in Staten Island, New York is an institution for the care of the mentally retarded. It housed 5,200 residents in 1972, with 3800 of them severely retarded, i.e. having an IQ of less than 20. Dr. Saul Krugman was appointed as consultant in pediatrics and in infectious diseases in 1954. He noted that several infectious diseases were prevalent within the institution, especially hepatitis and measles. In 1956, Dr. Krugman and his associates commenced research on hepatitis and did not stop their research effort until 1970. During that time period, four times each year approximately 12 to 15 children were admitted into the research unit, for a total of 700 to 800 children out of the 10,000 admissions to Willowbrook.

In order to gain a better understanding of the disease and hopefully develop a method of immunization against hepatitis, the researchers injected live hepatitis serum into the subjects to produce the disease. This research effort was approved by the Armed Forces Epidemiological Board, one of its funders, the Committee on Human Experimentation of New York University, and the New York State Department of Mental Hygiene. Justification was based on the grounds that (1) the children were bound to be exposed to the same strains under the natural conditions existing in the institution; (2) they would be admitted to a special, well-equipped, and well-staffed unit where they would be isolated from exposure to other infectious diseases that were prevalent in the institution—namely, shigellosis, parasitic infections, and respiratory infections—and thus that their exposure in the hepatitis unit would be associated with less risk than the type of institutional exposure where multiple infections could occur; (3) they were likely to have a subclinical infection followed by immunity to the particular hepatitis virus; and (4) only children with parents who gave their informed consent would be included. (Krugman, 1967)

The ethical issues in this "experiment" are numerous. Parents were placed in a difficult position by either having their children placed in unsanitary and poor social conditions or in the research unit, where high-quality health care and better social conditions existed. There was at least indirect if not direct coercion by Krugman and his associates. Should parental consent have been enough in this case? The fact that these subjects were children, mentally handicapped, and institutionalized made them particularly vulnerable. Why did these agencies fund such a project? Why was the money not diverted to improve conditions at Willowbrook so that disease would be less rampant for all children? If better conditions had existed within the institution, the justification offered by the researchers would collapse.

Veatch (1977) presents both extremes of ethical alternatives by stating

> At one extreme one could argue that the moral duty of any researcher encountering a group of subjects who will volunteer only because of their social condition is to improve that condition rather than take advantage of it. . . . One might argue from a morally rigorous position that there is always a duty to alleviate social conditions producing suffering when one has the skill and is directly involved with those suffering.

> At the other extreme is the argument that one can trade off a medical service to the general group in need of medical help for the privilege of experimenting. . . . This proposal has crassness, however, suggesting that the individual may be sacrificed for the good of the group. The end results might benefit the whole group, but the benefit to the subject certainly cannot justify the experimental risk. (p. 277)

Even when considering the moral trade-off, which occurs in some prisons and when individuals such as the mentally handicapped are incapable of consent, such a trade-off is difficult to support. Dr. Krugman and others at Willowbrook were dealing with two evils—poor social conditions within the institution and an intentional personal risk of harm.

Partially as the result of the Willowbrook incident, in 1974 Congress mandated the National Commission for the Protection of Human Subjects and Behavioral Research (hereinafter referred to as the Commission) to establish guidelines to protect vulnerable populations, including children, from exploitation as research subjects (McCartney, 1978). In brief, the Commission's recommendations to the Secretary of the DHEW in 1977 were

1. Research involving children is important and should be conducted according to these recommendations.
2. Research may be conducted providing that the Institutional Review Board (IRB) determines that the research is scientifically sound, has been conducted on animals or adult humans first (where appropriate), has minimal risks in design and procedure, provides for privacy of children and parents, and selection is in an equitable manner.
3. Research that does not involve greater than minimal risk to children may be conducted if the risk is justified by the antici-

pated benefit for the subjects; if the risk is no greater than alternative approaches; and, if consent is given by parents and
where possible by the children themselves.

4. Research that involves more than minimal risk and holds a
prospect of direct subject benefit may be conducted only if such
risk is justified by the anticipated results and the risk is at
least as favorable to the subjects as that presented by alternative approaches, and consent is given.

5. Research that involves more than minimal risk and fails to
hold out the prospect for direct benefit for individual subjects
may be supported if the IRB determines that such a risk is only
a minor increase over minimal risk, that generalizable knowledge about the condition will be obtained, that the anticipated
knowledge is of vital importance for understanding or amelio-
rating the condition, and of course that consent is given.

6. When research cannot be approved under the preceding conditions, it can only be conducted provided that it presents an opportunity to understand, prevent, or alleviate a serious problem
affecting children, that a national ethical advisory board has
reviewed the proposal and determined that it would not violate
respect for persons or the principles of beneficence and justice,
and that consent is given.

7. In addition to these recommendations, the IRB should solicit
the assent of both children and parents or guardians when appropriate, involve at least one parent or guardian in the conduct of the research, and accept a child's objection as binding
unless the intervention via research provides direct benefit to
the health or well-being of the subject.

8. Parental consent may be waived if it is not reasonably required
to protect subjects. However, there must be an adequate alternative mechanism for protecting the children depending upon
the nature of the research protocol.

9. Children who are wards of the state should be included in research only if it is related to their status as orphans, abandoned
children, and the like, or conducted in a setting wherein the
majority of the children are not wards of the state. An advocate
for each child must be appointed and given the same opportunity to intervene as would a parent.

10. Children who reside in institutions for the mentally infirm or
correctional facilities should participate in research only if the
conditions regarding research are fulfilled in addition to the
aforementioned conditions.

In 1978, the DHEW adopted all the Commission's recommendations
except: (1) a child's objection to participation as binding, (2) no spe-

cific age should be set for a child's consent to be mandatory, and (3) the Secretary may appoint an ad hoc panel rather than a national commission to review difficult proposals. While these exceptions may weaken the original proposal, adoption emphasizes that scientific research is important and can be performed ethically. The principles set forth in research on children should be transferred to other vulnerable groups used in experiments by health science investigators.

Informed Consent: Truthtelling and Deception

Informed consent essentially entails making the subject fully aware of the purposes of the experiment, the uses to which it will be put, all possible risks, and the credentials of the researcher. The requirement of informed consent is designed to protect the inviolability of the subject. Specifically, Capron (1974) views the functions of informed consent as (1) to promote individual autonomy, (2) to protect the patient-subject's status as a human being, (3) to avoid fraud and duress, (4) to encourage self-scrutiny by the researcher, and (5) to foster rational decision-making.

A classic case of research in which there was great disregard for informed consent is a doctoral dissertation by Laud Humphreys (Beaucham and Childress, 1979). He believed that the general public and law enforcement officials held several myths and misconceptions about homosexual males and their behavior in public places, especially bathrooms—known as "tearooms." To research behavior, he placed himself in various bathrooms and offered his services as "watchqueen," the person who watches out for police. Through this method of research he was able to observe hundreds of acts of fellatio eventually gaining the confidence of some of the regulars. To many of them, he explained his role as a researcher and persuaded them to disclose their motivations for tearoom sex and to talk about their lives in general.

In other instances, however, Humphreys was not so open, secretly following them outside where he copied the license plate numbers and thereby learned names and addresses. A year later he showed up on their doorsteps posing as a health services interviewer and questioned them about their lives, jobs, marriages, and so on. Overall, it was found that over one half of the subjects were married, living with their wives, and leading good lives. About 38% of the men were neither bisexual or homosexual but had poor marriages and subsequently sought sex without emotional entanglements and without jeopardizing their current community positions. These men felt masturbation was too lonely. Another group comprising 24% were bisex-

ual, happily married, and economically successful; still another 24%
were single and covertly homosexual; and only 14% were openly homosexual.

The research effort managed to eliminate many myths and did alleviate harrassment of homosexual men by police authorities. Nonetheless, informed consent was not obtained and the men did not know
they were part of a study. The research proposal had been reviewed
by dissertation committee members only and when the issue came to
light, the entire sociology department at Washington University was
in a furor. After publication (*The Tearoom Trade: Impersonal Sex in
Public Places,* Chicago: Aldine) in 1970 there was considerable out-
rage about research methodology, informed consent, and privacy.
While Carol's research in the case study may not be this explosive in
its topic, her dissertation committee will have to review the proposal
thoroughly.

As a result of a Canadian study (Pappworth, 1969) in which a University of Saskatchewan student suffered a cardiac arrest and subsequent decrease in memory and concentration during an experiment
to test a new anesthetic, the DHEW formulated the following guidelines for informed consent:

1. Fair explanation of the procedure to be followed, including identification of experimental methods,
2. Description of any attendant discomforts and risks reasonably to
   be expected,
3. Description of any benefits reasonably to be expected.
4. Disclosure of any appropriate alternative that might be advantageous for the subject,
5. An offer to answer any inquiries concerning the procedures,
6. Instruction that the person is free to withdraw consent and to
   discontinue participation in the project or activity at any time
   without prejudice to the subject.

> No such informed consent, oral or written, . . . shall include any ex-
> culpatory language through which the subject is made to waive, or ap-
> pear to waive, any of his legal rights, including any release of the or-
> ganization or its agents from liability for negligence. (U.S. DHEW,
> 1971)

While the guidelines provide a basis for informed consent, the researcher still faces several research and ethical dilemmas. For example, how much does the subject need to know before consent can
be given? If too much detail is given the subject may not understand
or perhaps may skew the data by acting the way the researcher

hopes. In some instances the researcher may not be aware of the potential discomforts that could occur even a year after the research, e.g. guilt from participating in sexual research so that it affects a marital relationship. How would you have altered Humphrey's study of homosexual males to incorporate informed consent? Should Carol have informed consent in her study? What are the pros and cons of informed consent in her research effort? If informed consent is to be present in her study, how should she go about it? What forms and procedures are required by your university to determine that informed consent has been fairly applied in studies dealing with human subjects?

Informed Consent and Double-Blind Studies

The design of double-blind studies is simple and logical. One half of the subjects are randomly selected to receive the experimental product and the other half is given a placebo, and the results are compared. Neither the researcher nor the subjects know who obtains the active substance or the placebo; hence the term *double-blind*.

Although the researcher values this methodology to earn accurate results, it possesses many ethical dilemmas. A study conducted by Goldzieher of the Southwest Foundation for Research and Education displays many of the ethical problems encompassed in double-blind research. (Veatch, 1971). The purpose of the experiment was to discover whether some of the reported side effects of the contraceptive pill were physiological or psychological. The subjects were primarily poor, multiparous, Mexican-American women who had come to a San Antonio clinic for contraception to prevent further pregnancies. Seventy-six of the women were given placebos and another group got various hormone contraceptives. None were told that they were involved in a research project or that they were receiving placebos. All were instructed to employ vaginal cream because the contraceptive pill might not be "completely effective."

The results of the experiment showed that the women taking placebos had many of the same side effects—depression, breast tenderness, and headaches—as those on the contraceptive pill. However, 13% (10) of the 76 women taking placebos became pregnant. Needless to say, these women were deceived; yet, a request for full, informed consent would have made the study impossible, because the women came to the clinic for pregnancy prevention. Could some information have been given without ruining the research? If deception is part of the research process, should the experiment be cancelled? In other words, what justification is required to approve deception? Were the results of the Goldzieher study worth 10 women getting pregnant?

Who is to decide whether the results of an experimental procedure are potentially worthwhile? Moreover, if such studies are even contemplated, how should the population for the study be chosen? In this case, why were poor, Mexican-American women selected, particularly individuals who could not afford medical care as clinic patients?

In short, the double-blind methodology is excellent for some research objectives, particularly if a placebo is employed; however, it is fraught with ethical dilemmas that should be addressed by the principal investigator.

Overall, recent trends indicate that the requirements for informed consent are becoming more and more rigorous. There are many special circumstances regarding persons who speak foreign languages and other minority groups. It is believed that a long consent form attached to a mail survey will reduce the number of returns. Just reading the form will take more time and thereby reduce returns, and the usual ominous tone is likely to decrease responses even further. Singer (1978) has shown that informed consent procedures lower response rates for interviews. Thorne (1980) in speaking about sociological research, has complained that federal regulations are based on the biomedical model of research and as such are not workable in for research that is observational field research. He states that

> The requirement that one obtain signed consent forms from everyone one studies may violate anonymity and actually increase risks for some groups of subjects. In the end the procedures may result in meaningless ritual rather than improving the ethics of field research. (p. 285)

The problem of informed consent for the reseacher is difficult, with the major problem being that of application—how much information, how much consent.

Right to Privacy and Confidentiality_____

All participants in human research have the right to privacy in that they have the right to request that their individual identities remain concealed. While the charge of invasion of privacy can be made in all methodologies, it is most likely to occur with survey research. The question of what constitutes invasion of privacy is quite subjective and may imply something different to the subject than the intent of the researcher. For example, in a drug survey the participant may have used cocaine but felt very guilty about it and not admitted it to anyone. Such a person may understandably feel that his or her privacy is being invaded when asked if cocaine had been taken at any time.

To insure anonymity it is important to explain to the subject that most researchers are interested in group data and that individual scores are compiled with others. Further, individuals are identified by number rather than by name. Perhaps most importantly, the subject needs to understand the importance of the data being gathered, if the project is deemed important enough the subject may be willing to sacrifice some privacy.

The principle of confidentiality is related to the right to privacy. Who will be able to see the data? In school systems both teachers and students are concerned that research data may be used to evaluate performance. The health science researcher should treat all data confidentially and ensure that (1) all data is returned anonymously and directly to the research office, (2) all data is rostered by number, and (3) unneeded material is destroyed upon completion of the project.

Of course, there are several other ways in which confidentiality could be broken. It may occur if a subject is a relative or friend of a member of the research team who has even limited access to the data. Research records can be stolen. A questionnaire may be found by a spouse, friend, parent, or colleague, or a telephone message could be taken that identifies the participant. Even the participant may break confidentiality by writing a name on the questionnaire that reveals the illicit use of drugs. These breaks may occur no matter how careful the investigator.

Reviewing the case study at the beginning of the chapter. What has Carol done to ensure the right to privacy and to maintain confidentiality? If her study was conducted as presented, might she violate the right to privacy? What suggestions could be given to Carol?

Responsibility for Harmful Consequences

Subjects have a right to expect the health science researcher to prevent harm from befalling them and to be sensitive to their need for human dignity. Further, as discussed under Informed Consent, DHEW guidelines require that each subject be told of any "attendant discomforts and risks reasonably to be expected." Once again, however, how much need be explained so as not to frighten the subject? What one subject finds disquieting another might not. The researcher must find a common ground for explanation and answer all inquiries honestly.

Dava Sobel (1981), a science reporter for the New York Times, described her experience as a subject in an experiment at Montefiore Hospital in the Bronx. The purpose of the study was to observe how certain bodily functions change in the absence of timing devices—clocks, calenders, natural light cues, and social regimentation. As the seventeenth volunteer and the first female she was placed in a special environment (room) and allowed to set her own schedule according to the dictates of her body for 25 days. Her account of informed consent from the subject's viewpoint is quite noteworthy but perhaps more so is her view of harm to the subject.

> Within hours, I realized that I had not quite understood what subjecthood entailed. First came the insertion of the catheter which was extremely painful. The procedure had to be done in both arms, since the doctor mistook the lack of blood flow from the right side for a defective or improperly inserted needle. [Blood samples were part of the experiment].
>
> . . . The frequency of those samples was my second shock. . . . I feel I should have been warned that the samples would be taken "very" frequently [every 20 minutes], interfering constantly with my work, my meals, and the time I expected to be alone in the bathroom. . . .
>
> Feeling tense, I wrote a letter to my husband dated "Day 1," stamped it, and gave it to the next white-coated technician who came in for a blood sample. He waved it almost tauntingly and said, "This will go out, but I won't say *when* it will go out. Maybe in a few days." I panicked. (p. 5–6)

There is no doubt that research of this nature will cause some discomfort, but how much? From Dava Sobel's vantage point, too much.

To complicate matters further, she was given very little help in reorienting herself to the "real" world. After 25 days in which she would sleep and eat at any desired interval, Sobel found her normal patterns so disrupted that she "might as well have been living inside a stranger" (p. 7). It took her approximately 2 weeks to readjust to her former schedule, and she missed work most of that time. Should it be the responsibility of the researcher to reimburse a subject who misses that much work? Overall, her account offers the researcher insight into harms, or at least risks, that the subject should be told of. As a point of note, these researchers did change their protocol somewhat.

Kolodny (1977) cautions of potential long-term consequences of study participation. In sexual research, a subject who is observed in some type of sexual activity may experience no problems while the study is underway, but may discover feelings of guilt years later. Perhaps, a potential spouse may refuse marriage when he or she learns of the participation.

In the case of Carol, could harmful consequences occur to any of her subjects? What would be the reaction of the middle-management executives if they discovered their work productivity was being monitored as part of a research project? What would happen to the trust level among the managers, Carol, and the CEO? Would future programs of health promotion be placed in jeopardy?

Though the health science researcher cannot hope to predict all risks and consequences, he or she should make an effort to communicate all known ones.

Research or Just a Look-See

A major question is, when does research become research or an experiment an experiment? Most researchers have "pet" ideas or theories they would like to test a "little bit" before taking on a full-blown study. However, when human subjects are involved, is it fair to include them in such tryouts without informed consent?

Further, what if data are collected when the health scientist is functioning as a clinical person and the data are later incorporated into research. For example, if a masters candidate serves as a counselor in local clinic for patients seeking an abortion and then records the anxiety and psychological trauma experienced by each patient for his or her own growth as a counselor, is that ethical? If at a later date the same candidate wishes to incorporate the patients' reactions into a masters thesis, is that ethical? The patients were not informed about the use of the data, because at the time a research project was not planned. Should consent be obtained even at this late date?

If you were a member of Carol's dissertation committee, would you consider her proposed effort as research or a look-see? Based on the first chapter of this textbook, what steps are necessary to comprise research? Just as important, should all the ethical issues thus far be applied to her proposal?

The Duty to Continue a Successful Research Effort

Researchers in the health science discipline frequently embark upon research efforts to improve the health of people suffering chronic conditions such as obesity, smoking, hypertension, and others. The underlying question is whether or not contemporary health scientists have an obligation to continue successful programs.

For example, if Carol finds that the stress reduction program does in fact lower physiological tension, improves work satisfaction, and augments productivity, should she continue the program for all workers? What if only two of the three variables are positive? Who would be responsible for continuing costs? The obligation of the researcher to the subjects subsequent to the research effort are debatable but should be addressed before the project commences.

Therapeutic and Nontherapeutic Research

If the research objective is to acquire information, should the justification be different than if the objective were to develop a cure or behavior pattern to improve health? In other words, is a different justification required for nontherapeutic research than for therapeutic research? In nontherapeutic research there may be no apparent benefit for the human subjects, while in therapeutic research at least the experimental group may benefit. Of course, in therapeutic research the question arises as to the right of the participant to request placement in the experimental group so that potential benefits may be obtained.

Is the nature of Carol's proposed study more nontherapeutic or therapeutic? If she is just attempting to gain knowledge about the affect of stress reduction techniques on physiologic, psychologic, and productivity variables, should her justification be different than if she were in fact planning a therapeutic study? Should health scientists who research in the behavioral field be held accountable for subjects' health behavior? All in all, therapeutic and nontherapeutic research efforts differ in objectives, but differences in justification are a moot point.

Sponsored Research

More often than not health science researchers cannot afford to pay for a project out of pocket. The myriad of expenses—drawing a large sample, training interviewers, postage, offices and overhead, computer time—must be met by a sponsor. Usually a government agency such as the U. S. Department of Public Health or a charitable foundation may provide funds and allow the researcher to conduct the project with no strings attached. However, previous examples throughout this chapter have illustrated how some agencies attempt to inflict their views on the project.

Bailey (1982) presents three major areas in which ethical conflict arises between the sponsor and the researcher. First, the sponsor may tell the researcher how to conduct the study or what findings are to be expected. Second, the sponsor may request suppression of findings that could range from total falsification to manipulation of statistics. Third, the actual sponsor may be concealed or the true purpose of the study hidden. The latter has occurred in several research efforts for which the Central Intelligence Agency served as sponsor (Sjoberg, 1959).

The sponsorship in Carol's dissertation is very subtle in that it is her employer. Has the CEO played a role in her objectives? methodology? How should she handle this situation? Should she risk termination of the study?

In writing grants or procuring funding from outside sources, the health science researcher must be cognizant of these potential ethical breaks. The researcher must be prepared for compromise in some instances, but in such cases should examine all ethical questions so as not to end the project with results that have been questionably attained.

Publication of Unethical Research

A research project does not become ethical because it produces valuable data; it is ethical or unethical from its inception. Subsequently, researchers, editors and editorial boards must look beyond the results of an investigation into all the ethical aspects involved in research. Only then can a fair and just decision be made about possible publication.

One option that may be chosen is the decision not to publish. Ingelfinger (1978), former editor of the *New England Journal of Medicine,* stated that "reports of investigations performed unethically are not accepted for publication" (p. 791). His belief is that researchers should not be involved in unethical acts, directly or indirectly. Subjects are not to be used as a means to an end. Moreover, failure to publish such research should serve as a caveat to other researchers. While some very worthwhile information will be lost to the profession, proponents of this position feel that more good consequences than bad will occur in the long run.

Beecher (1970) suggested a modification of this view by stating that "such material *ordinarily* should not be published" (p. 31). If unethical circumstances exist, Beecher believes that the researcher should report, in the text, where the dilemmas existed. In a parallel position, Levine (1973), former editor of *Clinical Research* and professor of medicine at Yale University, advocates that, "Manuscripts describing research conducted unethically but which satisfy the usual scientific criteria for acceptability should be published along with editorials on which the ethical deficiencies are exposed and criticized" (p. 763). This plan raises the ethical issues to a level of debate and still allows the results to be received by other professionals. Nevertheless it raises questions, too. Does such publication indicate that the editor or journal approves such actions or at best frowns upon them? Will it function as a deterrent to unethical research?

In essence, no matter what position is taken, the majority of the responsibility rests with the researcher. As a professional, the health scientist must conduct himself or herself in a fashion that is conducive to subject protection, profession and professional growth. Publication is both a responsiblity and privilege.

Summary

This chapter offered viewpoints on ethical dilemmas that confront the research effort. It was seen that unethical research has been conducted in the past with and without approval of recognized government bodies. One of the initial issues to be reviewed by any investigator is the justification to experiment on human subjects rather than animals or computer simulation. Frequently, justification revolves around (1) the interests of health sciences, (2) the interests of the subjects or patients, and (3) the interests of the community. All can be questioned.

Justification for research on vulnerable target groups, particularly children, was seen to be more complex. DHEW guidelines were reviewed because they are employed by IRBs.

Another major issue was informed consent involving truthtelling and deception. This area is of particular importance to both the researcher and the subject and is well scrutinized by professionals. Double-blind methdology presents unique problems to the informed consent issue.

Privacy and confidentiality are two highly regarded issues as seen by subjects. Concomitantly, fear of harm, albeit subjective, is a point of concern to subjects and researchers, alike.

Another issue was the degree of organization required to designate an experiment as an experiment. When an experiment or research effort has been proven to be successful, such as in the reduction of smoking, the question of whether or not it should be continued was discussed. This is particularly so if the nature of the study is therapeutic versus nontherapeutic.

Sponsorship and publication of results were also seen to be fraught with ethical decisions. Overall, the major responsibility rests with the researcher.

Suggested Activities

1. In coordinating patient education in a 350-bed hospital, give ethical reasons why you should or should not allow experimental education programs to be conducted? List guidelines for such experimental education if it was to be conducted.
2. Visit the research office on your campus and find out how they protect human subjects in campus research efforts.
3. Review the history of the IRB and the guidelines set forth for IRBs.
4. Being a promoter of health behavior change, you have decided to try something in your high school classes. For one of the classes you will teach the way you always have, with lecture-discussion and valuing exercises, examinations to test for knowledge, and a behavior inventory to check for pretest and posttest health behaviors. The other class will be taught the same way but behavior change will be emphasized by the use of behavior change contracts for grading—no change, the student fails; the more changes in multiple behavior, the higher the grade. At the end of the semester you will compare the two classes for behavior change and from that determine what you will do in the classroom in the future. Because this is just a little review of your own, you decide not to tell anyone, especially the students so their behavior will not be altered by the experiment itself.

   What ethical dilemmas exist in your plan? Is it fair and just to base grades on behavior change? What do you do for students who already have good health behavior? Should the students be informed at all? Is there a need to inform the administration the parents? Is coercion playing a role? How might this "experiment" be changed to improve the ethical status? Rewrite this miniproposal and address the ethical issues.
5. Working as a health consultant, you are confronted with a proposal drafted by a health educator in a clinic setting. Jon, the health educator, wants to mail a questionnaire to the clinic population who have been diagnosed as having genital herpes. Many of the medical facts he can pull from subjects' clinic records, however he wishes to investigate such things as current sexual life-style, romantic relationships, contraceptive techniques, and methods used to tell their sexual partners that they have herpes. He would have the secretaries in the office tabulate the data for each person and combine the questionnaire data with medical record date (via a code number placed on the questionnaire) for further information. The patients would not know about the code number or that he planned to publish the results without names.

   As a consultant, how would you advise Jon in regard to ethics in his survey research?

References

Bailey, K. D. (1982) *Methods of Social Research* New York: The Free Press.

Beauchamp, T. C. and Childress, J. F. (1979) *Principles of Biomedical Ethics* New York: Oxford University Press.

Beecher, H. K. (1970) *Research and the Individual: Human Studies,* Boston: Little, Brown & Co.

Biomedical Ethics and the Shadow of Nazism (1976) A conference on the proper use of the Nazi analogy in ethical debate, *The Hastings Center Report* 6(4) special supplement.

Brandt, A. (1978) Racism and research: the case of the Tuskegee syphilis study *The Hastings Center Report* 8(6):21–29.

Capron, A. (1974) Informed consent in catastrophic disease research and treatment, *University of Pennsylvania Law Review* 123(2):364–376.

Fromer, M. J. (1981) *Ethical Issues in Health Care,* St. Louis: C.V. Mosby.

Ingelfinger, F. J. (1978) Ethics of experiments on children, *New England Journal of Medicine* 288:791.

Kolodny, R. (1977) Ethical requirements: informed consent. In Masters, W.H., Johnson, V.E., and Kolodny, R. (eds.), *Ethical Issues in Sex Therapy and Research,* Boston: Little, Brown and Company.

Krugman, S. (1967) Experiments at Willowbrook State School, *The Lancet,* 1971, May 8, p. 321.

Levine, R. J. (1973) Ethical considerations in the publication of the results of research involving human subjects, *Clinical Research* 21:763.

McCartney, J. J. (1978) Research on children: national commission says "Yes, if . . . ," *Hastings Center Report* 8(5):26–31.

Pappworth, M. H. (1969) Ethical issues in experimental medicine. In Culter, D. R. (ed.), *Updating Life and Death,* Boston: Beacon Press.

Singer, E. (1978) Informed consent: consequences for response rate and response quality in social surveys, *American Sociological Review* 43:144–62.

Sjoberg, G. (1959) Operationalism and social research. In Gross, L. (ed.), *Symposium on Sociological Theory,* New York: Harper & Row.

Sobel, D. (1981) Time out of joint: 25 days in a sleep lab. *The Hastings Center Report* 11 (1):5–7.

Thorne, B. (1980) You still takin' Notes? Fieldwork and problems of informed consent, *Social Problems* 27:284–97.

U.S. DHEW (1971) The Institutional Guide to DHEW Policy on Protection of Human Subjects, 7 as amended by 39 Fed. Reg. 18914 (1974). C.F. 21 D.V.R. 130.37 (1973) FDA Policy on Informed Consent.

Veatch, R. M. (1971) Experimental pregnancy, *Hastings Center Report* 1:2–3.

CHAPTER 13

Ex Post Facto Research

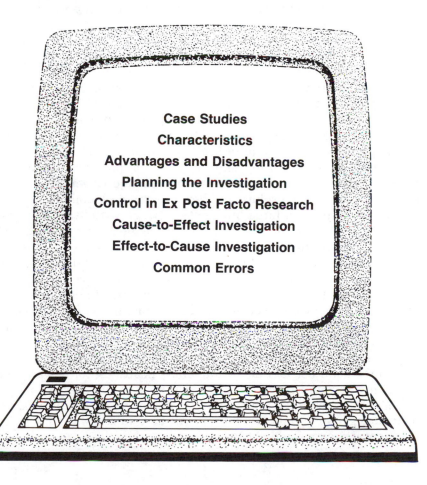

Case Studies_____

Mary Margaret, a health care professional at a large long-term care facility, was very interested in Alzheimer's disease. Her particular interest was the effect the disease and disease management process have on the children of those afflicted with Alzheimer's. For several years she has seen families attempt to cope with the problems presented when a parent has Alzheimer's. They have had to search for appropriate medical help and contend with the parent's daily problems such as giving up a job, managing money, loss of driving skills, poor personal hygiene, memory loss, wandering, incontinence, inappropriate speech and communication patterns, and a host of medical dilemmas. In many cases the problems have slowly exacerbated over a 10-year period and disrupted the lives of all those closely connected to the Alzheimer's victim.

Over the years she has watched several of the children, ranging in age from 25 to 50 years of age, make the decision to place their mother or father in the long-term care facility and then begin their visits. She felt that being witness to such a devasting disease for such a long period of time must have some impact on the children's perception and planning for later life, especially the retirement years. She wondered if such perceptions would be different from those of children whose parents were still quite healthy. Knowledge of such information might be beneficial in the development of programs at her residential facility. Her next, and most obvious inquiry was how should she go about finding a solution to her research problem.

Eric, a dentist in a large university setting, was always intrigued to find such a great difference in dental hygiene among his newly admitted adolescent patients. Some entered his office noting that they brushed and flossed frequently, and their dental check-ups supported their contention. However, many others confessed to brushing once or perhaps twice a day but rarely flossing their teeth. Dental caries and phyorrhea were evidence of their failure in dental hygiene. Although he conversed with his patients while they were in his office, his curiosity as to why some adolescents developed excellent dental hygiene behavior and others did not remained unabated. He decided to approach the administrator at the university health center to seek funding to investigate this problem. Moreover, he would seek help in establishing a research plan, because his background in research methodology was somewhat barren. All he realized was that an experimental design could not be used.

Characteristics of Ex Post Facto Research————————

Whenever possible, the health scientist will conduct experimental research to determine the relationship between two or more variables. However, in many instances this is not possible because the independent variable cannot be manipulated or the assignment of subjects to different treatments is not feasible. For example, one research group queried whether or not "public school students whose families are involved in tobacco production are more likely to smoke and to hold favorable attitudes toward smoking" than public school students whose families are not involved in tobacco production (Higgens, Whitely, and Dunn, 1984). The researchers were not able to assign certain children to tobacco-growing families and others to non-tobacco-growing families. Instead, it was necessary to locate children living in the two different types of home environments. In a study investigating the relationship between teenage client trust in confidentiality and contraceptive advice with subsequent use of contraception, the researchers were unable to offer "treatments" wherein one group of clients would develop trust and another group not develop trust (Nathanson and Becker, 1985). In other words, the independent variable had to occur naturally between the client and the provider.

It is virtually impossible to manipulate such variables as gender, race, socioeconomic status, marital status, level of education, and so on. Generally, hypotheses about the effects of individual attributes are not amenable to experimental research. This applies to Mary Margaret's intended research, also. A nonmanipulative variable is involved—the experience of having a parent with Alzheimer's disease. Because variation cannot be obtained by direct manipulation, she must select individuals in whom the variable is present or absent. Therefore, she must present children whose parent(s) has Alzheimer's disease and children whose parent(s) is healthy with an instrument to measure perception and planning for later life, especially the retirement years.

Similarly, Eric's study about dental hygiene proposes a difficulty in manipulation of an independent variable, because he is not even sure what the variable is. Thus far, he simply has groups of adolescents separated by their personal dental hygiene behavior. He must look back to the experiences they have had before becoming his patients in order to discover why they do what they do.

Studies such as Mary Margaret's and Eric's wherein subjects are sorted on the basis of some naturally occuring variable, are called *ex post facto* or *causal-comparative investigations*. According to Kerlinger (1964), ex post facto research is "that research in which the independent variable or variables have already occurred and in which the researcher starts with the observation of a dependent variable or variables. He then studies the independent variables in retrospect for their possible relations to, and effects on, the dependent variable or variables" (p. 360). Owing to the nature of health science, much of the research conducted in the discipline is ex post facto in nature.

Ex Post Facto and Experimental Research Approaches

In both the ex post facto and experimental research methods the focus is on the relationship between an independent variable X and a dependent variable Y. Both function on the same logic that two groups similar in all characteristics but one are compared in order to determine the effect of that one characteristic. Consequently, both approaches provide similar information. However, the evidence with an experiment is much more convincing than with an ex post facto study. This is because the extraneous variables in the experimental method are controlled through randomization and other techniques and there is active manipulation of the independent variable X. It can be assumed that Y varies as a result of manipulation of X. Note that the health scientist predicts from a controlled X to Y.

In the ex post facto approach, Y is observed before a retrospective search for X (antecedent variables) ensues. Once a plausible X is found, the hypothesis is tested by means of looking at the antecedent variable (X) to determine how it is related to the dependent variable Y. As the term ex post facto indicates, the changes in the independent variable X (the antecedent variable) have already taken place. Consequently, this lack of control of X and other possible X's make it more hazardous to infer that there is a real relationship between X and Y.

Concomitantly, in ex post facto research the subjects "assign themselves" to groups based upon the characteristic or behavior under study. For example, in Mary Margaret's study the subjects would "select themselves" according to being the child of a parent with Alzheimer's or not being the child of a parent with Alzheimer's disease, or in Eric's research, adolescent with positive hygiene or failing to have such behavior. Self-selection means that the groups being compared were not initially equivalent, which potentially influences their status on the independent variable. In short, when randomization is not possible, loopholes are created through which extraneous variables may pass. There is no doubt that ex post facto research lacks the degree of confidence that exists in the experimental approach.

Advantages and Disadvantages of Ex Post Facto Research

Including the two points raised in the previous section, causal-comparative or ex post facto research has three glaring limitations or disadvantages: (1) the inability to randomize or control extraneous variables, (2) the lack of power to manipulate independent variables, and (3) a high risk of misinterpretation. The first two limitations bring about the third.

As pointed out by Kerlinger (1964) one of the most dangerous fallacies in research is that known as *post hoc, ergo propter hoc*—after this, therefore caused by this. It is very easy, in fact too easy, to assume that one thing causes another simply because it occurred before the other. In looking for antecedent causes the researcher can be led to erroneous and misleading interpretations of data. For example, a health science researcher may ask why some students use marijuana and others do not. If he or she looks at two groups (users and nonusers) and moves backwards to seek antecedent causes (the independent variable X) several speculations could be made. Perhaps the marijuana users all smoked cigarettes first, or they all have low grades in school, or come from families with a domineering mother, or perhaps they were all bottle-fed rather than breast-fed. The plausability of many explanations for a complex event leaves the researcher open to error. This is particularly so when ex post facto research is conducted without hypotheses or predictions, i.e., data are just collected and then interpreted.

To overcome this limitation of interpretability, the researcher should develop and test alternative hypotheses (to be discussed later in this chapter). Another procedure is to use path analysis to examine the relationship between all the variables in the study (Cook and Campbell, 1979). Simply, path analysis is a technique to test theories about hypothesized causal links between variables (Rogosa, 1979). Except for the purpose, it is similar to such multivariate methods as multiple regression, canonical correlation, discriminant analysis, and factor analysis in that all are concerned with relationships between three or more variables. While these other techniques may be used occasionally to examine hypotheses about causal relationships, path analysis is much more powerful. Of course, even with these amendments, ex post facto research is not as powerful as experimental research in demonstrating causal properties.

Nonetheless, ex post facto or causal-comparative research is highly useful for identifying possible causes of observed variations in health behavior patterns. In fact, with some reflection on the variables in health science research—current health behaviors, home background, parental habits and upbringing, gender, socioeconomic status—it can be seen that they are not manipulable. Consequently, ex post facto research is not only necessary in many instances, but also allows for the opening of new avenues.

Planning the Ex Post Facto Investigation_____

As denoted previously, there are two types of ex post facto studies. Chapin (1947) referred to them as the cause-to-effect and the effect-to-cause approaches. In the cause-to-effect approach, the health science researcher may wish to study two or more groups, one of which has been exposed to the experience in question in order to determine the effects of that experience. For example, in Mary Margaret's proposed research, she would have one group whose parent(s) has been victimized with Alzheimer's disease and another group whose parent(s) is healthy and would then compare the groups of their perception of and planning for later life, especially the retirement years.

On the other hand, in the effect-to-cause approach the health science researcher may examine two groups that are different in one or more respects in order to discover the reasons why. As an example, Eric wishes to investigate why one group of adolescents has excellent dental hygiene behavior and the other does not to ascertain factors that may antecede one group's failure to engage in preventive dental hygiene.

It is necessary to determine which approach will be employed when the ex post facto investigation commences, because different procedures may be required.

Control in Ex Post Facto Research_____

Since the major weakness of ex post facto research is the lack of control over extraneous variables, the health science researcher should have a working knowledge of procedures to furnish some degree of control in the investigation. This section outlines techniques that may be appropriate to the researcher.

Matching

One of the most common methods to provide control in the ex post facto study is to match on a subject-to-subject basis. Herein, the researcher forms matched-pairs between the "experimental" and "control" groups on such items as socioeconomic status, level of education, family structure, and the like. To do this, of course, assumes that the investigator knows which factors may have some bearing on the dependent variable, i.e., correlation with the dependent variable. This problem in matching exists in experimental research, too.

Mary Margaret may attempt to match children of a parent with Alzheimer's disease with children of a healthy parent(s) on the variables of socioeconomic status, age, and level of education, because these variables may be related to perception of life and planning for retirement. Eric may match the two groups of adolescents on family structure and parents' level of education.

In addition to having knowledge about which variables to match, the researcher faces the problem of reducing the number of subjects that can be used for the final analysis. Chapin (1947) conducted one study with 1194 subjects and then decided to match them, ending up with twenty-three usable pairs. While matching may serve as a control factor, it does have inherent drawbacks.

Homogeneous Groups

Another procedure is to use groups that are as homogeneous as possible. In this approach, the health science researcher would select a sample in which all the subjects would be homogeneous on the variable in question. For example, if level of education was an extraneous variable, its effect could be controlled by the use of subjects who all have the same education. In this manner, the effects that are found can be justified as stemming from the independent variable more readily (Ary, Jacobs, and Razavier, 1972).

The use of homogeneous groups is not always available, however, because some of the extraneous variables either may not be identified or may not be present in large enough numbers to carry out the research. Further, if control is accomplished on only one variable, such as level of education, the researcher is unable to generalize findings to other levels of education.

Analysis of Covariance

A superior technique for control in ex post facto studies is analysis of covariance (ANCOVA). It is a post hoc method of matching on such variables as prior education, age, and socioeconomic status. Because

ANCOVA requires complex mathematical computations and demands several assumptions, the inexperienced health scientist is advised to consult a statistician and complete additional reading such as the volume by Hopkins and Glass (1970).

Control or Alternative Hypotheses

Like other research methods, the ex post facto study should begin with hypotheses. In addition to the principal hypotheses that explain the relationship between the independent and dependent variables, the health science researcher should develop alternative hypotheses. While this can be done for all studies, it is especially important in ex post facto research because this method, by its very nature, requires alternative explanations. That is, the researcher must always consider that forces other than the identified independent variable brought about the differences he or she is examining.

For example, in Eric's study, he may hypothesize that "parental teaching brought about the difference between those who demonstrate positive dental hygiene habits and those who do not." However, like other researchers using the ex post facto method, he would be unwise to accept the first plausible explanation. It may be that positive experiences with preventive dentists is the explanation. Each alternative hypothesis should be stated and tested.

The research results can confirm more than one alternative hypothesis, and this may be anticipated in ex post facto research because most health behaviors are often the result of several complex factors. Even when the existence of a relationship between two variables is demonstrated, it does not mean that one causes the other.

Intervening and spurious relationships show how a third variable operates in such a way to make the independent and dependent variables appear to be related. A spurious relationship is one in which two variables appear related because both are caused by a third variable. For example, a health scientist may find a strong positive correlation between the number of cases of herpes simplex and the size of city airports. The larger the airports, the greater number of cases of herpes simplex. Can it be concluded that those flying into larger cities are responsible for the incidence of herpes? It may be more realistic to comprehend that some third factor is bringing about both the incidence of herpes and some third factor is bringing about both the incidence of herpes and larger airports—simply, an increase in population density.

In examining two variables, X and Y, it may appear they are closely related when in fact the apparent relationship results from an intervening variable. In this instance, X and Y may be highly correlated but only because X causes a third variable, Z, which in turn causes Y. If it were not for the intervening variable, Z, there would be no relationship between X and Y (Bailey, 1982).

In some ex post facto studies, the researcher must contemplate the possibility that the reverse of the suggested hypothesis could also account for the finding. That is, rather than X causing Y, perhaps Y causes X. As all people in the health field know, there is a relationship between exercise and good health. The question is, does good health lead one to exercise or does the exercise bring about good health? Similarly, if the student of health explored the relationship between an acceptance of the holistic health philosophy and wellness-promotion activity, it could be asked whether those in wellness promotion developed this acceptance by being a part of wellness promotion or whether their involvement in wellness promotion came about because of their acceptance of the holistic philosophy. The hypothesis of reverse causality is very plausible in some health science investigations.

To rule out reversed causality, the health scientist could look for evidence that Y did not occur before X. In short, the time relationship may provide the necessary clues. Another approach is to obtain measurements of the same subjects at two different times—before they become involved in wellness promotion activities and after they have been involved for a period of time.

In summation, the health researcher should attempt to control the competing interpretations of a single relationship. Perhaps the best way is to state and to test any alternative hypothesis that might serve as a plausible explanation. To start, a list of all the possible independent variables should be drafted. Each one can be tested with the others held constant. If the investigator can eliminate the alternative independent variables, then the case for the principal hypothesis has gained support. In other words, to have more confidence that X is closely related to Y, the alternative hypotheses must be ruled out.

Procedure in the Cause-To-Effect Investigation

The first step to be taken by the investigator is to develop an hypothesis. In Mary Margaret's study, the hypothesis may be twofold in that "the children of an Alzheimer's parent (1) perceive a need to live life to the fullest each day and (2) plan ahead for complete medical care and disability insurance for the retirement years." When analyzing the data, Mary Margaret may find that her hypotheses are confirmed. However, because she is conducting an ex post facto investigation and not an experimental one, doubt still exists as to whether or not being the child of an Alzheimer's parent did in fact cause this perception and/or the planning for medical care and disability insurance. That is, perhaps another antecedent variable such as level of education brought about confirmation of the hypothesis. Because Mary Margaret cannot manipulate the independent variable X, being a child of an Alzheimer's parent, Mary Margaret must attempt to control extraneous variables in some other fashion.

Her next step is to select the two groups to be used in the study. The group whose parent has Alzheimer's disease can be randomly selected from the large facility in which she works. The comparison group can be selected from several of the organizations for the healthy elderly. In order to achieve some control, Mary Margaret could match the two groups on age and level of education and any other variables she deemed appropriate. To determine whether or not the two groups were initially similar in their outlook of life and/or planning for medical care and disability insurance, Mary Margaret could administer a questionnaire to gather data from which she could infer similarity or dissimilarity. Questions asked could include: How did you feel about work in relation to recreation before your parent contracted Alzheimer's disease? Did you have a tendency to procrastinate? How well versed were you in your health insurance plans?

Because matching can create problems, Mary Margaret could select analysis of covariance to compensate for the lack of equivalency in the groups initially. Further, she may wish to establish multiple comparison groups to provide more data for analysis.

In regard to data collection, Mary Margaret may employ any instruments she wishes to compare the two groups in terms of her hypotheses. Analysis of data, as in most ex post facto investigations, would be both descriptive and inferential.

Procedure in the Effect-to-Cause Investigation

The effect-to-cause approach requires the researcher to explore two or more groups that are different in one or more characteristics to discover the cause(s) for the difference. As in the cause-to-effect investigation, the first step is the development of an hypothesis. Eric's hypothesis denoted previously is an example: "Parental teaching brought about the difference between those who demonstrate positive dental hygiene habits and those who do not demonstrate positive dental hygiene habits." The need for an ex post facto study is indicated in that Eric is unable to manipulate existing positive dental hygiene habits nor assign the adolescents to groups. Instead, he commences with two groups of university student patients who already differ in dental hygiene habits.

Next, Eric must fully define what is meant by positive dental hygiene habits. It may be explained as brushing after each meal and flossing once a day. Ideally, he would then randomly draw from a larger group of university students who demonstrated positive dental hygiene habits and from a group who failed to exhibit such habits.

Because factors other than, or in addition to, parental teaching may have contributed to present dental habits, it is necessary to formulate alternative hypotheses. It may be that exposure to preventive dentistry through a dentist brought about the positive dental habits. Also, it may be hypothesized that the sight of family members with bad teeth caused some of the students to practice positive dental hygiene. Eric should look for all the variables that could influence positive dental hygiene and either match the groups on them or use analysis of covariance where possible so that each alternative hypothesis can be tested.

Once the groups are established and controls are designed, the researcher can begin data collection. Ex post facto research, particularly effect-to-cause investigation, collects biographical data to seek past causes for present behavior patterns. In Eric's study, knowledge of the student's parental relationship, dental health, interpersonal relationships, as well as self-concept and body image may be measured to reveal factors that played a role in the development of current behavior patterns. There are no limitations on the types of measuring instruments that can be employed in the ex post facto approach.

As Mary Margaret does in her study, Eric may conduct data analysis to show descriptive statistics for each group and inferential analysis to test the principal and alternative hypotheses. The technique chosen would correspond to the design and nature of the hypotheses to be tested.

Common Errors in Ex Post Facto Research

The health scientist must be careful not to make mistakes when conducting ex post facto research, especially some of the more common ones. One error that is often made is the belief that the results of an ex post facto study are proof of a cause-and-effect relationship.

Smoking studies have shown that such is not the case. A second popular error is failure to control for initial differences between groups. Third, the health researcher may not establish homogeneous groups or subgroups (age, gender, and similar variables) for comparison. A fourth mistake is using the wrong sampling distribution with small samples and a related fifth error is to use an incorrect t-test to compare independent means or correlated means. Failure to use a nonparametric test of significance when the assumptions necessary for parametric tests have not been met is a sixth common mistake.

Summary

Chapter 13 begins with two case studies that illustrate two types of ex post facto studies. The first study was the cause-to-effect approach and the second was the effect-to-cause approach. These were further illustrated in the discussion of characteristics of ex post facto research. Generally, it was seen that in ex post facto investigations the independent variable or variables have already occurred, and the health scientist studies retrospectively to determine the relationship between the independent variable and the dependent variable or variables.

Though ex post facto research is similar to experimental research in many respects, random assignment to groups and control of the independent variable are not possible in ex post facto research. It is this lack of control that gives ex post facto research less confidence than experimental research. In addition to these disadvantages, it was seen that there is a high risk of misinterpretation in ex post facto research. The problem of interpretability could be reduced through path analysis and other techniques to provide control.

The control techniques reviewed included matching, homogeneous groups, analysis of covariance, and the development of control or alternative hypotheses to be tested. Testing may reveal that relationships to exist because of intervening or spurious causes, and in some instances reversed causality may account for a finding.

Procedures in both the cause-to-effect and the effect-to-cause approaches were presented including comments on data collection and data analysis. As a final note, common errors in ex post facto research were presented.

Though ex post facto research has drawbacks, it is a technique with much potential in the health discipline. Like other research methodologies, it must be used appropriately and wisely.

Suggested Activities_____

1. Search professional journals and write an abstract from each journal demonstrating cause-to-effect and effect-to-cause approaches. Use the following journals: *Journal of School Health, Journal of American Public Health Association, New England Journal of Medicine, and Nursing Research*.
2. Prepare to defend or to refute the following statement: Ex post facto research and correlation research are one and the same.
3. List the commonalities and differences between ex post facto research and experimental research.
4. As a health researcher, what could you do to help overcome the possibility of misinterpretation that can occur with ex post facto methodology?
5. Develop three hypotheses for three different ex post facto studies. Formulate alternative hypotheses for each of the three speculative studies. Suggest how you would test each hypothesis and what inferential technique you might use.
6. Written below are abstracts from professional journals describing the research conducted. Read each abstract and determine the nature of the ex post facto study—cause-to-effect or effect-to-cause. If necessary, read the entire article.
    A. Effects of Unemployment on Mental and Physical Health (Linn et al., 1985)

    From a prospective study of the impact of stress on health in 300 men assessed over six months, men who became unemployed after entering the study were compared with an equal number, matched for age and race, who continued to work. Psychological and health data after unemployment were compared between the two groups by multivariate analysis of variance and covariance. After unemployment symptoms of somatization, depression, and anxiety were significantly greater in the unemployed than employed. Large standard deviations on self-esteem scores in the unemployed group suggested that some men coped better than others with job-loss stress. Further analysis showed those with higher esteem had more support from family and friends than did those with low self-esteem. Furthermore, unemployed men made significantly more visits to their physicians, took more medications, and spent more days in bed sick than did employed individuals even though the number of diagnoses in the two groups were very similar (p. 502).
    B. Cancer Risk in Adulthood from Early Life Exposure to Parents' Smoking (Sandler et al., 1985)

    We obtained data on smoking by parents from 438 cancer cases and 470 controls to investigate whether risk in adult life is related to transplacental or childhood exposure to cigarette smoke. Cancer cases were between ages 15 and 59 at time of diagnosis. All sites but basal cell cancer of the skin were included. Cancer risk was increased 50% among offspring of men who smoked. Increased risk associated with father's smoking was not explained by demographic factors, social class, or individual smoking habits, and was not limited to known smoking related sites.

Relative risk (RR) estimates associated with father's smoking tended to be greatest for smokers, males, and non-Whites. There was only a slight increase in overall cancer risk associated with maternal smoking. Mother's and Father's smoking were both associated with risk for hematopoietic cancers, and a dose-response relationship was seen. The RR for hematopoietic cancers increased from 1.7 when one parent smoked to 4.6 when both parents smoked. Although, they should be considered tentative, study findings suggest a long-term hazard from transplacental or childhood passive exposure to cigarette smoke (p. 487).

C. Does Race Affect Hospital Use? (Wilson et al., 1985)

Based on 1980 hospital discharges in areas in the State of Michigan, with substantial Black populations, Blacks use approximately 50% more hospital care than Whites, but about half this difference is associated with use in specific communities which affects both White and Black use. Black use is not associated with community size, per cent of Blacks, or available beds and doctors. After controlling for mortality and socioeconomic status, a small statistically non-significant difference in race-specific use remains for 23 Michigan communities. The elimination of race as an explainer of hospital use suggests progress in assuring equal access to hospitals, but differences in poverty, mortality, and some specifics of use remain (p. 263).

D. Smoking Behavior and The Tobacco Crop (Wilson and Higgins, 1984)

The purpose of the study was to measure the influence of the physical and economic presence of the tobacco crop on the smoking behavior and related attitudes of adolescents in tobacco raising regions. A stratified random sample of all grades five-12 from the schools in four Kentucky counties yielded a sample size of 1,322 students. A variable called Tobacco Crop Intensity (TCI) based on pounds of tobacco sold per population and land area was defined. It was determined that the counties were polarized on this variable; two counties have a much more significant crop. Students from the pairs of counties were surveyed and compared. Results indicated that young people living in the counties with high intensity tobacco production or whose parents grow tobacco were twice as likely to smoke cigarettes; some of their attitudes and beliefs indicate a greater predisposition to cigarette smoking. Implications for government agricultural and educational policy are discussed (p. 343).

7. You are a nurse working in a small rural hospital and would like to determine why some patients comply with physician's prescription orders and others fail to comply. Because you work with discharged patients as a follow-up, you have access to data and to patients from both sides of the compliance question. You would like to present your idea to the hospital administrator. In order to do so, complete the following:

a. Write out a problem statement.
b. Write out a common hypothesis and alternative hypotheses.
c. Design and plan the study to include selection of comparison groups, types of instruments for data collection, and suggested data analysis techniques.

8. You are a health educator in Appalachia teaching in a school with a mixture of very poor rural students and middle-class rural students. Recognizing that the poor students frequently lack for meals and the necessary health care, you hope to find out what effect this brings in school performance.

   What type of ex post facto research is indicated for this study? Outline and complete the necessary steps to conduct an ex post facto investigation.

References

Ary, D., Jacobs, L. C., and Razavieh, A. (1972) *Introduction to Research in Education,* New York: Holt, Rinehart and Winston.

Bailey, K. D. (1982) *Methods of Social Research,* New York: The Free Press.

Chapin, F. S. (1947) *Experimental Designs in Sociological Research,* New York: Harper and Row.

Cook, T. D. and Campbell, D. T. (1979) *Quasi-experimentation: Design and Analysis Issues for Field Settings,* Chicago: Rand McNally.

Higgins, C. W., Whitely, K. N., and Dunn, J. D. (1984) A comparison of smoking related attitudes and behaviors among Kentucky public school children whose families are and are not involved in tobacco production, *Journal of School Health* 54(5):185–87.

Hopkins, K. D. and Glass, G. V. (1970) *Basic Statistics for the Behavioral Sciences,* Englewood Cliffs, NJ: Prentice-Hall.

Kerlinger, F. N. (1964) *Foundations of Behavioral Research,* New York: Holt, Rinehart and Winston.

Nathanson, C. A. and Becker, M. H. (1985) The influence of client-provider relationships on teenage women's subsequent use of contraception, *American Journal of Public Health* 75(1):33–38.

Rogosa, D. (1979) Causal models in longitudinal research: rationale, formulation and interpretation. In Nesselroade, J. R. and Baltes, P. B. (eds.), *Longitudinal Research in the Study of Behavior and Development,* New York: Academic Press.

Sandler, D. P., Everson, R. B., Wilcox A. J., and Browder, J. P. (1985) Cancer risk in adulthood from early life exposure to parents' smoking, *American Journal of Public Health* 75(3):487–492.

Wilson, P. A., Griffith, J. R., and Tedeschi, P. J. (1985) Does race affect hospital use? *American Journal of Public Health* 75(3):263–269.

Wilson, R. W. and Higgins, C. W. (1984) Smoking behavior and the tobacco crop, *Journal of School Health* 54(9):343–346.

CHAPTER 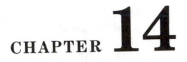 14

Writing a Research Report

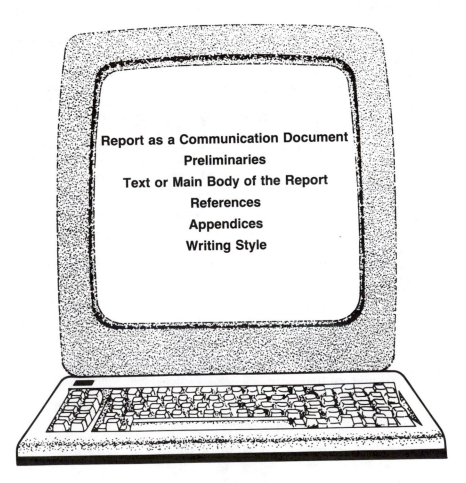

Report as a Communication Document

Preliminaries

Text or Main Body of the Report

References

Appendices

Writing Style

The preceding chapters have dealt with the many aspects of conducting research. Once the research study is complete, the project needs to be communicated to other interested professionals. The communication may take the form of a term paper, research report, manuscript for a journal article, master's thesis or doctoral dissertation. This chapter will provide some guidelines to help you prepare the research report. Keep in mind, however, that style manuals, university and college requirements, and each journal require different types of written preparation. Make sure to check the format that is required *before* you embark upon the writing of your study.

The Report as a Communication Document

Health science is exactly that: a science you have learned through many years of schooling. A good health scientist begins with a theory, devises hypotheses based on that theory, designs and carries out an investigation to test the stated hypotheses, and analyzes the collected data to ascertain if these hypotheses can be accepted (or rejected). The last step, which can be the most exciting, is to communicate this process to other health scientists and interested people. The study has been well planned and thought out, and carried through as expected. Usually, several obstacles have been faced and successfully dealt with. These obstacles and other problems undoubtedly alter the research process, therefore causing unexpected results. This is the exciting part! If the research project went as smoothly as planned, the report could have been written before the study was conducted. When you begin to think about writing the research report, you should probably start by thinking about the data you have collected and what these results actually mean. This process leads to finding unexpected results, which may lead to new, exciting, and extremely relevant information for the field of health science.

Some researchers are reluctant to report negative results or results that do not support their theories. All good research should be communicated; we have a responsibility to our colleagues to inform, reaffirm, and present new findings related to human health behavior. It is this communication that encourages others to conduct investigations that will help the growth of the health sciences.

The research report is generally divided into the following sections:

1. **Introduction.** An explanation of the problem and why it is important.
2. **Review of the Literature.** A review of relevant studies focus-

ing on the theory and its importance and implication for the study.

3. **Methodology.** A description of the procedures, subjects, and instruments employed in the study.

4. **Presentation and Analysis of the Data.** A discussion of the method used to analyze the data, a presentation of the findings, and a discussion of what the findings mean.

5. **Conclusions and Summary.** Conclusions and a brief summary conclude the report.

6. **References.** All cited sources are included here.

7. **Appendix.** If appropriate, this section may include instruments, letters of commitment, etc.

We cannot emphasize one point too much; remember, all journals have their own format, as do several style manuals used by different colleges and universities. The following material will enable you to write the research report, regardless of the format, because the information can always be rearranged to suit a particular format.

Preliminaries

We have outlined the many parts to the research report. However, certain *preliminary* pages might be necessary for a manuscript, journal article, thesis, or dissertation.

Title Page

The first page of the report is called the title page. The page usually includes the title of the paper, author, relationship of the report to either a course or degree requirement, name of the institution to which the report is submitted, and date of submission. The title of the report should be brief but specific in terms of describing the project. For example, if you were to conduct an experiment to compare the behavioral changes of tenth-grade students who completed a new health science course as compared to the behavioral changes of a matched group who were exposed to the regular health science instruction a good title might be: "A Comparison of Experimental and Regular Health Science Instruction on the Behavioral Changes of Tenth-Grade Students." A second choice: "Behavioral Changes of Tenth-Grade Students," is too short and does not really describe the experiment.

The title should be typed in capital letters, single-spaced, and centered. If there is more than one line in the title, it is divided so that each successive line is shorter, forming an inverse pyramid. Figure 14.1 is an example of a title page.

A COMPARISON OF EXPERIMENTAL AND REGULAR

HEALTH SCIENCE INSTRUCTION ON THE

BEHAVIORAL CHANGES OF

TENTH GRADE STUDENTS

BY

JAYNE A. ROBINSON

A Term Paper Submitted in Partial Fulfillment

of the Requirements in

HSS 400: Health Behavior

University of Illinois

March 6, 1987

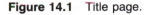

Figure 14.1   Title page.

Copyright

Most doctoral dissertations have a copyright. Theses and other reports may also be copyrighted, if you wish. To initiate this, the author must obtain a copyright authorization form, (usually available from university of college business offices) complete it, pay the fee, and include a copyright notice at the front of the dissertation or report: The notice appears, centered on a single page, as follows:

© Copyright by
(author's name)
(date)

If the author has received a great deal of assistance from a person or persons, an acknowledgment page is included at the beginning of the thesis or dissertation. This page should be kept simple and to the point. Usually, the student's committee members and family members are mentioned. In addition, it is considered correct to give mention to the participants and other site personnel.

If you are preparing a report or journal article, and there are groups or individuals that should be acknowledged, you can do so by providing a note to be placed on the first page (at the bottom) of the manuscript. The guidelines for acknowledgments here are slightly different from those used for theses or dissertations. The author would not acknowledge committee or family members, but might mention those who have helped in the data collection process, or those who have reviewed the manuscript previous to its being submitted for publication.

Table of Contents

The table of contents provides an outline of the contents of the paper. The major headings and subheadings are included along with the page number of each. Fig. 14.2 shows a table of contents for a research report. The table of contents for theses and dissertations will vary according to the style utilized by individual institutions.

List of Tables and Figures

When writing a report you may utilize figures and/or tables to supplement the manuscript. If you do, a separate list for each (tables and figures) should be included after the table of contents. The exact table titles and numbers used in the report are presented along with the pages on which they are located.

TABLE OF CONTENTS

Figure 14.2 Table of contents for research report.

Abstract

The abstract is a brief summary of the problems, methods, results, and conclusions of the study that gives a short rendition of the manuscript. This enables the reader to determine if it is necessary to continue reading the remainder of the report or article. Abstracts for theses and dissertations are usually presented after the table of contents. They are paginated in lower-case roman numerals, as are all preliminary materials mentioned in this section. An example of an abstract is shown in Fig. 14.3.

THE EFFECTS OF AN EXPERIMENTAL HEALTH EDUCATION CURRICULUM

KNOW YOUR BODY

Penelope Elaine Duff, Ph.D.

Department of Health and Safety Education

University of Illinois at Urbana-Champaign, 1982

The purpose of this study was to test the effect of an experimental risk reduction curriculum, Know Your Body, (KYB), on the traditional health outcomes of knowledge, attitudes and behavior. Also to be determined are the effects of the KYB clinical screening and the interactive effects of the KYB instruction and KYB clinical screening on the same health outcomes.

The subjects were 597 ninth grade students enrolled in health education classes in four senior high schools in Decatur, Illinois in Spring 1981. In the experimental 2x2 design each school represented one cell. Treatments were: School I had KYB instruction only, School II had KYB screening and traditional health education, School III had KYB instruction and KYB screening, and School IV had traditional health education only. All schools were pre- and posttested using the Seffring Health Knowledge Test and the KYB Health Attitude and Behavior Surveys. Clinical data collected included: height, weight, skinfold thickness, blood pressure, and resting and exercise pulses. Multivariate and univariate analysis of variance tests were employed.

Results showed that the main effects of instruction and screening had significant effects on the knowledge variable. For each main effect, School I and III scored significantly higher than School II. Significant differences were also associated with the interactive effects of screening by instruction. School I scores significantly higher than School II on the behavior variable. The attitude survey showed no significant difference amongst schools for each treatment effect. The clinical screening procedures must be further examined before conclusions as to their value can be determined.

Figure 14.3 Example of an abstract.

Text or Main Body of the Report_____

The main portion of the report consists of an introduction, review of the literature, methodology, presentation and analysis of the data, and conclusions and summary. Each of these sections serve as a communication of the study.

Introduction

The introduction serves to state the problem and coordinate that problem to the literature that has been published. Hypotheses or research questions are formed from reviewing the relevant literature. Delimitations, definition of terms, and assumptions are also part of the introduction. Finally, the importance of the research is described.

Statement of the Problem

The problem statement occurs within the first or second paragraph, setting up a rationale for the ensuing background literature. The writer should be sure that the problem is clearly and concisely stated, so that readers who may not be informed about the problem get true conceptual notion about the problem. When stating the problem, the author should cite those sources that have direct bearing on it and follow up with an in-depth review of the literature in a later section. This part of the introduction should begin with broad statements that become more specific until the study is introduced by means of stating the hypotheses or research questions.

Hypotheses or Research Questions

The next step in writing the research report is to formulate and state the hypothesis or research questions. Dependent upon the particular format you are required to use, the review of literature can precede the hypotheses, or serve as a rationale and hence be stated after the review of literature. In any case, the hypotheses should be reasonable and simply stated, consistent with known facts or theories, be able to be tested, and express the relationship between two variables.

There are some studies that do not lend themselves to formulation of research hypotheses. These are generally investigations that do not have experimental and control groups, but are considered experimental anyway.

Example of Research Questions

These research questions are taken from a study in which self-efficacy was used as a predictor of smoking in young adolescents (Lawrance, 1985).

1. Can we predict smoking behavior from the students' responses to the items on the self-efficacy scale?
2. Is there a difference in the response patterns of males and females to the self-efficacy items?
3. Do children of this age respond in a similar fashion 4 and 8 months later?
4. Which specific items on the self-efficacy scale discriminate the smokers from the nonsmokers?

Delimitations

Studies are usually conducted within certain boundaries and the results cannot be extrapolated to other populations. These are the delimitations. For example in a study entitled "Beliefs Associated with Smoking Intentions of College Women" (Roberts, 1979) the delimitations stated were:

> This study dealt only with freshman women enrolled at the University of Illinois who lived in Lincoln Avenue Residence, Busey-Evans Residence, Florida Avenue Residence, and Pennsylvania Avenue Residence Halls. (p. 9)

Definition of Terms

Some terms used in the literature and in studies may be ambiguous and thus cause confusion for the reader. To be sure that the reader does not misinterpret any terms, the writer devises a definition wherein the term provides a frame of reference for the reader. In addition, the variables that are being studied should be defined in operational terms. The following definitions of terms were from a study that examined the relationship between expectancy theory and student teacher's pre- and posttest scores (Tappe, 1985).

Expectancy Value Model. A model from motivational psychology that relates action to the perceived value of expected consequences. The primary components of the model are expectations and values that are utilized to predict action. For the purposes of this study the Vroom force model or job effort model was utilized.

Teaching Competency. One of fifteen teaching behaviors selected as germane to the practice of teaching.

Assumptions

There are some facts concerning the study that are established but the writer cannot prove these facts. In a study entitled: "The Health Belief Model and Contraceptive Behavior Among College Females" (Robertson, 1983), the following were listed as assumptions:

1. The design of the instrument would yield responses that were valid and reliable.
2. That self-report, as in the case of a self-administered questionnaire, is an accurate measure of actual behavior.
3. That individuals are able to project themselves into hypothetical situations and accurately assess their probable feelings and actions. (p. 30)

Significance of the Problem

The major purpose of conducting any study is to provide knowledge and insight into a particular theory or provide relevance for practitioners. In this section, the writer presents the possible implications of what the results of the study will mean to the specific area under investigation. A discussion of how these results will be useful in solving problems and answering questions in the general field is also included (Ary, Jacobs, and Razivieh, 1985). The significance of the problem should additionally include the applications of the results of the study to health science practitioners, if applicable. That is, if the findings of the investigation will benefit those in the field, then this should be stated. The problem's significance convinces the reader that the experiment is worthy and should be carried out by the investigator.

Review of the Literature

The literature review was discussed in detail in Chapter 2. Here we will explain, briefly, the importance of the review of literature, a suggested process for carrying out the task, and a summary of this particular section.

The review of the literature is intended to give the reader an understanding of *why* you have chosen to conduct your study. The relevant information is put together to give purpose to a question that is important, or that you may believe to be important. The writer uses mainly primary sources to support the previously stated hypotheses or research questions. The general themes to concentrate on in the writing of the review include: What previous theories are relevant to your problem? What is your knowledge about those previous works?

The process of conducting the search can at first look unwieldy and forbidding, especially if you have chosen a problem on which there has been much previous research. A good starting point, as was described in Chapter 2 is to conduct the search using note cards, prepare an outline of the major topics you have reviewed, and then provide order to those topics. You may have as many as twenty cards per topic and this is where the *writing* of the review of literature becomes difficult. Too often, writers abstract each source (article, book, and so on) and just write them down, paragraph after paragraph. This is *not* a good way to write the review: it is boring and provides no insight from the writer. Some studies that are considered the classics pertaining to your topic should be described in detail. Other projects should be mentioned and grouped together, to provide a coherent, well-integrated review. There are ways to handle this in your paper. You might write, "Findings of the above studies have been largely supported by a number of other studies that have employed similar approaches" (Borg, 1983). Then you can reference those other studies. Or you might write, "There are several other studies that support this notion (Smith, 1986, Jones, 1985, Johnson, 1987)."

As the literature review takes shape, i.e., the topics are well researched and referenced properly, you need to develop for the reader a sense of integration and insight into the knowledge that you have amassed. This is difficult because you must be thoroughly familiar with and have a complete understanding of the relevant literature. Interpretation of the findings of all of these studies becomes the most important part of the literature review.

The summary of the literature review should include a brief discussion of the findings and their implications for the study being proposed by the writer. These implications should indicate those areas of agreement and disagreement relevant to the problem, as well as any gaps in the existing literature.

Methodology

The methodology section includes a plan of how the study will be conducted so that the hypotheses or research questions can be ascertained. We have discussed in previous chapters the many research designs that are available for almost any type of study. The writer would choose one that best suits the hypotheses or research questions. The methodology section also includes a description of the subjects, the exact procedures utilized to collect the data, and an explanation of the instruments employed in the conduct of the study.

Subjects

The methodology usually begins with a description of the sample used in the study. Detailed description is necessary so that the reader can determine if the research sample is representative and can be generalized to other, similar populations. If the reader knows this, then he or she may be able to apply the results to another study, or even replicate the study. Information such as sex, age, educational level, social economic status, place of residence (urban, rural), and the like are important and should be included. In addition, a discussion of how the subjects were selected should be integrated into this section. Here the population from which the sample was drawn should be described and methods of selection mentioned, such as randomization or matching. These methods must be very carefully detailed and include the criteria, the number of lost cases, and the effect these lost cases might have on the study. The following is an example of the subjects' section from a master's thesis (Tunyavanich, 1975):

Example of Subjects' Section

The population defined for the purpose of this study included 412 cases from school unit superintendents and principals of middle, junior high school and senior high school attendance centers in the state of Illinois in 1975. Only 412 questionnaires were used from the original 871 cases collected by the Illinois Office of Education because the information on some of the questionnaires could not be accurately interpreted. (p. 21)

Procedures

In the procedures section of the paper, a detailed description of the procedures is written. A synopsis of the subjects, the setting, and the variables studied begins the section. One way to organize this part is to present the procedures in chronological order. You might begin by describing the research design with enough detail that a replication of the work could be attempted. Next, the writer gives a review of how the data were collected, again describing in detail any events that were unusual or that affected the study. A discussion of any steps taken to control or even to reduce errors (e.g., administering measures to all groups at the same time) should be delineated for the reader (Borg, 1983). This is necesssary so that the reader will be able to reconstruct the study, and perhaps avoid pitfalls that you encountered. All is done in the name of progress! If the procedures were complicated and had many variables, groups, and data collection methodologies, you can end this section with a one-paragraph summary.

Example of Procedure

PROCEDURE

The instructor of each section of the sex education and family life course administered the questionnaire on the first day of class to the students. The course was held on weekday evenings in the meeting rooms of university housing. The instructors were asked to have the students complete the questionnaire at the very beginning of the first class, prior to any instruction or introduction of materials for the course. Instructors were also asked to follow a guideline given to them when administering the questionnaire. Participation in completing the questionnaire was voluntary and anonymous. Students were asked to place the questionnaire, whether completed or not, in an envelope located in the center of the room. The last student was requested to seal the envelope. The sealed envelope was then returned to the mailbox of the investigator (see Appendix B). (Harmata, 1980, p. 56)

Instruments

In a research project, independent variables are manipulated and then studied for their relationship with the dependent variables. In order to accomplish this task, instruments or measures are used to assess achievement, behavior change, attitude, or some other construct. In this section of the report, a detailed description of instruments used to collect the data is given. If the instruments are standardized tests, then the description should be brief and include a description of the scores, a review of reliability and validity measures, a mention of each variable that was measured by the scores, and a statement of the relationship of the measure to the hypotheses or research questions (Borg, 1983).

Instruments can also be new or adopted from other standardized measures. If this is the case with your study, then the instrumentation section of the paper must be more detailed. Here the first construction phase must be explained. Types of items used are shown as examples, reliability and validity scores that have been obtained in pilot testing are revealed, and an explanation of the way the measure was constructed is offered. Finally, you should include, by example, the way in which the measure was scored. Usually, a copy of the instrument along with a key or instructions for scoring are included in the appendix of the paper or report.

Presentation and Analysis of Results

The presentation and analysis of the results of a study may be written together or separately. This depends upon format style and the type of paper, report, or thesis. In articles, again dependent upon the journal's format, the results and analysis (sometimes called discussion) sections are combined. In longer, more complicated studies, the results may be separated from the analysis, although the integration of the two is necessary throughout either section.

Introduction. At the beginning of the results and analysis section, the writer should present evidence that the study procedures actually tested the stated hypotheses or research questions. If, for example, you sent out a survey and obtained a low response rate, this may have influenced the results of the study. This fact must be mentioned in the results and analysis section. Also, if you had experimental and control groups you should be sure to indicate their homogeneity. If the groups did differ, then explain the procedures you took to deal with these differences. The next paragraph or so should explain the method of data analysis (the coding procedures used, how the raw scores were converted, combining responses, patterns of response, and so on). Included here should also be a discussion of the statistical analyses used. If you used ordinary or often-used methods, then the description should be brief, as in the case of analysis of variance. However, if you used more complicated and unusual analyses, then you need to fully explain the analysis and give a rationale for its use. (This is accomplished by citing a source for the reader).

At the end of this introduction section, it is recommended that you tell the reader how the results and analysis will be presented. One good method of organizing this section is to use the hypothesis or research questions as organizers. Each hypothesis is restated, one at a time, and the results and subsequent analysis regarding that hypothesis are discussed. This is an easy method to use, but certainly not the only one. You should discuss this matter with an advisor or someone who has had experience in writing reports on theses; their insights will prove helpful to you.

Presenting the Findings. When presenting the findings, you must be careful not to present so many numbers and tables that your results section is ignored. One method is to state the basic finding (related to a hypothesis or research questions) first, and then work to the more specific findings. The result should be communicated with words first, then numbers and statistics. It is also a good idea to provide brief summaries throughout the section because this maintains coherence and clarity for the reader.

Presenting the Analysis (or Discussion). This section on presenting the analysis has three main components: interpretation of the findings, implications of those findings, and application of the findings to practice. If this section is centered around the hypotheses or research questions and is combined with the results section, you do not have to restate the questions or hypothesis. You can begin by accepting or rejecting the hypothesis or giving the answers to the research questions. Here the writer should make some inferences from the findings and interpret the results in relationship to the theory and other research. This section is where the writer compares his or her results to other studies and states the possible flaws in the research. Reasonable explanations are expected; keep them brief and sensible. If, on the other hand, you might have developed a new theory, or link to a new or even old theory, you should explain that phenomenon as well. Again, even if this discussion is the most exciting event in your life, keep it brief and to the point.

The second part of this section deals with the implications that the results may have for the general field encompassed within your study. For example, you may have found that self-efficacy was a major predictor of smoking behavior among adolescents, but what are the implications for the health science field? Is self-efficacy, as a part of social learning theory, a good mechanism for determining program interventions in antismoking campaigns? These implications should suggest additions to theories and further research that may follow from the present study.

The final section of presenting the analysis should attempt to illustrate how these findings can be used by the practitioners in the field. Will these results provide a new administrative style, teaching method, or community organizer?

Conclusions and Summary

The last section of the paper or the final chapter of a thesis or dissertation is probably the one most often read. It provides a brief review of the investigation and clearly discusses the conclusions reached by the investigator. Many journals no longer require a summary because the material is covered in the abstract. Nonetheless, research papers, reports, theses, and dissertations still adhere, for the most part, to final conclusions and a summary.

Conclusions. In the conclusion, the investigator should indicate whether the findings support or do not support the hypotheses or what the findings mean in relationship to the research questions. The conclusions are actually the major *inferences* of the study based on the results of the experiment. For example, in one of our case studies, Jayne found that the new health science curriculum, "No Smoke" produced more changes in student's behavior regarding smoking than the old health science curriculum, "Smoking's Bad". This is an observed result based upon measurement scores and observations of students. Jayne could conclude by inference then, that the "No Smoke" curriculum is more effective in changing smoking behavior than the "Smoking's Bad" curriculum. This section may also include recommendations for further research and a discussion of new research questions that may have arisen.

Summary. The summary is usually the last section of the report and should briefly restate the problem, describe the procedures, and discuss the principal findings. The writer must be sure not to add anything new here because it is an account of what has already been written in the report.

References

All material that was cited in your report or article must appear in the reference list. The list begins with the word *References* centered at the top of the page. The works are arranged alphabetically by author's last name. The style manual that your institution has selected will provide exact details as to how to prepare the reference list. In this textbook, we have used the American Psychological Association's style manual, but there are others you can utilize.

Campbell, W. and Ballow, S. (1982) *Form and Style: Theses, Reports, Term Papers,* 6th ed. Boston: Houghton Mifflin.
The Chicago Manual of Style (1982) 13th rev. ed., Chicago: University of Chicago Press.
Mullins, C. (1977) *A Guide to Writing and Publishing in the Social Sciences,* New York: Wiley.

Appendices

The appendices include materials that were not appropriate to be included in the body of the paper, but will be useful to the reader.

These materials usually include copies of instruments, keys to those instruments, raw data scores, instructions to subjects, letters of support, and long tables or print-outs of secondary data analyses.

The appendix is usually noted by having a piece of paper precede it with the word "APPENDIX ," capitalized and centered. The first page of the appendix is titled *Appendix A,* centered at the top, and is numbered consecutively from the last pages of the manuscript. Each subsequent piece of material constitutes an appendix and is designated by B, C, D, and so on. Make sure to check your specific style requirements, because they may differ from our instructions.

Writing Style

The report, article, thesis, or dissertation need not be pedantic and dull, as so many have been. You should keep your writing to a minimum; it should be clear, concise, simple, and coherent. The main points to strive for when writing are clarity and accuracy (Kidder, 1981). Anything you add to enhance the text, such as humor, is acceptable if it is done in a professional manner. Many new writers want to make their reports flowery, including similies and alliterations. This type of writing style should be avoided in the writing of scientific papers.

Voice and Tense

Because scientific writing is supposed to be objective, writers have used the impersonal form of expression. For example, "the investigator observed" in place of "I observed." The good news is that many journals and style manuals for thesis and dissertations have relaxed this rule to enable the writer to have a more personal style. For example, "I instructed the data collectors" instead of "The data collectors were instructed." Though personal pronouns are now acceptable, do not overuse them in your report. The term *we* should be used if "we" really collaborated on the study. You may also use *we* occasionally when referring to yourself and the reader as in "We can see from Table 16. . . ."

The experiment must have been completed if you are now writing the report. Therefore, utilize the past tense throughout the paper. Be especially careful in the review of literature section, where there is a tendency to write: "Smith notes" instead of "Smith noted." The studies have been completed, therefore they should be reported in the past tense (Howard, 1985). There are occasions within the report where you can use the present tense, e.g., "Table 16 shows the relationship." In addition, when discussing the implications of your study you might write, "The data from the present investigation suggest."

Nonsexist Terminology

We are supposed to be an enlightened society and free from stereotypes. To reinforce this idea, writers are not to use sexist language, because it might convey attitudes and sex roles that perpetuate stereotypes. Therefore, in 1977 the American Psychological Association published guidelines for nonsexist journal writing. The manual does provide ways to use alternatives:

> *Improper:* The health scientist is the best judge of his attitude toward smoking.
> *Proper:* Health scientists are the best judges of their attitudes toward smoking.

In this example the use of the plural was used as an alternative to sexist language. At times, you might have to refer to an individual; this may be accomplished by using "he or she" or "him or her," if it is not done too often.

When describing your subjects, however, you must report numbers of males and females. This is done by using either female or male pronouns. Attempt to find sex-neutral terms: *flight attendant* rather than *stewardess, parenting* rather than *mothering,* and so on, to describe persons in your study. In addition, we should all attempt to avoid sex-role stereotyping when using examples (Kidder, 1981). Not all physicians are male, nor all dental hygienists female.

Rewriting the Report

When you first begin writing research reports it will seem an arduous and impossible task. But, as with anything else, the harder one tackles the problem, the less insurmountable that task becomes. This is very true with writing. As you write, you will find it helpful to have peers or faculty members review the drafts. Usually their comments will prove to be helpful, and you will learn something about the necessity for rewriting the original draft. Most, if not nearly all writers never submit a first draft, but rewrite various portions of a manuscript several times. This may seem tiresome, and it is, but it does produce good results.

The first draft is often written as quickly as possible, so that time and energy are saved for subsequent rewrites. You may realize after reviewing the draft (using the input of others as well) that the report needs more literature review or data analysis to support your arguments. Again, this is a difficult process. You may have to almost begin again but you will be much more satisfied with the results of your extraordinary efforts.

Summary

The research report, term paper, journal article, thesis, or dissertation is really a method of communication. As a health scientist you have the obligation to report the results of your investigation in a clear and concise manner. To accomplish this we have suggested that you first check with your local authority as to the type of style or manual that you should utilize. The second step in preparing a manuscript for a journal article, is to research that journal's specific style requirements.

A research report consists of several parts: introduction, review of the literature, methodology, presentation and analysis of the data, and summary and conclusions. Each section has several subheadings, which require attention to detail, clear and concise writing, and logical interpretations of the results of your study.

The writing style you grow into and eventually adopt will depend upon what you read and how often you read the literature, journal articles, theses, and dissertations. The style should be free of cliches, personal or sarcastic remarks, asides, and sexist language. Having others review your work before submitting it will be extremely helpful to you in preparing the manuscript. The finished product, with your name affixed to it, is well worth all the effort!

Suggested Activities

1. Determine the style manual your college or university requires you to utilize.
2. Prepare a detailed outline of a research report you are going to submit this semester.
3. Differentiate between hypotheses and research questions. Give examples of each.

References_____

Ary, D., Jacobs, L., and Razavieh, A. (1985) *Introduction to Research in Education,* New York: Holt, Rinehart, & Winston.

Borg, W. and Gall, M. (1983) *Educational Research,* New York: Longman.

Duff, P. (1982) *The Effects of an Experimental Health Education Curriculum: Know Your Body,* Unpublished doctoral dissertation, University of Illinois.

Harmata, J. (1980) *Differentiation Between Actual and Perceived Sexual Behavior Among College Students,* Unpublished masters thesis, University of Illinois.

Howard, G. (1985) *Basic Research Methods in the Social Sciences,* Glenview, Ill.: Scott, Foresman and Co.

Kidder, L. (1981) *Research Methods in Social Relations,* New York: Holt Rinehart, & Winston.

Lawrance, L. (1985) *Self-Efficacy as a Predictor of Smoking Behavior in Young Adolescents,* Unpublished doctoral dissertation, University of Illinois.

Roberts, S. (1979) *Beliefs Associated with Smoking Intentions of College Women,* Unpublished doctoral dissertation, University of Illinois.

Robertson, N. (1983) *The Health Belief Model and Contraceptive Behavior Among College Females,* Unpublished masters thesis, University of Illinois.

Tappe, M. (1985) *An Application of Expectancy Value Theory to Student-Teachers,* Unpublished masters thesis, University of Illinois.

Tunyavanich, N. (1975) *The Status of Health Instruction in Illinois Public Schools,* Unpublished masters thesis, University of Illinois.

Appendices

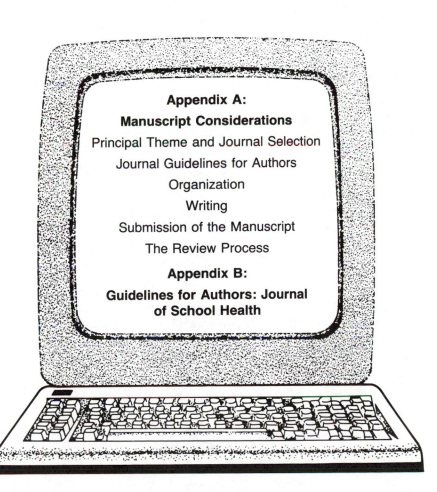

Appendix A:

Manuscript Considerations

Principal Theme and Journal Selection

Journal Guidelines for Authors

Organization

Writing

Submission of the Manuscript

The Review Process

Appendix B:

**Guidelines for Authors: Journal
of School Health**

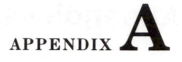

Manuscript Considerations

Health science researchers, whether in an academic, clinical, or field setting, should consider publishing their results in a reputable journal to assist others in their health work. This appendix is offered as a list of considerations for publishing your research.

Principal Theme and Journal Selection

One of the initial steps is to determine the principal theme of your research—clinical, school health, patient education, public health or a combination. Further, is the theme primarily theory or pragmatic in nature? In other words, which audience would be most interested in reading about your research endeavor?

Exploring the many journals in the health profession, you can quickly discover which journal is most appropriate for your manuscript. For example, the *Journal of School Health* is likely to be more receptive to manuscripts about children's health than some others. If your research effort was highly specialized, perhaps a journal such as the *Journal of Sex Education and Therapy* or *Journal of Human Stress* might be most appropriate. Similarly, some journals cater to an audience that is especially interested in theory, and still others prefer manuscripts that offer practical tips for teaching or field work. Based upon your principal theme, select the journal that serves an audience best suited to the theme and orientation of your research.

Journal Guidelines for Authors

Once the appropriate journal has been selected, the researcher should obtain a copy of its guidelines for authors by either writing the journal or obtaining one from a recent issue. Appendix B offers an example of the guidelines from the *Journal of School Health*. The suggestions contained in the guidelines should be followed closely by the author. In some instances, the guidelines will indicate that the journal has multiple sections, each of which involves a speciality area. Submission requirements, manuscript length, title page, style, abstract, visuals, and tables are all addressed in these guidelines.

Organization

It is important that you examine articles in recent copies of the selected journal to ascertain the usual organization. Generally, it will be found that four major sections are contained. The first section, frequently titled *Introduction,* addresses related studies, references to any theoretical propositions or interventions (when fitting), as well as the justification and purpose of the study. This section should be brief and the related literature segments should contain only those studies which are pertinent to your efforts.

The next section explains what you did and how you did it. This part, named *Methodology,* should offer the reader information about the setting, sample, instrumentation, and procedure. Only a few statements about the setting are usually required, with more elaboration on the sample and sample selection. If the instrument was borrowed, full credit should be given and the instrument's reliability and validity noted. If the instrument was designed by you, then you should give information as to how reliability and validity were obtained. This is not necessary if the instrument was developed by someone else. Be certain to discuss how the data were collected and who collected it—there is no need to mention names.

The procedure segment may be contained within the preceding segments or can be separate. This is simply a presentation of the steps taken by you and/or others to complete the study.

The third major organizational component describes what happened. This is the *Results* or *Findings* section. Herein the results must be stated very clearly and in a fashion understandable to the reader. Be certain to provide the eligible sample size and the number who did not participate and why, when applicable. Present the most important results with a notation of the statistical techniques employed. Tables may be used to condense the data. Realize that more data may exist than can be printed in one manuscript; if this is the case, use only the information applicable to the principal theme.

The fourth and final section, referred to as *Discussion,* may include conclusions, implications, and recommendations for further research. Explain the meaning of your findings as they apply to the health field and in particular to the readership. If contradictions to other studies exist, attempt to clarify the issues. In some instances, you may be able to suggest some alterations to improve the study or intervention.

Writing

The finished manuscript should be clear, concise, and consistent. There should be a coherent and logical flow from start to finish. Language should be simple, free of jargon, and, of course, nonsexist. It may be wise to put the manuscript aside for a day or two and then reread it to check your writing. If you are satisfied, give it to a colleague to critique. Then, if you accept any recommendations received, make the appropriate changes and have it reread again before submission.

Submission of the Manuscript

Be certain to follow the guidelines of the selected journal in regard to the number of and type of copies to be forwarded. In addition, pages should be in the order requested—usually an abstract followed by the text with references and then the illustrations and tables. Also, list the author or authors on a separate page, indicating the corresponding author and address. Do not forget to include a cover letter explaining why you have selected this journal.

Most journals will send you an "acknowledgment of receipt" form letter or card so that you know it has been received. However, if this is not the usual practice of the journal, it is suggested that you enclose a stamped, self-addressed postcard that can be returned by the editor. In any case, if after 2 weeks you have not been notified, contact the editorial office in case the manuscript was lost in the mail.

The Review Process

For most journals, the editor will forward the manuscript to at least two (and usually three) referees for review. These peer-referees are asked to give an appraisal of your manuscript in terms of applicability to the journal; importance and timeliness of the content; organization and flow of the material; appropriateness of information in the methodology, instrumentaton, and findings section; meaningfulness of the discussion section; and overall writing. When there are discrepancies among reviewers, the editor may make the final decision or send it out for further review. This process may take 2 months and in some journals up to 6 months.

Eventually, you will receive a letter from the editor. It may indicate full acceptance, acceptance with minor revisions, the need for extensive revisions with another peer review, or rejection. Usually the suggestions for revision are very good and will improve the manuscript considerably. If the manuscript is rejected, explore the reasons. Many times, it may be because the materials were inappropriate for the particular journal and you then may make modifications and forward it to a more appropriate journal. Please keep in mind that all authors receive rejections from time to time and that you should not cease future attempts at publishing your research.

References

Day, R. A. (1979) *How to Write and Publish a Scientific Paper,* Philadelphia: ISI Press.

Huck, S. W., Cormier, W. H. and Bounds, W. G. (1974): *Reading Statistics and Research.* New York: Harper & Row Publishers (Chapter 1).

Relman, A. S. (1981) Journals. In Warren, K. S. (ed.), *Coping with the Biomedical Literature,* New York: Praeger Publications 1981.

Sadler, D. R. (1984) *Up the Publication Road: Green Guide No. 2,* Sydney, Australia: Higher Education Research and Development Society of Australia.

Tornquist, E. M. (1983) Strategies for publishing research, *Nursing Outlook,* 31(3):180–183.

Guidelines for Authors: Journal of School Health*

A Note to Authors

These guidelines are provided to assist prospective authors in preparing manuscripts for the *Journal of School Health*. Failure to follow the guidelines completely may delay or prevent consideration of the manuscript. Contact the *Journal* office for assistance: *Journal of School Health,* P.O. Box 708, Kent, OH 44240, (216) 678-1601.

Features

Manuscripts may be submitted for publication in five categories. **Articles** address topics of broad interest and appeal to the readership. **Research Papers** report the findings of original, stringently reviewed, databased research. **Commentaries** include position papers, documented analyses of current or controversial issues, and creative, insightful, reflective treatments of topics related to or affecting health promotion in schools. **Teaching Techniques** present innovative ideas concerning health instruction. **Health Service Applications** are practical papers of interest in school nursing, medicine, denistry, and other aspects of school health services. The JOSH editorial staff determines placement of accepted manuscripts within the five categories. Letters to the editor about subjects relevant to health promotion in schools also are welcomed.

---

*These Guidelines have been printed with permission from the *Journal of School Health,* a publication of the American School Health Association, P.O. Box 708, Kent, OH 44240.

Submission Requirements

Submit a cover letter with the original manuscript and four copies to Managing Editor, *Journal of School Health,* American School Health Association, P.O. Box 708, Kent, OH 44240. Poor quality copies will not be considered. Manuscripts must be typed on white, 8½" × 11" paper and double-spaced throughout, including the abstract and references. Number the manuscript pages consecutively with the first title page as page one followed by the second title page, abstract, text, references, and visuals.

The cover letter should include the name, mailing address, and telephone number of the corresponding author. The cover letter also should state that the manuscript or its essence has not been accepted or published previously and is not under simultaneous consideration for publication elsewhere. Rejected manuscripts will not be returned unless accompanied by a pre-addressed envelope with adequate return postage. Authors interested in submitting manuscripts on floppy disks may contact the editorial department for details.

Manuscript Length

Manuscript length requirements are based on standard margins and the equivalent of about 25, 10-pitch lines per page. Commentaries, Teaching Techniques, and Health Service applications should not exceed 5–6 typed pages not including a maximum of 10 references and two visuals. Articles should not exceed 10–12 typed pages not including a maximum of 20 references and three visuals. Research Papers should not exceed 10–12 typed pages not including a maximum of 25 references and four visuals.

Title Pages

The first title page should include the manuscript title, the category to which the manuscript is being submitted, and the names, academic degrees, current positions, professional affiliation, and mailing address for **all** authors. For jointly authored works, indicate the corresponding author and include a telephone number. Joint authors should be listed in the order of their contribution to the work. A maximum of six authors for each manuscript will be listed. The second title page should include the manuscript title and the category to which the manuscript is being submitted.

Abstract

A 150-word abstract must accompany Articles and Research Papers. The abstract should provide sufficient information for the reader to determine the purpose and relevance of the work.

Style

Prepare manuscripts using the AMA Stylebook (1981), *Manual for Authors and Editors: Editorial Style and Manuscript Preparation.* Manuscript titles should be brief and specific. Manuscripts normally should be written in the third person, avoiding sexist language. Spell numbers one through ten, and use the % symbol to report percentages. Research manuscripts should include the year and timeframe in which the data were collected. Unfamiliar acronyms should be preceded by their full title following first usage with the acronym or abbreviation in parentheses. Funding sources may be recognized, but personal acknowledgments will not be printed. Footnotes should be eliminated or incorporated into the text where feasible. Outlines and multi-part manuscripts normally are not considered.

Cite references in the text in numerically consecutive order. List the references as they are cited; do not list references alphabetically. Abbreviate journal titles according to *Index Medicus.* Journal citations should include author, title, journal abbreviation, year, volume, issue, and pages. Book citations should include author, title, city, publisher, year, and pages. Authors are responsible for the accuracy of all references.

1. McClary DG, Bauer JH, Chang CL: Smoking cessation strategies in review. *J Sch Health* 1985;55(3):102–110.

2. Wilson T, Steiner AR, Lopez JM: *Health Promotion in Schools,* Chicago, Professional Publications, 1958, pp 120–126.

Visuals

Use visuals only when necessary. Incorporate basic information into the text in narrative form where feasible. Each chart, graph, diagram, table, figure, and photograph should have a brief, self-explanatory title. Submit each visual on a separately numbered page at the end of the manuscript.

Authors may furnish camera-ready art for visuals, or the *Journal* can prepare the visuals and bill the author. Submit original line art, professionally prepared in the required *Journal* format, using Helios Condensed typeface or the equivalent. Center visual titles in 9 pt Helios Bold Condensed. Depending on the size of the visual, use a width of 19 picas unless the visual contains six or more separate columns, in which case, use a width of 40 picas to accommodate the *Journal* column format.

Editing

Manuscripts are edited for length and clarity. An edited copy of the manuscript is sent to the corresponding author for proofing before publication. If the corresponding author does not respond as requested, the article is printed as it appears on the proof. Costs for changes requested after the proofing period are billed to the author.

Reprints

Authors and co-authors receive two complimentary copies of the *Journal* in which their article appears. Authors also receive a form for ordering reprints. Additional copies of the issue may be purchased from the *Journal* office.

Copyright

In accordance with the Copyright Revision Act of 1976, Public Law 94–553, the following statement must be submitted in writing and be signed by all authors and co-authors before a manuscript will be considered:

> "In consideration of the JOURNAL OF SCHOOL HEALTH taking action in reviewing and editing my submission, the author(s) undersigned hereby transfer, assign, or otherwise convey all copyright ownership to the JOURNAL OF SCHOOL HEALTH in the event such work is published in the JOURNAL."

Failure to provide the statement will delay consideration of the manuscript. Following publication, an article may not be published elsewhere without written permission from the *Journal* publisher.

Peer Review

Contributed manuscripts normally receive a blind peer review from at least three reviewers. Major reasons for rejection include insufficient relevance to health promotion in schools, lack of originality and uniqueness, improper format and style, faulty research design, poor writing, and space limitations. The *Journal* editor makes the final decision concerning acceptance of manuscripts.

January 1986

Figure A-1 Summary of Manuscript Requirements

Category of Manuscript	150-Word Abstract Required	Maximum Page Length[1]	Maximum References Allowed	Maximum Visuals Allowed	Number of Copies Required[2]	Copyright Release Required
Commentaries	No	5–6	10	2	0/4	Yes
Teaching Techniques	No	5–6	10	2	0/4	Yes
Health Service Applications	No	5–6	10	2	0/4	Yes
General Articles	Yes	10–12	20	3	0/4	Yes
Research Papers	Yes	10–12	25	4	0/4	Yes

[1]Assumes standard margins and 25, 10-pitch lines per page
[2]Original and four copies

Checklist for Authors

- The manuscript topic is appropriate for the *Journal.*
- Names and mailing address are provided for the senior author and all coauthors.
- The corresponding author is designated clearly including name, mailing address, and telephone number.
- A copyright release statement signed by the senior author and all co-authors is included.
- The AMA stylebook (1981) was followed for format, references, and documentation.
- The manuscript is written in the third person, avoiding sexist language.
- Personal acknowledgements are not included, and footnotes are minimized or deleted.
- Two title pages are enclosed.
- Both title pages indicate the category to which the manuscript is being submitted.
- Manuscript length and number of references and visuals conform to requirements for the category.
- The manuscript title is brief and specific.
- The original and four clear copies are enclosed.
- A 150-word abstract is included for Articles and Research Papers.
- All pages are numbered consecutively from the first title page.
- Visuals are prepared on separately numbered pages and placed at the end of the manuscript.
- Adequate return postage is enclosed, if desired.
- The manuscript has been checked thoroughly for style, readability, and quality of writing.

Author Index

Subject Index